CONTENTS

INTRODUCTION

No doubt you can think of at least a hundred-and-one good reasons for not bothering too much about your health. Perhaps you reckon you're in pretty good shape anyway. Perhaps you're too busy to worry about such trifles. Perhaps you'll think about it when the time comes. Or perhaps you'll leave it to the doctors to bail you out. Maybe you think being concerned about your health is unmanly. Or self-indulgent. Or counterproductive. Or too depressing. Or just plain boring. Perhaps you take a fatalistic view, and see your life, and health, as a sort of lottery — you have to take the rough with the smooth, and if your number's up, that's it. Perhaps your philosophy on health and illness is to live now and pay later. Or perhaps you would simply rather not think about it at all and leave health to the health freaks.

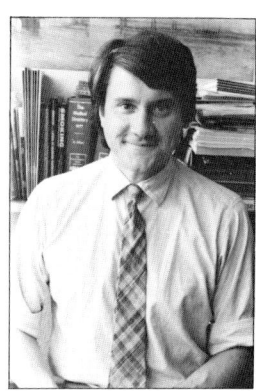

Dr Alan Maryon Davis

For whatever reason, the fact is that most men tend not to bother much about their health until they start to lose it. True, some men make an effort to keep themselves in shape through physical fitness, but they are in the minority. Most think the time and place for exercise is Saturday afternoons on the television. The irony is that the average man spends more time and trouble on his car's bodywork than on his own. But whilst the car can always be traded in for a newer model, his body has to last a lifetime. Regrettably, in far too many cases, it doesn't go the full distance.

Far too many men die before their time from diseases which are largely preventable: heart disease, lung cancer, chronic bronchitis and emphysema, bowel cancer, cirrhosis of the liver — the list goes on and on. Other men escape an early death only to suffer years of discomfort or disability from these very diseases. The sad fact is that in nearly every case the risk of disease is linked to the way a man leads his life. Lifestyle factors, such as an unbalanced diet, lack of exercise, stress, cigarette smoking, misuse of alcohol, and others, account for most of the ill-health affecting men under the age of 65.

Heart disease is a classic example. It is the biggest mankiller in the western world. Heart attacks or disabling angina strike one man in five before the age of 65, killing half the victims outright. A man in his late forties is about five times more likely to succumb to heart disease than is a woman of the same age. Of course, you can't help the fact that you are male; nor can you influence other risk factors such as increasing age or a family history of heart disease. But you *can* do something about the other major risk factors — by looking hard at your way of life and making a few wise adjustments here and there.

The average male smoker, for example, can halve his risk of a heart attack by giving up the habit — and that huge benefit will apply within a year or two of stubbing out his last cigarette. Men who exercise regularly, moderately vigorously, over a period of years, can also reduce their risk of heart attack by about 50 per cent. Similar risk reductions can be achieved by staying slim and cutting down on saturated fat in the diet.

But the important point is that, because the underlying disease process — fatty deposits in the arteries of the heart — starts 10, 20 or even 30 years before symptoms appear, it is crucial to make the necessary changes as early in life as possible, whilst you are feeling perfectly fit and well. To leave things until trouble sets in is, literally, fatal.

So much for gloom and doom. But good health is much more than the mere absence of disease. In the same way that tuning a car engine can make it run sweetly, so too can a few adjustments to lifestyle help a man to a state of ultra-health — a feeling of positive physical and mental well-being.

This is not mere metaphysical mumbo-jumbo. There is increasing evidence, for example, that regular aerobic exercise tones up the body and mind in a whole variety of ways, inducing a feeling of euphoria and helping to fight off disease. The male body is built for action. We still have the same body that evolved in the great grasslands at the dawn of human history — designed for strength of arm and fleetness of foot. Now, in our push-button world of labour-saving micro-chip automation, too many of us have become the all-too-willing victims of inertia — a factor which is thought by many doctors to contribute more to male stress than any of the so-called pressures of modern-day life.

In this book you will find a practical guide to positive health, mental and physical. We look not only at the main threats to the well-being of men of all ages, from the preoccupations of tentative youth to the mature concerns of older men, but also at ways of positively enhancing a man's potential across the whole spectrum of health. By separating fact from fiction, and recommending the simple steps to be taken, along with the reasons for doing so, we hope to encourage more men to make the most of their lives, and hence their families' lives, by taking the trouble to take care of themselves.

Dr Alan Maryon Davis

MANPOWER

Being healthy and feeling fit are not necessarily the same thing. If you ask the average man if he is healthy, he will probably immediately think in terms of his physical health. He may review any recent illnesses or aches and pains he has suffered, and if he has no actual problems, he will probably say, 'Yes, fine, I'm really healthy.' What he may really mean, however, is, 'No, I'm not actually sick at the moment.' This is because for most men, health is simply the absence of disease.

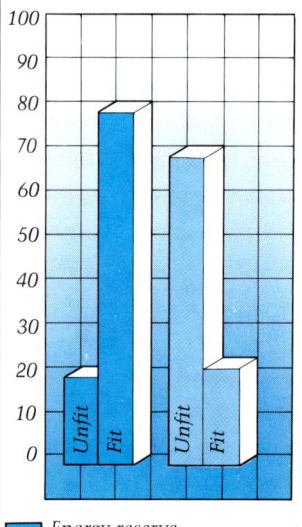

Energy reserve

Energy used for identical type of work

0-
100
Acquired physical capacity (%)

A person with a low physical capacity uses up all his energy reserve and more, whereas a fit person doing the same task uses only a portion of his energy reserve.

But is this the best we can expect from our bodies and our minds? Must we really expect our health to be at risk from a constant battle against disease and maintained only by medical assistance?

All our views on health are coloured by our 'medical' definition of the word - indeed, many people actually glory in discussing the intimate details of their own or other people's illnesses. Instead, however, we should think about 'positive' health or well-being. We should also consider what are reasonable expectations for health. Feeling healthy when we are 20 is very different from feeling healthy when we reach the age of 75. For a young man, positive health may mean feeling fit and full of physical energy. For an older man in a difficult working environment, feeling healthy could mean rather that, as well as feeling physically fit, he feels mentally alert and ready to face problems. And for an elderly man, feeling healthy might mean feeling relaxed and happy, with no serious health problems and looking forward to years more life without worries, pressures or responsibilities. All this makes it very difficult to define 'good health'. An athlete will understand good health in a very different way from a pensioner.

We in the world's advanced economies have access to good medical care, and 'good health' in the traditional sense can be well looked after by the doctor. But to be well in the fullest sense of the word and to be able to demand more and expect more from our health, we have first to be aware of our own bodies. This is an area of domestic life where men have tended to abdicate responsibility. Traditionally used to being administered to, most men have quietly sat back and relied on their womenfolk to hand round the medicine, suggest a diagnosis and ladle out the sympathy. Although most men are sensible enough to go to the doctor when they suspect something may be going wrong or to undertake their own minor treatment for simple problems like headaches or colds, when it comes to promoting *positive* health, few men know what needs to be done or where to turn for advice. The solution lies with you, to take an active role in

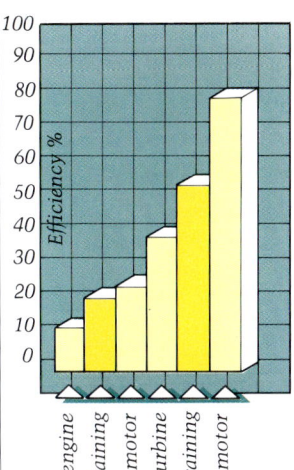

The efficiency of an unfit human body compares badly with modern machinery. However, a fitness programme can greatly improve efficiency.

promoting your own health. *You* are responsible for monitoring the way you feel and for taking the steps needed to produce the real glow of positive health.

In many ways, physical health, in its positive sense of being something more than the absence of disease, is easier to cultivate than some of the other mancare measures discussed in this book. But it is only one aspect of true health: there is no point in cultivating a god-like physique if your emotional life is a mess.

So what can you expect from achieving positive physical health? Think of it in terms of a car. If your car is kept in a cold, damp garage, unused for months on end, it will gradually deteriorate. The bodywork rusts, wiring deteriorates, engine oil thickens, and when it is driven out for a dash down the motorway on the annual holiday, it is likely to break down. At the very least, it will not perform at its peak.

Your body is much the same. Constant inactivity means that muscles waste and become flabby, so that you lack strength and stamina. Like the car wiring and engine oil, your systems can deteriorate through under-use. And also like the car, regular maintenance helps to overcome the problems, keeping you fit and ready to go.

It's quite easy to prove that regular exercise improves physical health, and athletes have taken the process even further by 'fine-tuning' their bodies with exercises specifically designed to improve their performance in a particular sport. But it's not so easy to prove, scientifically, that exercising regularly also improves our sense of well-being, thus enabling us to achieve our target of positive health.

Yet few men doubt that exercise *does* give you that positive glow of well-being, provided it is accompanied by other improvements in lifestyle, such as adopting a sensible diet and avoiding obvious health hazards such as smoking and over-indulgence in alcohol.

If you are naturally active, you may already be doing enough to keep your system reasonably healthy. But you probably won't be exercising sufficiently or in the right way to give you that necessary physical edge. Don't use the fact that you are not by nature an energetic person or that you don't have the time as excuses for not taking more exercise. There are *always* a few minutes in the day when you can carry out some form of physical activity, for your expectations of physical health are not necessarily those of a man who aspires to be an athlete!

Pulse and blood pressure readings indicate the general condition of the heart and blood vessels. An inflated cuff stops the blood flow, the pressure is released slowly and a reading taken when the pulse is first heard and when the blood again flows freely.

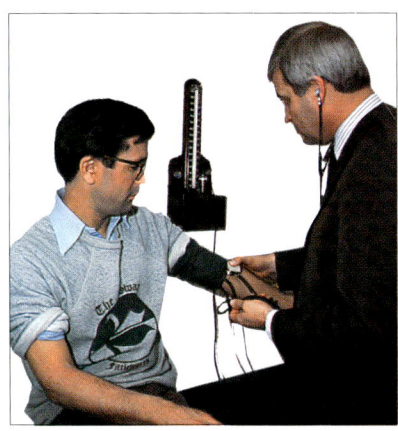

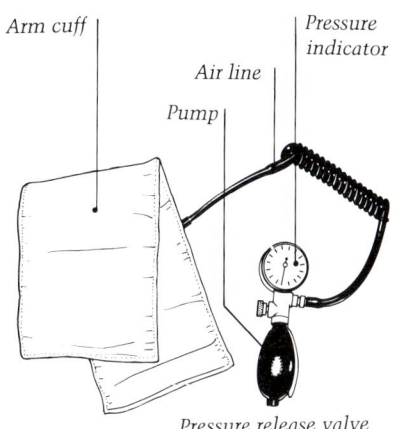

Arm cuff

Air line

Pump

Pressure indicator

Pressure release valve

HEALTH AND EXERCISE

The traditional view of the word 'health' as a struggle against disease is also important when considering physical fitness.

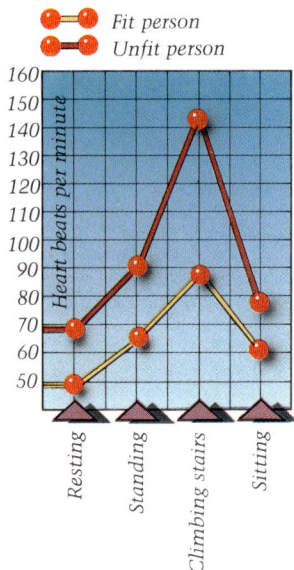

Fit person
Unfit person

Heart beats per minute

160
150
140
130
120
110
100
90
80
70
60
50

Resting
Standing
Climbing stairs
Sitting

Everyday activities increase your heart beat. The heart of a fit person is very efficient and can circulate enough oxygen around the body to cope with the extra demands of the working muscles by increasing the pulse by 30 to 40 extra beats a minute. The less efficient heart of an unfit person does not shift the same volume of blood with each pump, therefore it has to beat up to 100 beats more each minute to circulate sufficient oxygen.

Lack of exercise can cause disease - very serious disease in some instances - - and there is increasing evidence that men who take the right type of regular exercise are likely to be less prone to diseases such as heart attacks and strokes and, because of this, tend to live longer than those who take little or no exercise. So you could look on achieving physical fitness as a cheap form of life insurance, and one where *you* are the beneficiary. Later in this chapter we will be considering in detail ways of working out sensible yet effective exercise routines. But, in addition to these, it is worth looking at the small yet effective adjustments you can make to your everyday life to promote self-health. For example, a simple change like taking a brisk 20-minute walk at lunchtime instead of going for the obligatory drink, can maximize your work performance as well as make you feel more in tune with your body.

The parts of the body most liable to deteriorate through inactivity are those responsible for carrying the blood around the body, particularly to the muscles, which are the key to physical activity. This system of heart and blood vessels is known as the circulatory or cardiovascular system, and it is necessary to understand how physical activity can protect and improve the system.

One of the main purposes of the circulatory system is to supply oxygen to the muscles, brain and other parts of the body. This gas, which is extracted from the air we breathe, is required by all the cells of the body, and the more active these cells are, the more oxygen they need to carry out their vital life processes. During exercise the muscle cells have to work harder and we breathe more deeply, or pant, to get more oxygen into the body. Blood can only hold a limited amount of oxygen, so the heart must pump harder and faster to get more blood and the oxygen it contains to the parts of the body where it is needed.

The system is critical both for health and for life itself. Like some other systems in the body, the circulatory system adjusts itself according to the demands made on it. For a person in vigorous physical health and with plenty of stamina, the circulatory system can cope easily with extra demands made on it during exercise; for a sedentary person, on the other hand, the system will have adjusted to lesser demands and may not be able to cope with prolonged heavy exercise. Regular physical activity involving large groups of muscles in rhythmic activity causes the circulatory system to build up its efficiency so that it can cope with extra demands.

THE CIRCULATORY SYSTEM

The heart and its blood vessels may be regarded as relatively simple mechanical devices. Their main function is to collect oxygen from the lungs, pump it round the body in the blood, from which it is extracted as needed, and at the same time to remove waste products produced by the cells. Just as oxygen demand is greatest during exercise, so are the quantities of waste produced by the hard-working cells.

The heart is a simple pump, about the size of a clenched fist, and positioned in the centre of the chest (*not* on the left, as is popularly supposed). An average man's heart is about ten per cent heavier than a woman's to compensate for his larger frame. The heart actually contains two quite separate pump mechanisms, each constructed in the same way. Each has a collection chamber for blood, the atrium, at the top, and a large muscular pumping chamber, the ventricle, at the bottom.

Blood, with its oxygen used up, is returned to the heart from the body. It fills one atrium, then flows into the ventricle, which contracts sharply, forcing blood through a one-way valve into a blood vessel leading to the lungs. Here the blood vessels divide into a network of tiny, twig-like capillaries, vessels so fine that oxygen in the lungs can enter the blood, and be carried away again, back to the opposite side of the heart. Here the same pumping process takes place, this time forcing the blood, now containing oxygen, out and around the whole body.

Blood leaving the heart passes along arteries, thick-walled vessels that

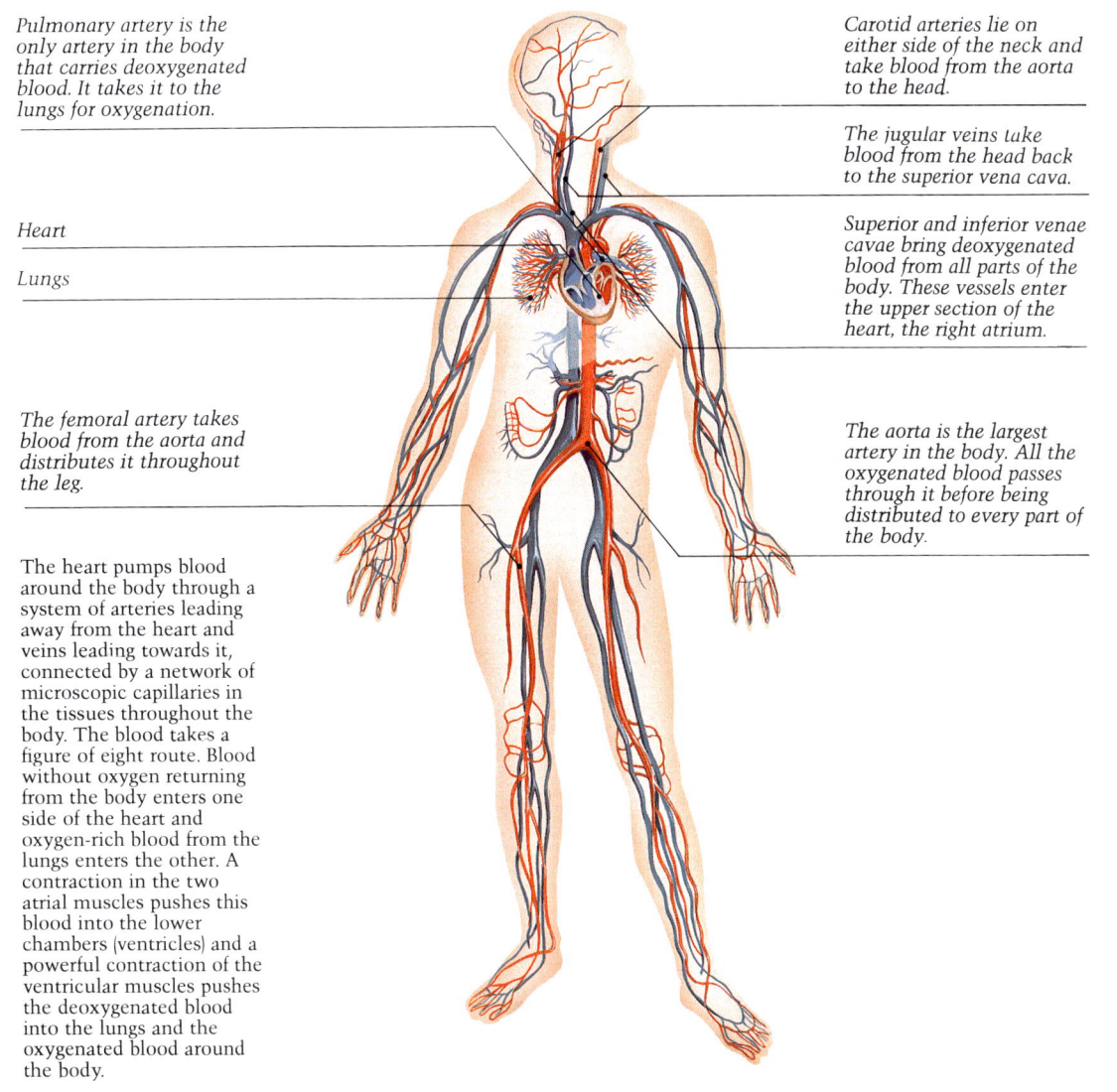

Pulmonary artery is the only artery in the body that carries deoxygenated blood. It takes it to the lungs for oxygenation.

Heart

Lungs

The femoral artery takes blood from the aorta and distributes it throughout the leg.

The heart pumps blood around the body through a system of arteries leading away from the heart and veins leading towards it, connected by a network of microscopic capillaries in the tissues throughout the body. The blood takes a figure of eight route. Blood without oxygen returning from the body enters one side of the heart and oxygen-rich blood from the lungs enters the other. A contraction in the two atrial muscles pushes this blood into the lower chambers (ventricles) and a powerful contraction of the ventricular muscles pushes the deoxygenated blood into the lungs and the oxygenated blood around the body.

Carotid arteries lie on either side of the neck and take blood from the aorta to the head.

The jugular veins take blood from the head back to the superior vena cava.

Superior and inferior venae cavae bring deoxygenated blood from all parts of the body. These vessels enter the upper section of the heart, the right atrium.

The aorta is the largest artery in the body. All the oxygenated blood passes through it before being distributed to every part of the body.

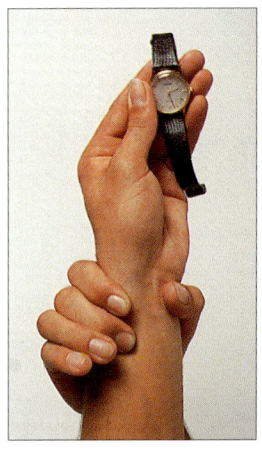

The radial artery lies near a bone of the forearm, the radius. By compressing the artery with two fingers a pulse can be felt. The pressure waves are caused by the contractions of the heart.

can withstand the pressure of the blood and that, because of their elastic walls, smooth out most of the pumping impulses of blood leaving the heart. Despite this, there is still a distinct pulse with each pumping stroke of the ventricles, and this can be felt over the artery in the inside of the wrist, or heard by the doctor when he uses a stethoscope to measure blood pressure. It is useful to learn how to check your own pulse rate so you can monitor the progress of your improved fitness.

Blood passes from the arteries, which branch and sub-branch into the minute capillaries that penetrate almost all the body, then drains back into veins, which return the de-oxygenated blood to the heart to begin the process again. By now, the blood is no longer under great pressure, having travelled all round the body, so the veins do not need to have very thick walls. Indeed, the blood moves so sluggishly through veins that the largest veins need one-way valves to stop it flowing back or 'pooling' in the legs.

Blood in the arteries is always under pressure, and this is normal and necessary if it is to be pumped through the arterial and capillary network against the resistance caused by friction. But it must be at the correct pressure. Too low, and you would faint from lack of blood and oxygen reaching the brain. If your blood pressure is too high, there are serious health hazards to the brain, kidneys, and to the heart itself.

Most of the heart, and especially the powerful ventricles, is composed of muscle, which pumps tirelessly throughout life. Just like any other muscle, the heart muscle needs adequate supplies of oxygen, and it has its own blood supply, along the coronary arteries. These arteries can become partly blocked, which cuts down the flow of blood and causes the crippling pain of angina. If the vessels become completely blocked, a heart attack or 'coronary' results, when the lack of oxygen causes a whole section of heart muscle to die - the size of the area affected determines how serious are the effects of the attack.

THE BENEFITS OF EXERCISE

What does physical fitness mean to you and will it give you any real benefits? Here are some of the positive advantages you can expect from being fitter - that is, the sort of fitness you can achieve by taking regular exercise.

● You will have more physical stamina to work hard and continuously, both at your normal day-to-day work and at home when you undertake some DIY work.
● You will be able to give a better account of yourself in activities such as sport or leisure pursuits, without feeling exhausted or suffering aches and pains the following day.
● You will have more physical energy, so you can better cope with occasional vigorous exertion, like chopping wood, mixing cement, using a pickaxe in the garden or running for a bus.
● You will become so physically well-tuned that you will be less likely to suffer aches and pains, and your joints will be kept more flexible so you should be able to stretch and turn without feeling stiff.
● You will help to improve the health of your circulatory system, provided you also look after your diet and take other sensible health precautions.
● Your sex life will be improved.

Some of these benefits have been scientifically or statistically demonstrated by looking at the health records of very large groups of people over many years. Studies of many thousands of men have compared those with physically energetic jobs or leisure activities with those who do not take any regular exercise. The results of these studies have made it apparent that men who exercise regularly are much less prone to heart attacks. As with all 'scientific' research, there are alternative explanations, of course. It is possible that men who took up jobs requiring physical strength or stamina were already healthier and thus less likely to suffer ill-health in later life. Yet a study of men who had been college athletes and who were presumably at that time supremely fit, found that in later life they were no healthier than non-athletes, *unless* they had kept up their exercise since college days.

The evidence that exercise has a protective effect on the body is compelling, even if not 100 per cent proven. It certainly does not seem worth gambling your health on the small chance that the evidence based on studies of thousands of men over many years is completely mistaken.

ARE THERE ANY DISADVANTAGES IN EXERCISE?

Like almost every human activity, exercise has its risks, but these have to be kept in perspective. The hazards are *very* small. When you start physical exercise programmes, the most common hazard is injury - usually very minor and caused by overdoing things early on.

Obviously, the more vigorous the exercise, the greater the chance of injury. Each type of activity has its own particular injury hazards, and these are discussed later in this chapter. In running, for example, the most likely problem is a sprained ankle. As in all physical pursuits, a slow and gentle start to training allows you to build up your strength and suppleness so that muscles and joints become progressively less liable to injury, as the improvement in your heart and circulation gives you more stamina.

Heart attacks and other forms of sudden death do sometimes occur during exercise - but many more take place while the victims are relaxing at home or even while they are asleep in bed. Obviously if you know you are suffering from heart trouble or any other potentially serious health problem, you should consult your doctor before taking up a vigorous activity or exercise programme. Even if you do have a medical problem, exercise can be beneficial *provided* it is taken under the guidance of your doctor. What is known to be dangerous is for a man to pursue an inactive life and then occasionally to take part in a sport or activity where explosive effort is needed. Squash is the classic example: more men have dropped dead playing squash - a potentially valuable form of vigorous exercise enjoyed by millions - than any other sport, probably because it has become fashionable among unfit yet highly competitive executives, who play only occasionally. They would be better off taking a short walk away from the office each lunchtime.

If you are in any doubt at all about your health, it is obviously advisable that your doctor checks you over before you embark on any of the more vigorous forms of exercise or sport.

The Royal College of Physicians and the British Cardiac Society recently commented:

"Most people do not need a medical examination before starting an exercise programme. There are no risks in regular rhythmic exercise as long as the programme begins gently and only gradually increases in vigour."

But there are some obvious risk factors which should make you check with your doctor. Most are common sense. If you suffer from any of the following, see your doctor before you begin your exercise programme: heart disease; bronchitis; asthma; high blood pressure; diabetes; chest pains; fainting spells; dizziness; arthritis or cartilage problems; any chronic or debilitating disease.

A relatively new but still fairly unusual problem is addiction to exercise. For some people, this addiction is important in that it keeps them working very hard at a vigorous pursuit, but for others exercise becomes an obsession which takes precedence over all else in their lives. It has been suggested by some doctors that an obsession with running in middle-aged men is the equivalent of anorexia nervosa in adolescents. An exercise obsession is thought to be related to some recently discovered substances called endorphins, powerful drugs that are produced in the brain, especially during vigorous exercise. Endorphins seem to be the natural equivalent of narcotic drugs such as morphine and heroin, and they have similar effects. The result is that sustained vigorous exercise becomes enjoyable, as the endorphins work on the brain, producing a 'high' or 'buzz', which is greatly sought after by the dedicated keep-fit fanatic. Endorphins have other effects too; they reduce the pain caused by over-exercise, often allowing runners to continue until they become totally exhausted or even do themselves serious injury, presumably because the endorphins have masked the natural warning signals of an over-worked system. The presence of endorphins, acting as natural analgesics or pain-killers, is probably also the reason why minor injuries during sport or other exercise are often not noticed until some time after they have occurred.

So are all these potential problems any reason to postpone your physical fitness programme? Of course not. Very few people have problems, and avoiding them is simply common sense.

DO YOU NEED TO GET FIT OR FITTER?

Almost certainly, you could be fitter. You can soon prove this for yourself by doing a simple exercise that causes you to exert whole groups of muscles in a regular manner. The exercise increases the demand for oxygen, causing your heart to beat faster and your lungs to work more efficiently.

The simplest test for physical fitness is to walk up and down a flight of 15 stairs, 3 times. You should be able to do this without getting breathless and at the same time carry on a normal conversation. If you do become breathless, you know what needs to be done!

A more accurate indication of your physical fitness is to measure how long it takes for your heart rate or pulse to settle back to 'normal' after exercise. First, take your pulse rate, as described earlier in this chapter, preferably when you wake up in the morning and before you have the chance to become active or to start worrying about the day's activities. This will give you your 'resting' pulse rate. It will vary with age, and should become lower after regular exercise has improved the health of your circulatory system. If your resting pulse rate is faster than 100 beats a minute, you may require treatment and should consult your doctor.

If your resting pulse rate is below 100, you can now easily test your heart recovery time. Step up on to a 20cm (8in) standard stair with one foot, followed by the other, then step down again, moving both feet. Repeat this 24 times a minute for 3 minutes then stop and wait for 30 seconds and take your pulse rate. You can check the results against the chart on page 10.

You should find that, after a few weeks of regular exercise, both your resting pulse rate and heart recovery time decrease noticeably, as your heart and circulation become used to the extra work and operate more efficiently.

WHAT SORT OF FITNESS?

Just as there are many ways to keep physically fit, so there are many forms of fitness. You will have to decide what your objectives are before you begin any serious exercise programme. There is little point in taking up the training routines of an Olympic sprinter if all you need is the stamina to go for long country walks. Let us make clear what we mean by fitness in its various forms.

Stamina   Most men understand stamina as meaning staying power or having the ability to carry out vigorous physical activity for long periods, without over-exertion and without becoming too tired. This is the sort of fitness you would require for hiking or swimming, cycling and jogging, sustained for more than a few minutes. These kinds of pursuit are well suited to the middle-aged man who wants (or needs) to take up some form of regular physical activity. Developing stamina means that the major muscle groups become more efficient at using oxygen so that during vigorous exercise the 'strain' on the heart is reduced. Stamina is improved through achieving a series of lesser objectives. For example, if you go swimming, you should try to achieve a few extra lengths of the pool each week. Exercise leading to improved stamina involves the rhythmic use of large muscle groups such as the major muscles of the legs, arms and trunk.

Suppleness   Muscles that are under-used gradually shorten, restricting the amount of movement in the joint. Frequent exercise of the right sort continually stretches these muscles, keeping the joints supple. Without this suppleness painful muscle tears can occur during strenuous exercise.

The ability to flex and bend the body is needed for everyday activities as well as for sports or other active pursuits. All the dozens of joints in the body need regular use if they are to function freely and to continue to function well into old age. Yoga, dancing and swimming are the kind of activity that will improve suppleness.

Strength   Muscles respond to extra demands placed on them by becoming larger and more powerful. The reverse is also true – the less they are used, the smaller they become. You can see the effects of inactivity on muscles when the plaster is removed from a broken limb, which will have become wasted and weak. But with physiotherapy - using strengthening exercises - the limb quickly recovers its usual size and strength.

Any form of exercise intended to improve stamina will also improve the strength of your muscles, but there are, of course, many other exercises

The trapezius muscle moves the shoulder blade and maintains the posture of the head.

The deltoid muscle is the main muscle for raising the whole arm.

The triceps muscle contracts to extend the arm.

The brachioradialis muscle helps to flex the arm and turn the palm of the hand upwards.

Latissimus dorsi connects the back to the arm and is a powerful muscle used for pulling the arm downwards.

Gluteus maximus is the large muscle of the buttock. It extends the hip joint.

Semitendinosus is one of the hamstring muscles which bends the knee.

Biceps femoris is another hamstring placed on the outer side of the thigh.

Gastrocnemius is a paired muscle making up the bulk of the calf. It is attached to the achilles tendon and points the foot.

Sternomastoid connects the head to the chest and contracts to twist and flex the head.

Pectoralis major is the main muscle on the front of the chest and brings the arms forward.

Biceps brachii makes up the bulk of the front of the upper arm and is the strongest flexor of the arm.

Rectus abdominus is the longitudinal stomach muscle used for bending the trunk forward and helps maintain back and stomach posture.

Sartorius is the longest muscle of the body stretching from the hip to the tibia and helps to bend the hip and knee.

Quadriceps muscle has four parts forming the bulk of the front of the thigh. It extends the knee.

Over 650 muscles move the body and help to maintain its posture. Each muscle is attached at points to the bones of the skeleton and when the muscle contracts the bones move through a joint. However, even the simplest movement is a result of the action of groups of muscles. Each muscle anchors a bone and contracts or relaxes (depending on the movement) like a system of pulleys and levers. The muscles responsible for movement are called voluntary muscles and have a different structure from the muscles of the heart and the involuntary muscles of the bowel, the blood vessels and the bladder.

that have a more direct effect on muscular strength. Some forms of weight-lifting, for example, develop enormous musculature but with very little improvement in stamina, and many competitive field sports require great strength. We also need extra strength for occasional, unexpected events like pushing a broken-down car.

In practice, to be reasonably fit, you will need all of these attributes: stamina, suppleness and strength. You will need them in varying degrees, depending on your objectives. And of course, however fit you are, you will need to coordinate the different aspects of fitness if you are going to use them for sport. To play any competitive sport successfully you must be able to integrate all the aspects of fitness, together with rapid and instinctive thinking.

THE STRUCTURE OF FITNESS

To understand how your body can be improved by exercise, it is necessary to look at the structures we will be working with and how they operate. We are primarily concerned with the musculo-skeletal system - that is, the interaction of bones and muscles needed to move the body.

The skeleton is the framework that gives the body support and shape, and protects the delicate internal organs. The skull is made up of 22 interleaved bones. The skeleton provides a system of levers for the muscles to work on, and in order to provide a full range of movements, different types of joints articulate the bones with one another. The *hinge joint* provides extensive movement in one direction, but none in the other as in the knee and elbow *1*. The *ball and socket joint* provides a much wider range of movement and articulates the hip and shoulder *2*. The head is able to twist round from side to side and it is a *pivot joint* that gives this full range of movement *3*.

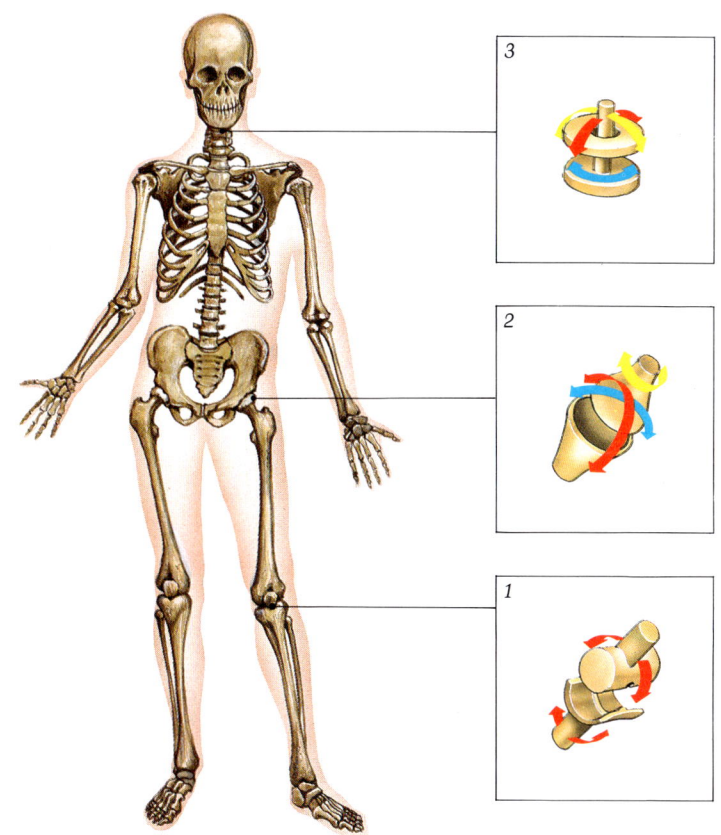

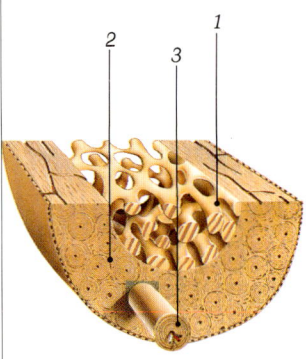

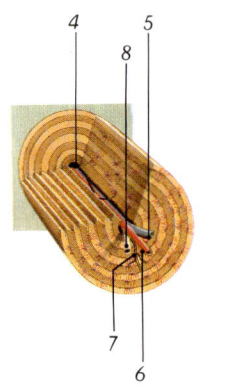

A cross-section through a long bone shows the dense, compact bone surrounding a porous centre of spongy bone. This design means that bones are strong but flexible and light. The bone is living tissue which receives its blood supply through a network of canals within the Haversian system.

1 Spongy bone *2* compact bone *3* Haversian system (*Detail*) Central canals run through each Haversian system *4*. Every canal carries a vein *5*, artery *6*, nerve *7* and lymph vessel *8*.

Bones form the main support of the body. They are rigid, and joints are needed to allow our bodies to move freely. Bones are composed of mineral material, but they also contain living cells and are therefore capable of repair if damaged. Once we reach adulthood, our bones will not lengthen but they can become stouter and stronger. Bones are constantly being re-modelled, depending on the demands made on them. Exercise makes bones stronger; look at the bones in a tennis player's racket arm and compare them with the bones in the other arm.

A healthy bone is immensely strong and, weight for weight, is actually stronger than steel. Living bone is composed of 50 per cent water, the rest being mostly calcium salts. The hard, stone-like outer layer of a bone gives the bone its strength, while the spongy and porous bone beneath keeps it rigid yet light. The structure is very complex, and the layers of bone are precisely placed to spread and distribute loads, especially in the vulnerable areas around joints.

The long bones of the arms and legs are hollow and filled with marrow, a jelly-like material in which blood cells are produced. The hollow shaft of the bones helps reduce their weight. Blood vessels run into and throughout the living bone, nourishing the bone cells. Bone is covered by a thin layer of tissue, which contains the cells that help to repair damaged bone. This layer is very sensitive, and it is this that causes such pain when deep bruising affects a bone such as the elbow or shin that is near to the body's surface.

Bending and Twisting   Joints have a special relevance to physical fitness. Suppleness depends largely on the health and effectiveness of the joints, and joints can be improved by exercise. They can also be damaged relatively easily if they are misused.

Wherever two bones meet, there is a joint. Some joints, like those in the rounded cranium of the skull, lock bones together immovably; usually, however, joints allow bones to move against each other.

In a movable joint, the ends of the bone that are in contact are made from a milky-white, rubbery substance called cartilage, a springy material that cushions the bones and stops the hard bone material from wearing away. Lubricating fluid contained within its cavities exudes into the joint, making the surface of the cartilage very slippery and reducing friction as the joint moves. As a living tissue, cartilage can, to some extent, repair itself from the ravages of normal wear and tear but, if cracked or broken, pieces of cartilage may become trapped in a joint and cause long-term problems, sometimes requiring surgical treatment.

Between the cartilage at the bone-ends is a fluid-filled bag called the synovial capsule. This contains a lubricant that is an even more efficient lubricating mechanism for the joints than the fluid contained in cartilage. Synovial fluid is, however, more complex and more liable to damage. The synovial capsule can be badly affected by arthritis (see Chapter 4).

Joints are stabilized by ligaments; strong fibres that define the limits of joint movement. For example, ligaments stop your knee-joint from folding forwards and they also hold bones together, so that joints cannot pull apart.

There are many types of joints, and each is designed to work in a particular way, so it is important to understand how each joint is supposed to function before you try to force it into an inappropriate exercise to

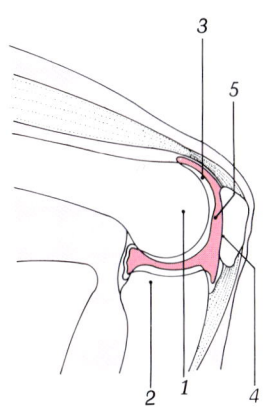

Joints are able to move freely because the ends of the articulating bones are covered with a frictionless synovial membrane. This produces a lubricating synovial fluid which surrounds the working part of the joint.

1 Femur 2 Tibia 3 Cartilage
4 Synovial membrane
5 Synovial fluid

improve its suppleness. Fingers and elbows, for example, are simple hinge joints, working in only one direction and allowing little side-to-side movement. But the wrist joint and the joint at the base of the thumb have a different design, allowing movement in any direction. Hips and shoulder joints, too, are extremely mobile, the ball and socket arrangement allowing limbs to rotate to almost any position. The hip joint, which carries tremendous loads during running and jumping, is especially large and strong.

Probably the most complex set of joints are those in the spine. Vertebrae are basically ring-shaped bones, with elaborate spines and spurs on to which muscles are attached. Many parts of each vertebra are in contact with other parts, all cushioned with cartilage, and they allow a limited amount of movement so that the spine can flex smoothly without damaging the vulnerable spinal cord it contains.

Very few joints work in isolation, and several types work together in certain sorts of movement. As your head moves, for example, one joint allows rotation, and a different type of joint allows it to rock back and forth.

If you stress a joint that is not supple, or overflex a supple joint, you are likely to tear a ligament or muscle, causing pain or inflammation. If you dislocate a joint, the bones are levered apart and the ligaments and other tissues torn. They will repair themselves gradually, provided they are rested and the bones supported during the healing process.

POWER TO MOVE

All your movement is powered by the muscles. Nearly all muscles are anchored to bones, which they move by a system of leverage. The exceptions are some of the muscles in the scalp and face, those in the internal organs and those that move the hairs in the skin when we experience 'goose-flesh'. These muscles are all anchored to soft tissue.

Muscles are made up of bundles of fine, hair-like fibres, up to 30cm (12in) long, depending on the length of the muscle itself. A muscle can contain two thousand or more of these fibres, arranged in small bundles, wrapped in protective membranes, and well supplied with blood-vessels and nerves.

Muscle fibres will shorten when they receive an electrical signal from the nervous system, and when many fibres shorten together, the whole muscle becomes shorter, moving the bones to which it is attached. Muscle is fastened to the bone by a rope-like cord of tendon - a material similar to ligament - which is firmly anchored to the surface of the bone.

Some tendons are very long. The tendons that you can feel on the inside of your wrist when you move your fingers run right up the forearm, where the muscles moving the fingers are positioned near the elbow. All tendons are covered by a slippery lubricated membrane, which allows the same free movement as the other moving parts of the musculo-skeletal system.

If you gradually build up an exercise programme, you will strengthen the tendons and their attachments to bones. A tendon sometimes tears away from its long anchor, causing a very painful injury. Such tendon damage is associated with some types of athletic event such as sprinting, where sudden physical exertion is used.

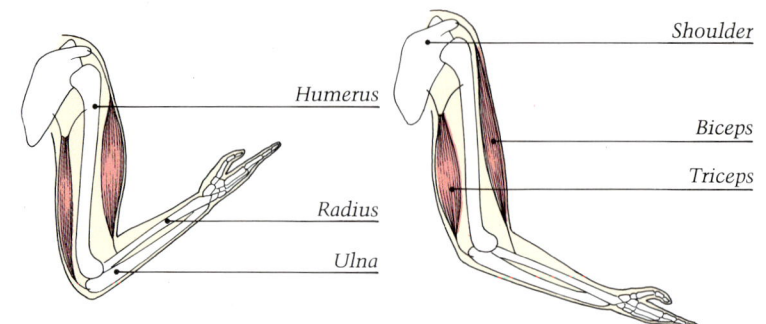

Movement is produced by opposing muscles. The biceps muscle is attached to the shoulder and the radius, the triceps to the shoulder and humerus at one end and the ulna at the other. When the biceps contracts it thickens and shortens and the triceps relaxes to allow the forearm to come up. To straighten the arm the reverse occurs.

To work efficiently, muscles need fuel, and the harder they work, the more fuel they need. Muscle contractions (and other body processes) are fuelled primarily by glucose and to a lesser extent by fatty acids (see Chapter 2). Glucose is stored in the muscles in the form of glycogen, which is 'burned' or broken down by enzymes using the oxygen carried in the blood to release energy, thus powering muscle contraction. The harder you work, therefore, the more oxygen you need to keep going, so you breathe more deeply and your heart works harder to pump more oxygen-bearing blood to the working muscle.

Glycogen is stored in the muscles, ready for use, but only in limited amounts. After a couple of hours of vigorous exercise, therefore, it will probably be used up, and you will feel totally exhausted and incapable of further work. Your body can then switch to a different form of energy release: burning fatty acids. Fatty acids are normally burnt on only a minor scale, but as you train on a regular basis, energy from burning fatty acids can provide the power you need to continue running, cycling or whatever else you are attempting. Fatty acid metabolism will also mean that you are beginning to burn up stored body fat, which is another key objective in striving for physical fitness!

While these activities are taking place, waste products are being produced by the muscles. These are carbon dioxide, water and lactic acid. Carbon dioxide is removed from the bloodstream as it passes through the lungs. Water is removed via the kidneys and by sweating. Lactic acid is removed by the blood and broken down by enzymes, but vigorous exercise can produce lactic acid in such large quantities that it cannot be removed quickly, which causes muscle pains and tiredness. The improvement in the blood circulation that results from taking regular exercise means that the lactic acid is rapidly flushed out of the muscles and endurance improves.

AEROBIC ACTIVITY OR ANAEROBIC HYPERACTIVITY?

The whole body works on the basis of aerobic activity: the use of oxygen to burn up fuel to provide energy. Aerobic exercise is exercise that makes you breathe harder, so causing you to take more oxygen into your system. Aerobic training both improves the efficiency with which you get oxygen into your system and the efficiency with which your muscles use that oxygen.

Effective aerobic training should involve activity at above-normal levels but below the levels that cause you to become too tired or breathless. As your aerobic capacity or stamina improves, so you can step up the level of training.

But what about anaerobic activity? During very vigorous activity your muscles may use energy so rapidly that not enough oxygen can be supplied quickly enough. They go into a state called 'oxygen debt', during which waste lactic acid builds up to very high levels. This happens with sprinters, who require explosive energy for a very short time; no one can keep up this form of energy expenditure for more than a minute or two, however. The build-up of lactic acid is painful and the muscles tire rapidly. Oddly enough, the stated objective of many so-called 'aerobics' classes is to achieve the 'burn' or muscular pain caused by this build-up. In fact, the 'burn' is actually a warning signal, telling us to desist before causing real damage through muscle spasm and injury.

THE ROLE OF OXYGEN

The whole aerobic system depends on the use of oxygen to burn the 'fuel' that powers the muscles, so the amount of oxygen used is a good measure of how well the system is functioning. Although you cannot measure your oxygen consumption directly without special equipment of the sort used in the training of top-level athletes, an increase in oxygen consumption does demonstrate how regular exercise changes the way our bodies work. Lungs, heart and muscles all work more effectively than in pre-exercise days.

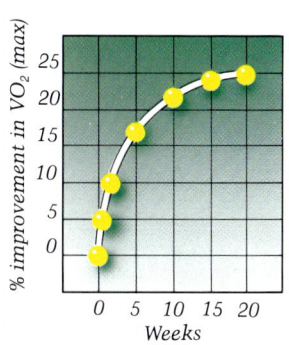

Fitness training aims to help you improve your maximum capacity for oxygen uptake known as VO_2 (max), and to be able to use a larger percentage of that capacity. Your improvement eventually levels off and you should aim to stay on this higher level.

A special term is used to describe maximum oxygen consumption - VO_2 (max). This figure will be proportional to your bodyweight, as a large man, who should have more muscles, will have a greater energy consumption, and hence consume more oxygen, than a man who weighs less.

An unfit, sedentary man will have a low VO_2(max) figure, for he cannot be using much oxygen; a trained athlete might have a VO_2(max) figure that is four times greater. As you follow an exercise programme, your VO_2(max) will steadily improve, until it reaches a maximum figure which is limited by heredity. This is why most men, however hard they try, will never reach the VO_2(max) figure achieved by an Olympic athlete, who has probably inherited the ability to use oxygen in the most efficient way.

The changes that allow the increased usage of oxygen and that are caused by regular exercise take place in various ways. The heart and blood vessels become more efficient at transporting oxygen-rich blood; in the muscles themselves, the number of tiny capillary vessels carrying blood to the individual muscle fibres increases; the muscle fibres thicken and contract more powerfully; and the whole muscle increases in size in response to the increased demands placed on it. In addition, microscopic changes take place within the muscle fibres themselves so that they can use the oxygen more efficiently. As you continue to exercise regularly, these factors work together to improve your stamina and strength.

As getting oxygen into the body as efficiently as possible is absolutely crucial, it is obvious that any activity that compromises the working of the lungs must have a deleterious effect on aerobic performance. The greatest avoidable hazard to aerobic efficiency is cigarette smoking. The irritant effects of tobacco smoke damage and thicken the delicate tissues through which oxygen is absorbed into the lungs, and also cause the smallest air passages to narrow, thus impeding the flow of air and oxygen. In addition, the carbon monoxide present in tobacco smoke becomes permanently attached to the red pigment haemoglobin, impairing its oxygen-carrying capability. All these factors combine to reduce the amount of oxygen reaching the muscle. Moreover, substances absorbed from smoke also have a damaging effect on the heart and circulation, so, even apart from the well-known health risks associated with smoking, it is clear that the habit is *not* compatible with positive health, well-being and, especially, with aerobic fitness.

A CLOSER LOOK AT MUSCLE

Most of the muscles in our bodies are called voluntary muscles because we can consciously control their movement. In many internal organs, including the heart, the muscles are involuntary, working automatically to perform their functions.

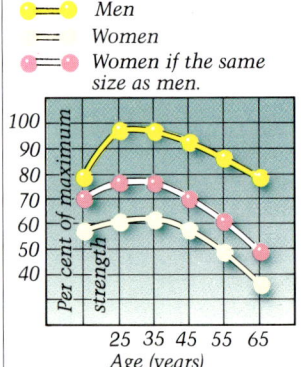

Men
Women
Women if the same size as men.

Strength varies with age and sex. As the graph shows, men are not stronger just because they are bigger than women.

Voluntary muscles contain contractile fibres of two sorts, which are called slow-twitch and fast-twitch fibres, depending on how they respond to a 'contract' order from the nervous system. Each bundle of muscle fibres contain a mixture of the two types, and the proportion of each type affects the way our muscles behave.

Usually the slow-twitch, or slow-to-respond, fibres predominate. These are the fibres that give stamina and work well for long periods without tiring. They are aerobic and need adequate oxygen supplies if they are to work effectively. The leg muscles of a good long-distance runner will contain up to 90 per cent of these slow-twitch fibres. Although the proportion of slow-twitch fibres in your muscles is largely a matter of heredity, you can increase their relative size and efficiency by exercise.

In a sprinter or squash player, on the other hand, the fast-twitch fibres will predominate. A sprinter may have 75 per cent fast-twitch fibres in his leg muscles. They are responsible for the explosive effort needed for sports of this type, working aerobically, but only for very short periods. As with the slow-twitch fibres, specific exercises can increase the size and efficiency of the fast-twitch fibres.

HEALTHY MUSCLE?

Muscles keep working even when we are inactive. The nervous system sends occasional signals to a few muscle fibres at a time to make them contract. At any one time, therefore, some of the muscle fibres will be contracting, and the muscle will be lightly contracted. This gives the muscle its tone.

Most muscles work in opposition; that is, if a muscle moves a bone in one direction, another muscle will move it back again. Muscle tone means that these muscles are always pulling slightly against one another, even when no movement is taking place, so that they do not waste away completely through inactivity.

The effect of inactivity on muscle is, however, very important. There are more than 600 muscles in the body, making up nearly half of our bodyweight, so it is important that they remain healthy. Lack of use impairs muscle tone, and this can cause various problems. Back pain, for instance, can be caused by weak muscles in the back, while a flabby stomach results from poor tone in the abdominal muscles.

BODY CHANGES

The changes resulting from regular exercise are not just in oxygen consumption, fitness and improved well-being. Some fundamental alterations occur in our physiology - the *way* the body works.

As well as improvements in the efficiency of the heart, increasing its output, there will be changes in the volume of blood in the system and in the amount of haemoglobin it contains. Haemoglobin is the red pigment that gives blood its colour and that carries oxygen to the tissues. As the chart below shows, the differences between sedentary men and athletes for all these factors are marked.

The benefits to the system do not occur only *during* exercise. Even when resting, a physically fit person uses less energy than before he began training, for the basic chemistry and physiology of the body has improved.

While exercise training is beneficial for both men and women, there are several basic differences in structure and physiology which mean that men have a greater potential in terms of strength and speed. Therefore men will generally excel in sports requiring these attributes, while women may be superior in sports involving co-ordination and suppleness, and where the larger size and weight of a man could be a disadvantage.

EXERCISE FOR EVERYDAY LIVING

Now that you have made the sensible decision to start an exercise programme, you will need to select an appropriate type of exercise or combination of exercises. Re-examine your lifestyle, and decide how great a commitment in terms of time, convenience and expense you can make to exercise.

Taking up mountaineering may not be too practical if you live in a flat area; golf may be very expensive; formal weight training programmes may need the availability of a gymnasium. Balance your resources against your objectives. You are going to have to enjoy your exercise training, otherwise you will soon begin to find excuses for dropping out, first occasionally, then completely. For this reason, it is best to take up a form of exercise that involves social contact with other people, which will provide a dual motivation for continuing beyond those periods when you just don't feel like physical work.

The various types of physical training that you may consider taking up have different effects on the body, and it is important to understand these before you select the type of activity that will best meet your particular needs. You may hear technical terms bandied about between fitness fanatics, who use the terms to define the type and function of their exercise programmes.

Isometric exercise   Particularly effective at building up muscle bulk as well as strength, isometric exercise involves little or no actual movement. It encourages muscle development by exerting a muscle against a static resistance, which can be an opposing muscle. For example, if you sit in a chair, and push one leg down very hard against the floor, you are actually exercising your leg muscles isometrically. Similarly, an isometric exercise for the forearm could involve the continual clenching of the fists. Isometric exercises are available to develop most of the major muscle groups of the body, and these are the means used by body-builders in conjunction with weight-lifting.

However, although isometrics can be carried out almost anywhere, and with little or no equipment, this form of exercise does not have much benefit for an all-round fitness programme. It burns off little energy, so there is no accompanying improvement in the circulatory system associated with other types of exercise - indeed, blood pressure can actually increase during isometric exercise. Isometrics can develop specific muscles, and this may be useful in particular types of sport. Used alone, however, isometrics cannot be recommended as a means to promote physical fitness, although in combination with dynamic, rhythmic exercise, isometrics could be a useful adjunct to improve your strength and build.

Dynamic exercise involves movement and falls into three categories:
• aerobic exercise, such as running, jogging, swimming or cycling
• indoor exercise such as yoga or dance
• sport, which can mean competitive sport, or pursuits like mountaineering or long-distance walking.

Some of the implications of the most common and accessible forms of exercise are discussed later in this chapter.

Aerobic training   As we have seen, aerobic exercise involves the effective utilization of oxygen, and its main benefits are on the cardiovascular system. To be effective, aerobic training must involve moderately vigorous exercise of the major muscles in the body - as many as possible together - over periods of at least 20 minutes. It is intended to raise your pulse rate and breathing rate. To achieve benefits, such aerobic training must take place at least twice a week over a long time — preferably indefinitely!

Long slow distance (LSD) training   A form of aerobic exercise that involves moderate exertion over a long time, such as jogging or walking (as opposed to running), it encourages the development of slow-twitch muscle fibres and improves stamina.

Tempo training   Activities such as running or cycling may be carried out for longer durations at a faster pace and under competitive conditions.

Interval training   Exercise that involves changes in the level of operation required is known as interval training. Jogging gently for a couple of miles may be followed by a short sprint which would, in turn, be followed by

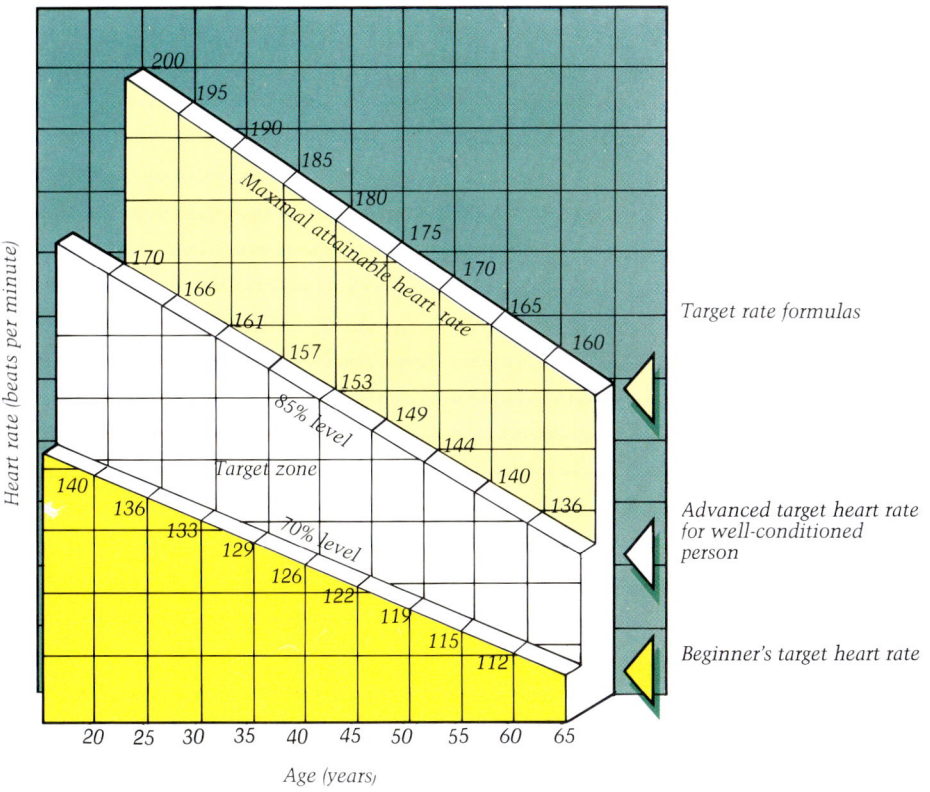

Heart rate (beats per minute)

Maximal attainable heart rate

85% level

Target zone

70% level

Target rate formulas

Advanced target heart rate for well-conditioned person

Beginner's target heart rate

Age (years)

At rest the average man's heart beats at around 70 times a minute, but it can speed up to 200 beats a minute during vigorous exercise. This maximum attainable heart rate drops steadily as you grow older. It is dangerous to keep your heart pounding away at its maximum level for any length of time, and the chart shows the heart rate you should aim to maintain during your exercise sessions, so check your pulse regularly as you work out.

another period of more gentle jogging. Usually, the period of more vigorous activity is gradually stepped up.

Isotonic training   This is a form of dynamic exercise during which the muscles are moved rhythmically, as opposed to isometric training in which the muscles are made to work against resistance and do not move appreciably; eg, holding up a weight. The most common forms of aerobic training, such as swimming and jogging, fall into this category.

Isokinetic training   Training, available in specialized gymnasiums and health studios, that combines the benefits of both isotonic and isometric activity by subjecting the muscles to relatively high loads of isometrics, but with the movement and flexibility associated with isotonics. This is a very effective way of developing all-round physical fitness, but it really requires regular access to the proper equipment and training.

Calisthenics   A system of regular rhythmic exercises, similar to the traditional 'keep fit' or modern dance exercises, it is not usually sufficiently energetic to be classified as truly aerobic, and such exercises do not necessarily raise the heart rate enough to build up stamina. However, they do improve suppleness. Recently, however, a considerably more vigorous type of calisthenics has achieved wide popularity and can have the desired effect. Most of the exercises are so energetic that they are actually anaerobic, and there is some risk that this type of exercise in particular can cause muscle damage if embarked upon before a more gradual improvement in fitness has been achieved.

Spend two or three minutes on each of the following exercises to limber up your muscles before exercising hard. For side bending place your hands on your hips and lean slowly to the right, come back up again then lean to the left. Try not to let hips and shoulders twist, and do not bend further than is comfortable for you.

With feet apart, stretch your arms in front of you and concentrate on keeping your shoulders relaxed and low. Keep your eyes on your right hand, swing your right arm to the right as far as is comfortable, but keep it straight and high. Return to the front and repeat with your left arm.

Stand with feet apart, arms stretched out in front with fingertips touching. Raise your arms above your head and press them back past your ears. Bring your arms down to the sides of the body, take them back past your hips and press each arm upwards and backwards at the same time.

Place your hands on your hips, raise your right leg up to your chest. Bend the other knee to maintain balance. At the same time bend directly forward at the waist without twisting so that your forehead touches your knee. Return to the upright position, and repeat the exercise with the other leg.

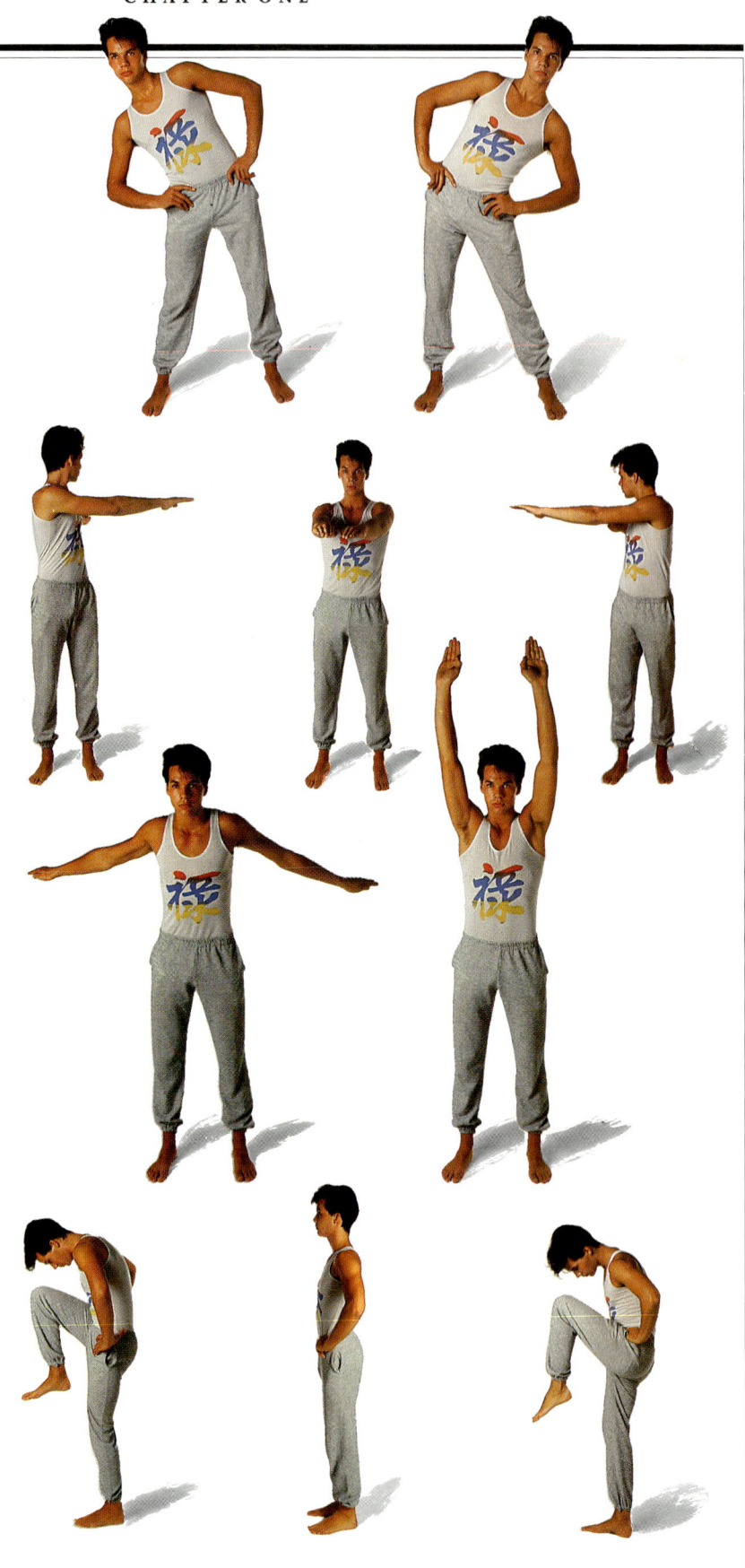

EXERCISE AND INJURY

Just about every physical activity has its risks, and fitness training is no exception. Of course it is possible to jog into the path of a moving car or to trip over a football and sprain your ankle, but these are simple accidents for which *you* are responsible. Your fitness programme would not be at fault if you were unlucky enough to have an accident of this type.

Temperature in degrees

Although 98.4°F is regarded as normal body temperature, this fluctuates throughout the day and night. As you exercise your temperature rises because the release of energy in the muscles produces heat. The body of an unfit person has a less efficient cooling system and the body temperature can rise dramatically. As you get fitter you may notice you sweat more profusely and stay cooler.

In general, fitness training carries its own warning signals. Provided you never push yourself to the point of discomfort and remember to build up your strength, suppleness and stamina gradually, you should experience no problems. This is particularly important if you are unfit or only moderately fit when you start your programme. It is only too easy to rush into training or overdo exercise and injure yourself or become thoroughly exhausted. At first, it is natural to feel muscular stiffness after exercise, but this is short-lived and should disappear quickly as you continue to exercise.

In general, the best guide to the amount of exertion you should be putting into your exercise is that at first you should never exert yourself past the point of being able to hold a fairly normal conversation, even though you may be a bit breathless. And you should *never* push yourself to the point of pain. Once you are into the swing of physical exercise, you will soon recognize the warning signs of over-exertion. Pre-exercise warm-ups are important. You should get your muscles working properly before you begin to exercise them in earnest, and for muscles to work properly, their blood supply must be working well; gentle exercise will start off this process. Paradoxically, the fitter you are, the larger your muscles will be, and the longer they will take to warm up.

If you are going in for a moderate form of exercise, it probably doesn't matter if you don't warm up. Gentle jogging is itself a form of warming up, and most exercise classes incorporate a warm-up period at the beginning of each session. But if you were to begin sprinting without warming up first, you would certainly not perform at your peak and would also run the risk of damaging a muscle or tendon. The hamstring injury is a classic example of damage caused by over-exertion of powerful muscles.

The sort of warm-up exercises you should use will depend to a large extent on the type of activity you will be carrying out. A few simple stretching, turning and flexing movements, carried out for just a few minutes before the exercise proper, are generally sufficient.

Just as important as warming up properly is knowing how to stop. Even if you are tired after your day's exercise programme, don't just stop dead. Your whole system has been keyed up to peak performance during the exercise with your heart, respiratory and hormone systems working hard. If you stop suddenly, it will 'over-run' before it can return to normal rest working. In particular, your blood flow will be increased for a while. So repeat some of the warming-up exercises to taper off your physical efforts for a few minutes, by which time your system will have settled down. If you just rest straight away, your muscles will contract and become stiff and sore. A hot bath will ease the stiffness that may follow the first stages of fitness training.

Body temperature is an important consideration during exercise. Here commonsense should prevail. A trendy tracksuit may look very professional, but on a hot day it is only too easy to over-heat; heat exhaustion is particularly common among marathon runners in the summer. As we have seen, energy for exercise is produced as the body's fuel is burned by oxygen, while the excess is released as heat. This is got rid of partly by panting, which allows some excess heat to escape from the lungs, and partly, and more importantly, by perspiring, which cools the body by the evaporation of sweat. It is important to allow air to reach the body in hot weather so that the evaporation of sweat can continue, and this usually means running or exercising in light clothing such as a cotton T-shirt and shorts.

Salt is lost from the body in the perspiration, together with large amounts of water. It is important to drink plenty of water before or after prolonged exercise in hot weather and to add extra salt to your food or to take salt tablets to replace that lost in perspiration.

If it is cold or wet, wear several layers of light clothing rather than a single heavy sweater or tracksuit. The layers provide better insulation as air is trapped between them, and separate items of clothing can be removed if you begin to feel too hot. If it is really cold, wear gloves and some form of headgear, for 20 per cent of body heat is lost from the head.

If you get wet you may not feel uncomfortable as long as you continue to exercise, but as soon as you stop you will begin to feel cold, and you should change into warm, dry clothing immediately. Drops in body temperature can be dangerous, especially while your circulatory system is re-adjusting after exercise, so keep warm while you are doing your 'cooling-off' exercises.

These general rules apply to almost all types of fitness programme, but some types of activity have special problems, and these are discussed later in this chapter, under the individual types of fitness programme.

WALKING

If you are going to take your aerobic fitness programme seriously, you will probably aim to take up running, swimming or some other similarly energetic pursuit. As you will have to build up to these gradually, however, it would be sensible to start off with something a little less strenuous, and walking is probably the easiest and most convenient form of aerobic exercise there is.

If you are not particularly fit, you would probably not be able to commence running training without first undertaking a period of 'conditioning' by walking to improve your stamina. Walking has the distinct advantage of not requiring any special equipment, other than sensible footwear and clothing. You probably won't need the specially cushioned running shoes used by joggers, and under most conditions, ordinary trainers will do. Your footwear and the clothing you wear during walking will depend greatly on *where* you walk. Light clothing and trainers may be fine for a few laps of the local park, but if your idea of walking is a hike over the moors, boots and weatherproof clothing are far more appropriate.

This is probably going to be your first attempt at a fitness programme, so please be careful to get it right. Don't start your walking until at least a couple of hours after a meal. And of course, never push yourself to the point of discomfort or exhaustion. There is nothing to be ashamed of in cutting short your exercise in the early stages. Be especially cautious if you are not feeling fully recovered, for virus infections in particular can leave you feeling weak for quite a while, as you will find out if you push yourself too hard.

Of all forms of aerobic activity, walking is the one best suited for the whole family, including young children, although you may have to adjust your stride to accommodate their shorter legs. A simple walking programme is outlined here, which shows you how to build up your exercise and your fitness, starting with a short walk of only a mile or a 15-minute walk. You should easily be able to increase your performance in the stages shown in the chart. If not, don't worry; just stick at the same level for a little longer, then try again.

Once you have completed this programme, you may want to move to something more energetic, such as running or a sport. If not, you will need to keep up your level of fitness by walking at least five miles, three times each week. Thinking twice before using the car could be all that's necessary! Another possibility, if you want to stay with walking, is to switch to race walking, a very rapid form of walking achieved by developing a strange rolling movement with the hips, which is rather ungainly but very good for the lower back. The object is to achieve a walking speed so rapid that it would be more comfortable to break into a trot, and at that point the amount of energy consumed is probably as great as that used in running.

WEEK		1	2	3	4	5	6	7	8	9	10	11	12
Minutes		15	20	23	26	30	30	30	30	28	28	35	34
		OR	OR	OR	OR	OR	OR	OR	OR	OR	OR	OR	OR
Distance	km	1·6	2	2·4	2·8	3·2	3·2	4	3·2	3·2	3·2	4	4
	mls	1	$1\frac{1}{4}$	$1\frac{1}{2}$	$1\frac{3}{4}$	2	2	$2\frac{1}{2}$	2	2	2	$2\frac{1}{2}$	$2\frac{1}{2}$
Alternative time for any distance									60	60	60	60	
Alternative distance in any time	km						4	4·8					
	mls						$2\frac{1}{2}$	3					
Repeats per week		5	5	5	5	5	3	3	4	4	4	4	4

A simple walking programme shows you how to build up your exercise and fitness starting with a short walk of only a mile or a 15-minute walk. You should be able to increase your performance in the stages shown in the chart, but if not stay at one level for longer then try again. To keep up your level of fitness, walk five miles three times a week.

RUNNING

Most men think of running when exercise is suggested, and in some social circles today, it is almost abnormal *not* to run. Your running could take the form of a solitary trot through the streets in late evening or it could be the mass run in the marathons and half-marathons that have become a feature of city life.

As with other forms of exercise, you can grade your running according to your level of fitness. You will probably start off with jogging, but, as your fitness builds up, you will automatically find yourself slipping into a more powerful stride.

An extra attraction of running is that you can achieve a greater expenditure of energy with only a short run than you can with walking or any other less strenuous pursuit. If you wish, you can cram your day's exercise into a short lunch break. Running is permitted, and accepted, almost anywhere.

As has already been emphasized, it is important that you wear appropriate clothing. You will soon warm up, so don't wear anything too heavy, and don't wear anything that will trap perspiration and prevent it evaporating to cool you. Otherwise, the type of clothing you wear for running is not important and will probably be dictated by style and vanity.

More important than your clothes is your footwear, for the stresses and strains on the feet are more extreme in running than in walking, especially if you are pounding the pavements. There are several important points to consider when you are buying running shoes, and it will not pay to economize. Remember that each foot hits the ground about 800 times for each mile you run, and your running shoes should be tough enough to last for 1000 miles of running - so you can work out for yourself how hard they will be working.

WEEK		1	2	3	4	5	6	7	8	9	10	11	12
PROGRAMME 1 *Minutes*		17	22	16½	26	21½	25½	21½	34½	21	34	25	34
Distance	km	3·2	4	3·2	4·8	4	4·8	4	6·4	4	6·4	4·8	6·4
	mls	2	2½	2	3	2½	3	2½	4	2½	4	3	4
Repeats per week		3	4	4	4	4	4	4	4	4	3	3	3
PROGRAMME 2 *Minutes*		—	45	35	55	44	65	63	75	44	60	—	—
Distance	km	4·8	any distance	6·4	any distance	8	any distance	11·2	any distance	8	any distance	8	12·8
	mls	3		4		5		7		5		5	8
Repeats per week		2	1	1	1	1	1	1	1	1	2	2	2

Running (or jogging when done at a slower pace) is one of the most accessible ways to improve your fitness. It carries very little risk provided you begin gently and build up gradually, and two alternative intermediate level programmes are shown here.

However, if you are middle aged or elderly it would be sensible to have a check-up before starting a fitness programme. You can check that you are within your capabilities by taking your pulse or making sure that you are not uncomfortably out of breath. In fact, you should be able to carry on a conversation with someone running alongside you. The running programme is not designed to help you acquire physical speed. This requires long and very specific training because it is a specialized form of fitness for serious athletes.

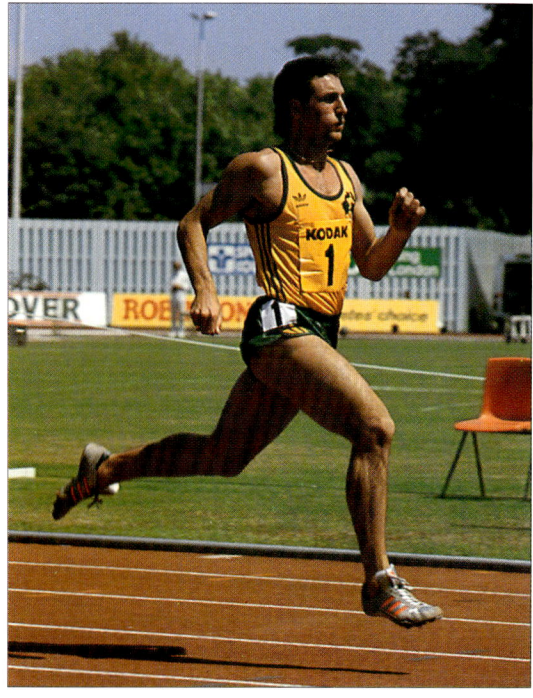

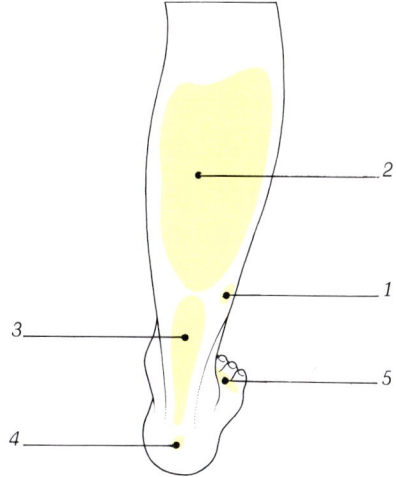

Start running in a relaxed, easy stride that you feel you could keep up for a while without getting too tired or breathless. Keep your body upright, with your arms relaxed, your fists loosely clenched and your shoulders relaxed and loose. Make sure that your heel strikes the ground first, so that your foot can roll forward, enabling you to spring off the ground with a thrusting push from the ball of your foot. Don't try to breathe through your nose alone, but breath through your mouth as much as you need.

Minor injuries can result if an incautious running programme is embarked upon and many can be avoided altogether by using correct footwear, warming up the muscles by brisk walking prior to running and increasing endurance gradually. The commonest are outer shin muscle strain or peroneal tendon strain 1 caused by running on uneven ground or adopting a gait which puts weight on the outside of the foot. Calf pain 2 is caused by overuse of the calf muscle which cannot expand in its tight sheath. Achilles sheath pain 3 may result from the heel tab of shoes pressing against the tendon, and heelbone lumps (bursae) 4 are caused by shoes rubbing. March fractures 5 were first described by soldiers (hence the name) and produce pain in the central bones of the forefoot caused by stress fractures of these small bones following excessive road running.

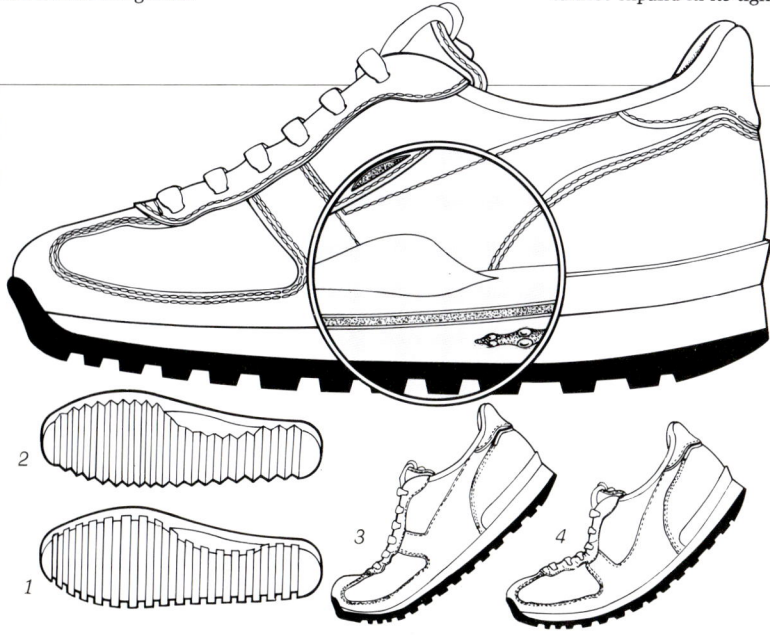

Footwear is all important for running. Your foot hits the ground 800 times for each mile you run and your shoes should last for 1000 miles of running. Choose a shoe that has a layered cushioned sole with an instep support. If most of your running is to be on tarmac go for the waffle-patterned tread 1 which cushions the impact, but buy a zigzag tread 2 for soft surfaces. Make sure the shoe bends at the ball of your foot 3, not at the arch 4. Wear the socks you will run in when you go to try on your shoes. The shoe uppers should be of a natural fibre such as leather, suede or canvas.

SWIMMING

If you review the primary objective of physical exercise - improving your stamina, strength and suppleness - swimming must be the best all-round choice to enable you to improve in all three areas. Because water supports you, the pull of gravity plays no part in swimming, and the amount of effort you need to move your body is, therefore, determined wholly by how energetic *you* want to be. This can mean anything from floating, to soothe away the day's aches and pains, to energetic sprinting or race training.

Swimming can be a particularly good way for older men or those who are normally sedentary to become fitter. Even obese men or those with hip or knee problems can swim gently, effectively freed from the weight of their bodies.

Many men regard swimming as a social event, often with the family, which may involve no more than just splashing about and swimming the occasional 'length' between the chatting and the horseplay. This is not going to do much for your stamina or strength, although any form of 'exercise' in the water will at least start to improve your suppleness. The other extreme is out-and-out racing, for which specialized coaching is essential. Before you rush to take *this* up, consider the age at which competitive swimmers peak. Most start their career in their early 'teens and are over the hill by the time they reach their early 20s. You would have little or no chance of catching up with them, either in a race or in terms of fitness.

For most men, as with other forms of aerobic exercise, the middle course is most sensible. If you can't swim or don't swim well, it's never too late to learn, and many people take up swimming after they have retired. Most councils and many clubs run swimming classes in which qualified instructors take you through the basic steps.

WEEK		1	2	3	4	5	6	7	8	9	10	11	12
PROGRAMME 1 Minutes		5	5	7½	7	10	12	10	12	11½	14	16½	16
Distance	m	200	200	300	300	400	500	500	600	600	700	800	800
	yds	219	219	328	328	437	547	547	656	656	435	497	497
Repeats per week		5	3	5	3	5	5	3	5	3	5	5	3
PROGRAMME 2 Minutes		5	8	7½	13	10	12	16	12	17	14	16½	22
Distance	m	200	300	300	500	400	500	700	600	800	700	800	1,000
	yds	219	328	328	547	437	547	435	656	497	435	497	1094
Repeats per week		5	2	5	2	5	5	2	5	2	5	5	2

A swimming training schedule, like any other fitness programme, should be started at a comfortable point. Two alternative programmes, both at an intermediate level suitable for the reasonably fit, are outlined here. However, as previously emphasized, don't over-do things in the early stages. Check the length of the pool to make sure of the distance you are swimming. Aim to be moderately breathless or use your pulse rate as a guide to check whether you are swimming vigorously enough. Allow a two-hour gap between eating a meal and swimming.

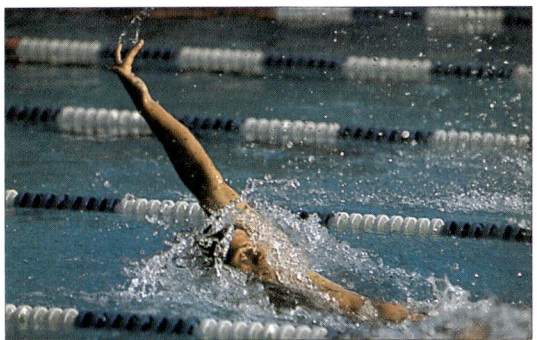

BACKSTROKE

Although the face is out of the water, concentrate on developing a regular breathing pattern. Let the water carry the weight of your head. Your hand enters the water little finger first and is then driven backwards. Your cupped hand pulls forwards, bending at the elbow and finishing underneath the hip as the other hand enters the water. For the kick, keep the ankle flexible and whip the foot upwards as if you are flicking a football off the surface of the water. Muscles used: latissimus dorsi; pectoralis major; deltoids; trapezius; gluteus maximus; hip flexors; quadriceps; abdominals.

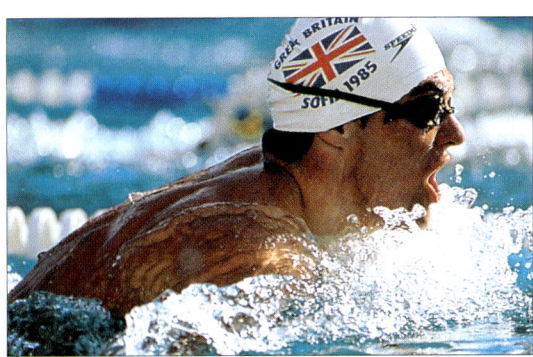

BREASTSTROKE

Swum correctly, this can be as demanding as the crawl. From the central position your arms scull outwards as if parting the water for your head to pass through and pulling the water back behind your body. Short, sharp movements give maximum power. Keep your knees high for the frog kick. As your feet snap together and your arms begin their circular motion again, exhale explosively under water so that you can take a deep breath in the short time your face is above the water. Muscles used: triceps; latissimus dorsi; quadriceps; adductors.

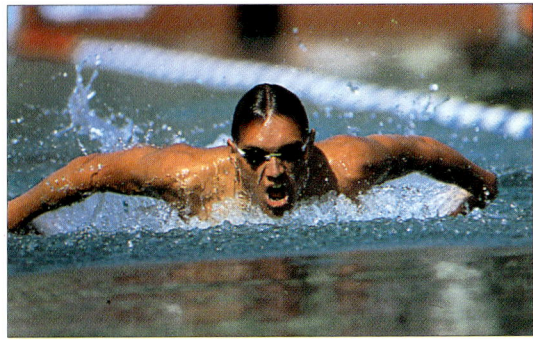

BUTTERFLY

This gruelling stroke is the most difficult to master. Your hands enter the water like a double crawl action and at the same moment the feet kick down to begin the undulating, dolphin-like kick. You begin to exhale under water as your hands press backwards. Your hea comes out of the water at the end of the arm pull and you take a deep breath before plunging the head below the surface again as the arms come up. Muscles used: latissimus dorsi; pectoralis major; deltoids; trapezius; gluteus maximus; hip flexors; abdominals; quadriceps; erector spinae.

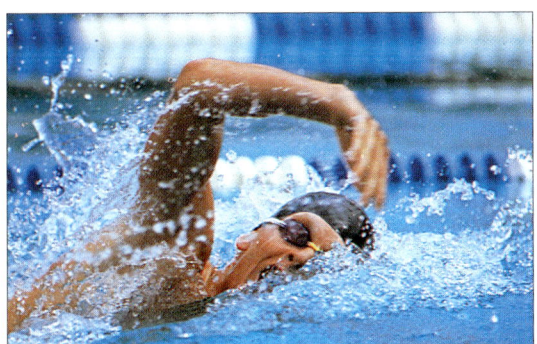

CRAWL

Most men would like to swim the crawl, but the breathing pattern is difficult to master. You must start to breathe out through your mouth at the beginning of the stroke cycle and continue to exhale as your face swings under the water. As the stroke cycle ends and the first arm leaves the water again, turn your head back towards your shoulder and take a controlled breath from the pocket of air in the bow wave formed by your head pushing through the water. Muscles used: latissimus dorsi; pectoralis major; deltoids; trapezius; glueus maximus; hip flexors.

Leisure or 'fun' pools are ideal for family recreation, but not really suitable for serious training. The traditional, deeper pool, divided into lanes, reduces the risk of collisions with other swimmers, especially if you can exercise early, before the pool becomes crowded.

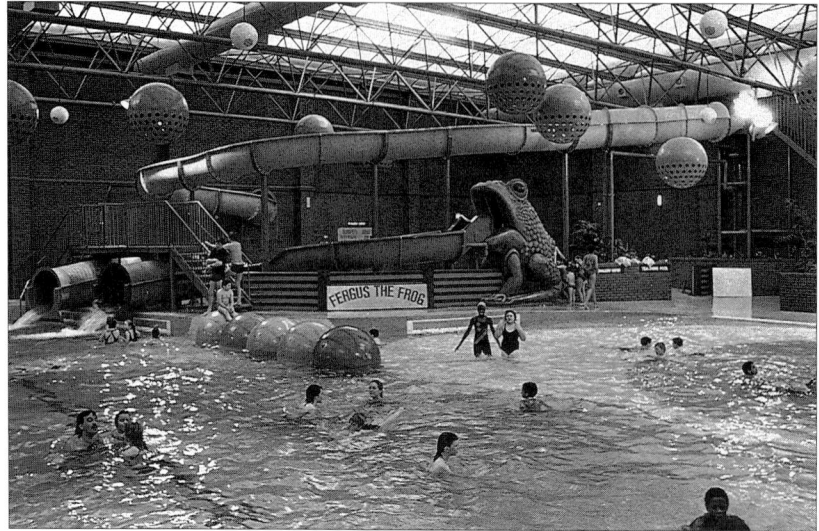

Most of your swimming will be done in public pools. It is not a good idea to swim in unheated pools, rivers, streams or the sea. At the low water temperatures you will encounter, you will not be able to swim for long enough to help your fitness training, and these low temperatures will mean that your body will not respond normally to the exercise. Very cold water can also be extremely dangerous once your body temperature starts to drop.

If swimming is your chosen exercise type, you will need to use your local heated pool on a regular basis. In many areas there are large leisure or 'fun' pools, but these are not really suitable for training as it is seldom possible to swim for more than a few strokes before bumping into another swimmer, and if you swim back-crawl or butterfly you are liable to injure someone else with a flailing arm. The traditional rectangular pool, divided into lanes, is much better for serious training, especially if you can use it at a time when it is not too crowded. Most pools now open quite early to allow serious swimmers to exercise early in the day, before the pool fills with family groups and people splashing about.

Swimming pools are heavily chlorinated to minimize the spread of disease in the water, and some people find this irritating to the eyes, causing itching and redness - 'swimmers' conjunctivitis'. If you have sensitive eyes, wear proper swimming goggles. They are very small and will fit snugly into your eye sockets, so that they will not be dislodged by knocks or diving. Read the instructions carefully so you can fit them properly, and adjust them to ensure they do not leak.

Ear plugs and nose clips are sometimes worn, but unless you have a specific medical condition for which your doctor has advised their use, you should avoid them. Ear plugs especially can be dangerous if you dive under the water, as the pressure may force them deep into the opening to the ears and damage the ear drum.

A few health hazards associated with swimming arise because of the wetness and the high humidity that continue even after you leave the water. Ear infections are quite common, as the organisms causing them thrive on dampness. Always dry your ears thoroughly. A small passage called the Eustachian tube leads from the back of the throat to the inner part of the ear, and if you dive under the water, the increased pressure may push bacteria from the mouth up the tube and into the ear, so causing an infection. Both types of ear problem need medical treatment, but they clear up very quickly.

Foot problems are quite common, and, once again, the dampness of the pool area is the cause. Athlete's foot, which is caused by a microscopic fungus, generally attacks the soft skin between the toes, causing itching and peeling. Verucas are flat warts that affect the soles of the feet and can become painfully in-growing. Both conditions can be picked up at the swimming pool or changing rooms, and although they may be easily treated by the doctor, it is advisable to keep your shoes on as much as possible when changing to reduce the chances of infection.

Diving can be an exercise in its own right. It is particularly good for improving suppleness but has little effect on the other aspects of fitness, and cannot properly be considered an aerobic exercise.

Another activity associated with swimming is life-saving. This obviously has important humanitarian aims, but it has considerable benefits in terms of physical fitness. Built up through a series of grades, training for life-saving includes excellent fitness programmes that are designed to improve your strength and stamina, so you are able to support and recover anyone who is drowning.

FITNESS ON WHEELS

Cycling is another easily accessible aerobic activity and, in some ways, it is the most convenient, for many men combine their cycling exercise with their daily journey to work. Cycling is another of the exercises that can involve the whole family, and it is more appealing than running to some older men, as it produces less wear and tear on the feet.

But cycling in busy streets can be so stressful that it undoes all the physical benefit that you derive from the exercise. However, if you live in the country or can easily reach a country area or a park, cycling can be both relaxing and fun. It tends to develop different muscle groups than other forms of exercise such as running because of the rather static position of the body, and it does little to improve your suppleness. It is very good for the legs, however, and of benefit to the circulatory system.

If you are thinking of buying a bicycle you will certainly not need an exotic machine with innumerable gears and a featherweight frame. In fact, if exercise is your *only* criterion, you could be better off with an old-fashioned, sit-up-and-beg boneshaker, which would be extremely heavy and hard work to pedal. Most men find that a perfectly standard, 3-speed bike is quite adequate, and even this is an extremely efficient way to convert your energy into movement - so efficient, in fact, that you will find yourself travelling for considerable distances with little effort, as you achieve your exercise targets.

Wind resistance is the principal hindrance to speed on a bicycle, which is why racing cyclists crouch down, a position that also helps them put more power into pedalling. Drag from air resistance increases enormously as your speed increases, and it will affect the effort you have to put into pedalling, making it difficult to be precise about the targets you should attempt in your cycling exercise programme. The effect of even small gradients is equally dramatic.

The only sensible way to check if you are putting the proper amount of effort into your cycling is to pedal hard enough to get moderately out of breath, but not so hard that you become too breathless to hold a conversation. Just like any other exercise, you should always slow down for a while if you get tired.

Of course, if you don't want to cycle outdoors, you can always buy an exercise bike to use at home. To be effective, the bike must be adjustable to suit your body frame, and must have an adjustable load approximating to the resistance against which you would be working if you were cycling along the road. This load can be increased as your fitness improves. Exercise bikes are convenient and you won't be knocked off them by a car, but they are even less effective than a normal bike at exercising muscles other than the legs and lower back, as your body remains completely static. However, they can be useful as training for 'real' cycling or as part of an indoor fitness programme.

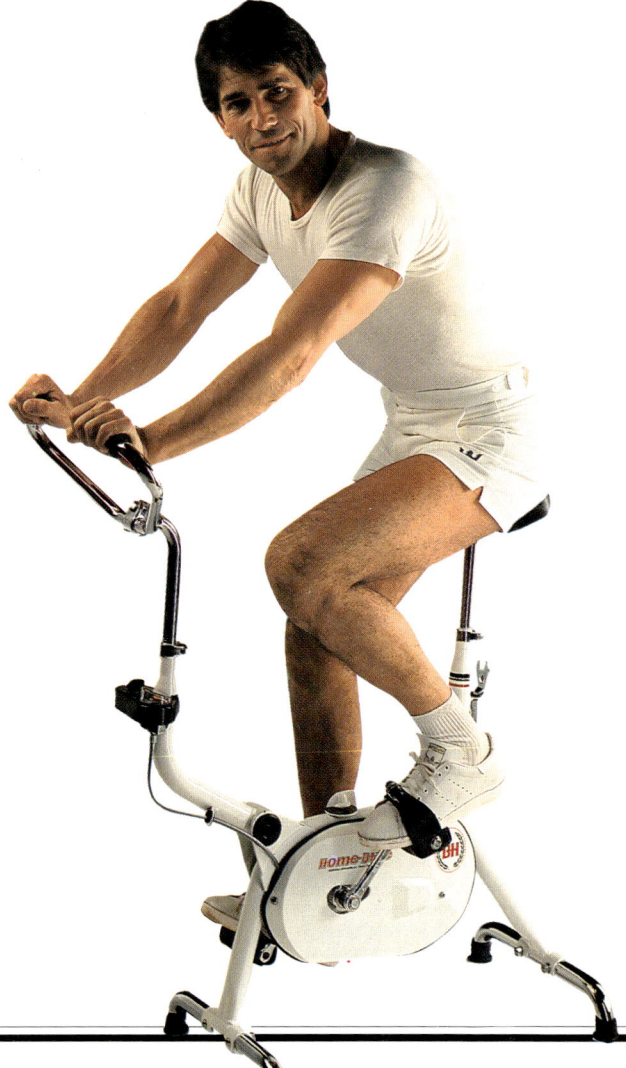

A good-quality exercise bike can be expensive, but at least that factor provides an incentive to use it. Bikes are a particularly useful form of exercise for people who would find a weight-bearing exercise such as running uncomfortable — for example, those who are obese, arthritic or back and foot sufferers.

WEEK	1	2	3	4	5	6	7	8	9	10	11	12
PROGRAMME 1 Minutes	20	16	20	24	16	28	18	26	14	22	17	10
Distance km	8	6·4	8	9·6	6·4	11·2	8	11·2	6·4	9·6	8	4·8
mls	5	4	5	6	4	7	5	7	4	6	5	3
Repeats per week	3	3	3	3	3	3	3	4	3	4	3	2
PROGRAMME 2 Minutes	55	40	50	—	48	58	45	—	53	—	42	—
Distance km	16	12·8	16	19·2	16	19·2	16	24	19·2	32	16	48
mls	10	8	10	12	10	12	10	15	12	20	10	30
Repeats per week	2	2	2	2	2	2	2	1	2	1	2	1

To undertake the cycling programme outlined here, it is not necessary to have a smart, 10-speed bike. Since the terrain and the relative wind speed make such a difference to cycling energy levels, the times and distances in these two intermediate level programmes are less accurate than in the running and swimming programmes. Go by time not distance, and keep up a reasonable level of effort, cycling hard enough to sweat a little, but easily enough to continue a conversation.

INDOOR FITNESS

You may have good reasons for wanting to carry out your fitness programme indoors, but don't be fooled by glib advertising suggesting that you need spend only a few minutes each day with a particular type of exercise equipment to achieve peak fitness. Whether you exercise indoors or out, you will need to expend around the same amount of energy to achieve the same ends.

Indoor exercise does have the advantages that you are not subject to changes in the weather and that you can exercise when it most suits you. Indoor exercise is probably best used combined with one of the outdoor forms of exercise already discussed, or the other types of physical pursuits reviewed later in this book.

Probably the greatest problem with undertaking a programme of indoor exercise at home is motivation - or lack of it. It can be very lonely on an exercise bike or rowing machine, and many people quickly abandon this form of exercise, which is why so many of these devices are offered for sale in the classified sections of local newspapers or end up in the attic. This is a pity, especially as all that is required is twenty to thirty minutes two or three times a week. If you have a low boredom threshold for this type of indoor exercise, try listening to the radio or watching television while you exercise - time will fly. On the other hand, peace and solitude are positive advantages for disciplines like yoga, which combine both physical and emotional or spiritual exercise.

Many men find that they perform indoor exercise best when they are part of a group in a club or gymnasium. There are, of course, social benefits from joining a club, but more importantly, you will be much better motivated by a coach or leader encouraging you and monitoring your progress. There is always the incentive to push yourself just that little bit harder or to continue for longer when you want to keep up with the group. And if you allocate a regular time each week to exercise with a group at a gymnasium or club, you will not be distracted by the thought of wanting to watch a special programme on the television, as you might be if you exercised alone at home.

There are so many different forms of clubs and organizations dedicated to physical fitness that everyone should be able to find the sort of exercise that will interest them sufficiently to keep up the motivation throughout a complete exercise programme. Clubs range from those that specialize in calisthenics or dance exercise and often meet in school halls, for no special equipment is required, to martial arts clubs, which may need little but an exercise mat. At the other extreme are the well-equipped gymnasiums, which specialize in isokinetic training and cater largely for businessmen, who choose to exercise at lunchtime and in the early evening. These are relatively expensive, but they are very effective. If you are spending a lot of money on getting fit, you will be extremely conscientious about carrying out the exercises!

Well equipped specialist gymnasiums are relatively expensive, but very effective in providing the motivation to keep fit and the means of monitoring your progress.

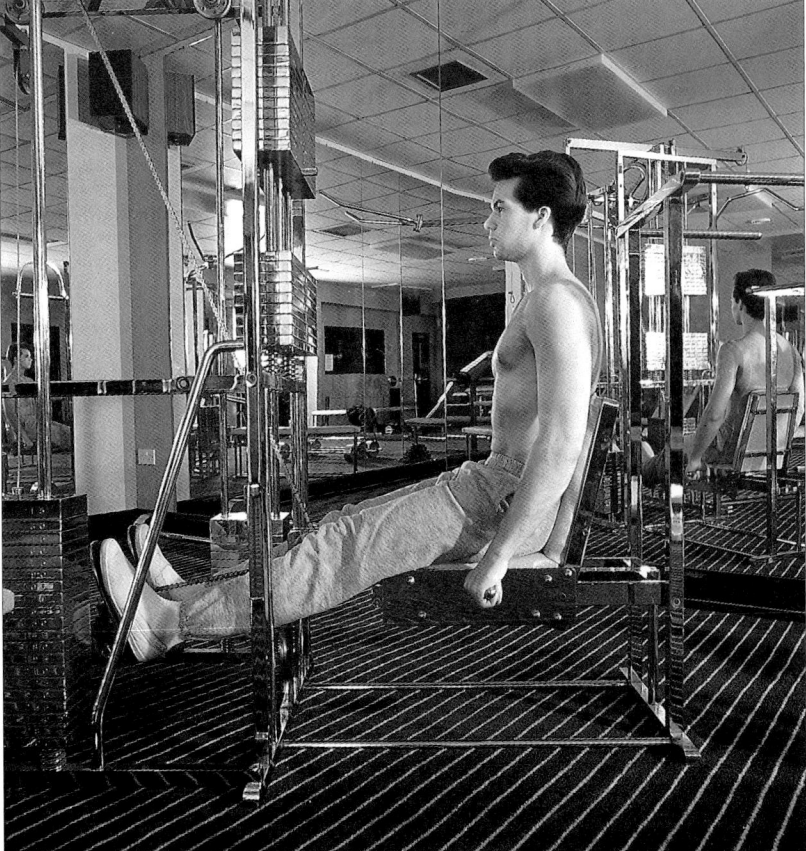

Here is a simple schedule for a skipping programme. Begin with Programme 1 and work up towards Programme 2, stepping up the work rate gradually and resting before you get too tired.

WEEK	1	2	3	4	5	6
PROGRAMME 1						
Minutes	5	$5\frac{1}{2}$	$5\frac{1}{2}$	6	$6\frac{1}{2}$	7
Repeats	3	3	4	4	4	4
PROGRAMME 2						
Minutes	10	$11\frac{1}{2}$	12	13	14	15
Repeats	5	5	5	5	5	5
WEEK	7	8	9	10	11	12
PROGRAMME 1						
Minutes	7	8	9	10	11	12
Repeats	3	4	4	4	5	5
PROGRAMME 2						
Minutes	15	16	17	18	19	20
Repeats	6	6	6	6	6	6

FITNESS ALONE

If you decide to keep fit at home, you may be able to persuade other members of the family to join you, to give you that extra encouragement to keep at it. Your chosen exercise programme may require only minimal equipment or you may wish to fit yourself out with a home gym.

Skipping is one of the simplest yet most effective forms of aerobic exercise. Not just a child's game, it forms an important part of the training for boxers, footballers and others. Skipping is a powerful form of aerobic exercise, and in its more energetic forms, involves most of the major muscle groups of the body - not just those of the legs.

The range of exercise equipment available for use in the home is very large, but much of this apparatus - treadmills and rowing machines, for example - is not only expensive but bulky and is not easily accommodated in most modern homes. Some of the simple devices such as spring-loaded grip developers are very effective isometric aids to muscle development but, as we have seen, isometrics alone do not improve overall fitness, though they can play a part in your fitness programme by increasing your strength.

One type of 'exercise' device does need special comment. A series of pads are stuck on to 'overweight' parts of the body, and electrical stimulation from the pads causes muscles to twitch and, supposedly,

Continued on page 42

The choice of sports available today is enormous, so that everyone can find one or more activities to suit them and help them become fitter. This table rates each type of sport according to its physical criteria and its social side, for quick and easy reference.

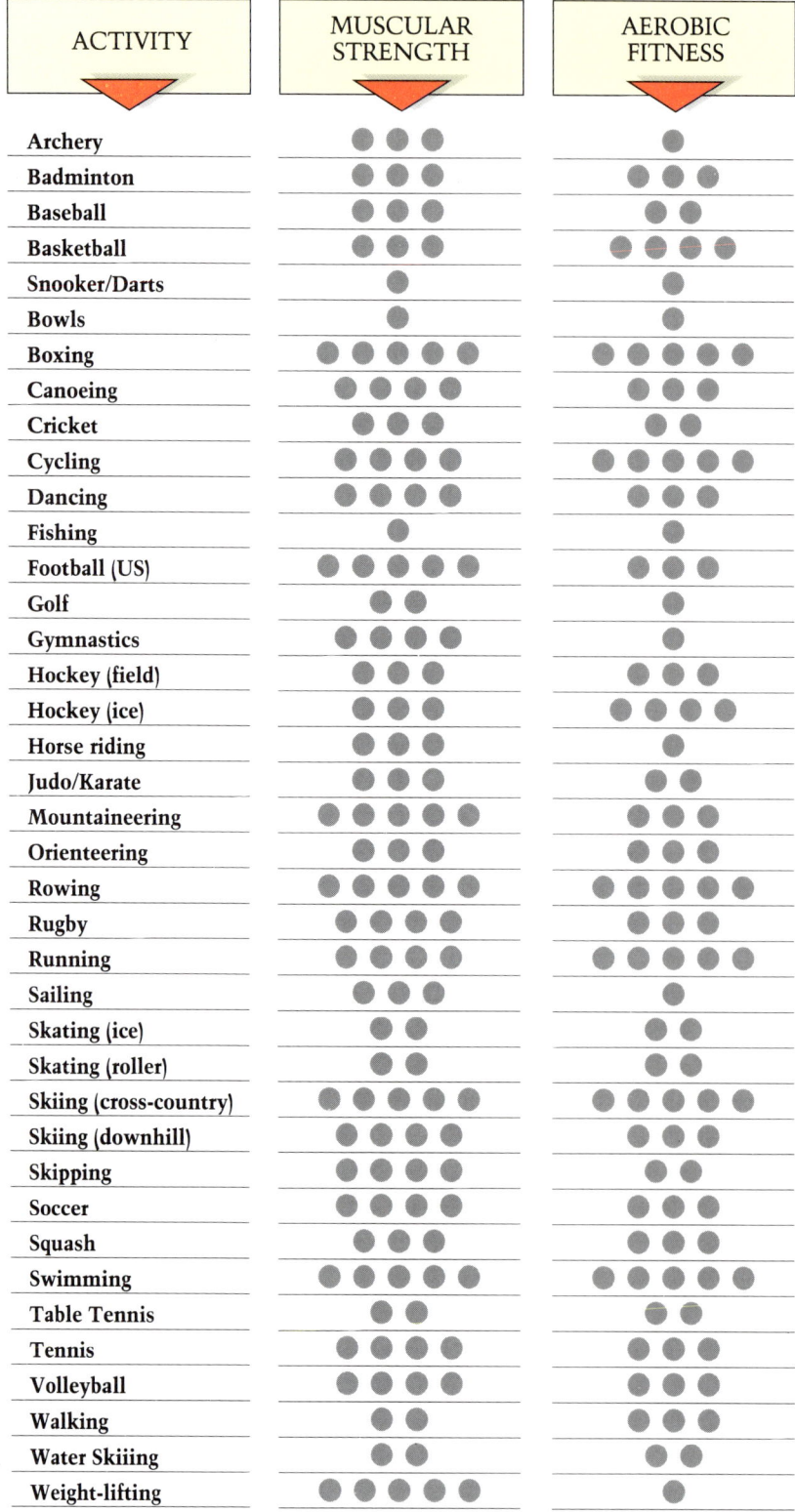

ACTIVITY	MUSCULAR STRENGTH	AEROBIC FITNESS
Archery	●●●	●
Badminton	●●●	●●●
Baseball	●●●	●●
Basketball	●●●	●●●●
Snooker/Darts	●	●
Bowls	●	
Boxing	●●●●●	●●●●●
Canoeing	●●●●	●●●●
Cricket	●●●	●●
Cycling	●●●●	●●●●●
Dancing	●●●●	●●●
Fishing	●	●
Football (US)	●●●●●	●●●
Golf	●●	●
Gymnastics	●●●●	●
Hockey (field)	●●●	●●●
Hockey (ice)	●●●	●●●●
Horse riding	●●●	●
Judo/Karate	●●●	●●
Mountaineering	●●●●●	●●●
Orienteering	●●●	●●●
Rowing	●●●●●	●●●●●
Rugby	●●●●	●●●
Running	●●●●	●●●●●
Sailing	●●●	●
Skating (ice)	●●	●●
Skating (roller)	●●	●●
Skiing (cross-country)	●●●●●	●●●●●
Skiing (downhill)	●●●	●
Skipping	●●●	●●
Soccer	●●●●	●●●
Squash	●●●	●●●
Swimming	●●●●●	●●●●●
Table Tennis	●●	●●
Tennis	●●●●	●●●
Volleyball	●●●	●●●
Walking	●●	●●●
Water Skiing	●●	●●
Weight-lifting	●●●●●	●

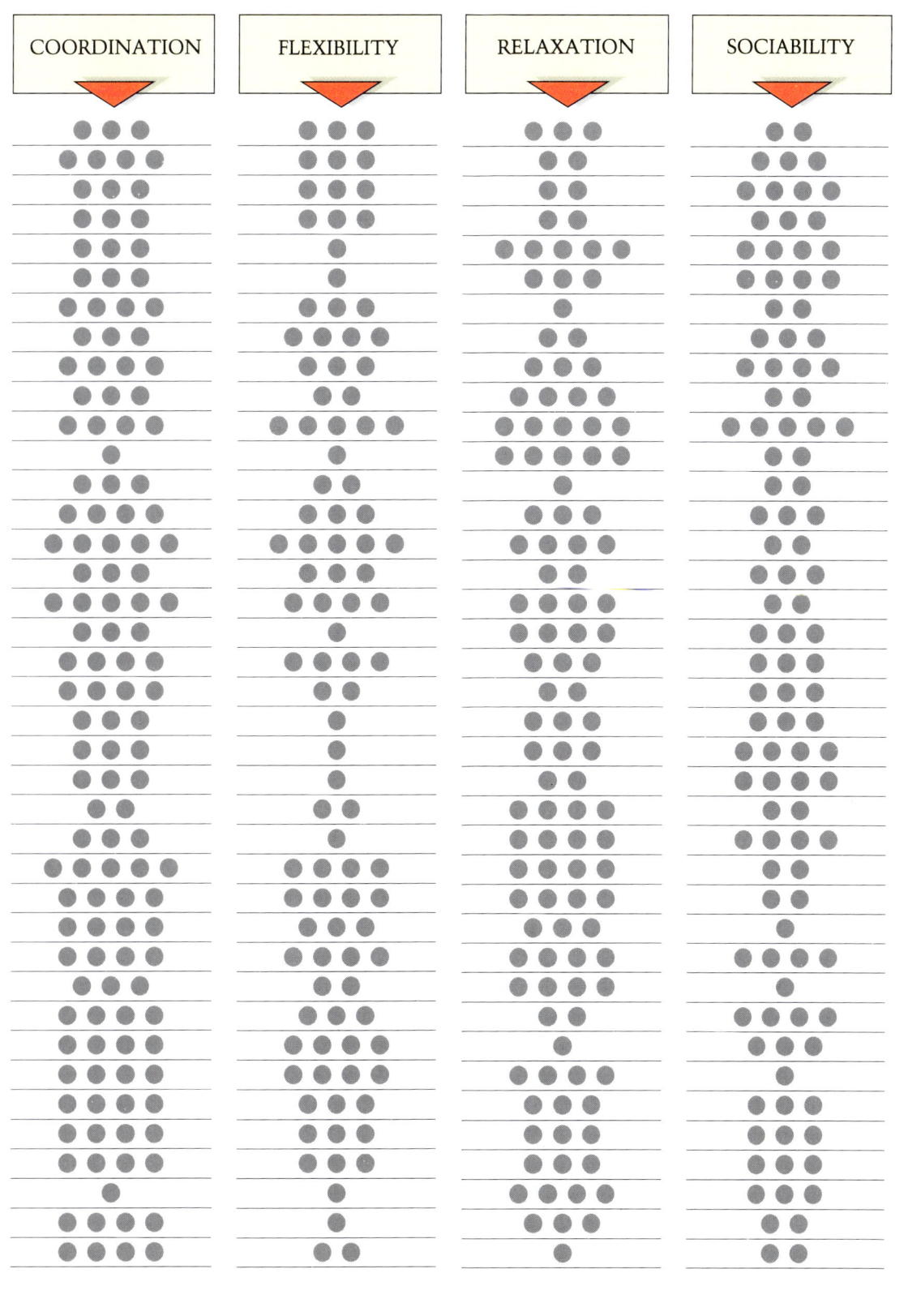

Continued from page 39

transforms fat into muscle. The whole concept is based upon a misconception of how the body uses fat, and such devices have absolutely no place in a fitness programme.

Weight-training can be carried out at home quite easily, with small weights used to increase the load on the limbs while you exercise. Small ankle and wrist weights can be purchased, and these simply increase the effort you put into other types of exercise.

More vigorous weight-training, involving heavier weights, requires proper coaching. It is easy to injure yourself by lifting heavy weights, and the training machines available in gymnasiums and health clubs are designed to overcome these problems by adjusting the effort required according to the muscles involved.

STAYING FIT

After all the effort and when you have achieved your chosen level of fitness, what then? You can't just settle back into your former unhealthy lifestyle and, in any case, you probably won't want to, now that you are feeling good.

Once your body is toned up by a proper programme of exercise, a short period without exercise won't matter at all. But if you stop for more than a few weeks, your body will begin to revert to its former condition, and within about six to eight weeks you'll be back where you started!

Stamina is the first to go, slumping by about 25 per cent quite quickly, then declining more slowly. If you stopped exercising altogether, your muscles would gradually reduce in size, and with them your strength, but this happens quite slowly. Unfortunately, what also happens is that, if you continue to eat the same amount but are no longer burning off the energy by exercising, the energy is converted into fat - hence the large numbers of middle-aged ex-sportsmen with pot bellies, which are made even worse as their abdominal muscles become flabby through lack of exercise.

•Capacity for oxygen uptake, known as VO_2, see chart, page 21

The obvious answer is to keep up your exercise programme at a sensible level. As we have seen, oxygen uptake - VO_2 (max) - reaches a peak during exercise training and cannot normally be pushed higher. You should aim to exercise sufficiently to maintain a reasonable VO_2(max), although you need not continue to follow such a concentrated programme. It isn't necessary to push oneself to peak VO_2 (max) in exercise training to achieve a moderate beneficial level of fitness, unless one is training for some competitive sport. But, whatever intensity of training you choose, you will have to maintain the effort in order to maintain the achieved level of fitness. If you slacken off, your fitness will fade too. You might switch to an energetic leisure pursuit or take up football or tennis. Now is the time to exercise for enjoyment and to take advantage of your improved physical fitness. For example, if running was your chosen method of getting fit, you might want to try orienteering, which combines running with map-reading and various other skills. Or you could go in for the fun-runs and half-marathons that are now so popular. Look upon your improved fitness as a foundation on which you can build a new range of physical activities, either competitively or purely for leisure. Enjoyment is the key to physical fitness. If you don't choose activities that you enjoy, you are unlikely to keep exercising as a way of life and hence you will lose all the benefits you have gained. You may decide to take a holiday that will involve physical activity or sport. Skiing, windsurfing and dinghy sailing are all excellent aerobic activities, but if you are to make the best of them, you should be fit *and* trained before you arrive at your holiday destination. Training is available for these and almost all other leisure pursuits and will ensure you get the best from your short annual holiday. It will also mean you are less likely to injure yourself by overdoing an unfamiliar form of exercise.

RELAXATION REVIEW

The choice of sports and activities available to you is almost infinite, although some will be inaccessible or too expensive, but their potential benefits vary very widely, and it is worth looking at the chart below to find if an activity you may never have considered could be both useful and enjoyable.

Before you begin a programme of exercise, you should consider the wider implications - the accompanying social life, for example, as well as the amount of time you are able and willing to invest in your physical fitness. If you choose an outdoor activity, you may need to find an alternative for the winter months. Before you embark on any of the activities listed, try them out without the expense of kitting yourself out fully or joining a club. Many organizations will accept a guest on a trial basis, and you may find that sampling a new activity gives you the impetus to participate in earnest, or it could help you decide that this is not for you.

It is probable, too, that a single type of activity will not be sufficient for all-round fitness, all year round. The chart below covers many leisure, sporting and domestic activities. If you can't find the particular one you are looking for, look at the details given for a similar pursuit, as this will give you a very good idea of the benefits you could expect to achieve. Remember, too, that pursuits such as fishing and sailing, which generally do not rate very highly in terms of *physical* benefit, may be extremely beneficial for mental relaxation and relief of stress.

EATING FOR HEALTH

What does eating mean to you? Do you enjoy food, or is eating simply an inconvenience, like an itch that needs to be scratched? The answer probably depends on where you live. For a peasant in a third world country, eating is the most important aspect of life. There is never enough food, so the question of whether a particular food is good for health is academic; he is eating to avoid starvation.

Western man, on the other hand, is unlikely to starve. Although malnutrition can and does occur through eating the wrong types of food which in turn adversely affects the body and the way it works, true hunger is seldom a problem. If you analyse your own responses to food, you will probably find that your hunger pangs are satisfied after the first few mouthfuls. So why do we continue to eat?

We eat largely for pleasure, not just to fill our stomachs. This is why we have developed meals with several courses, each of contrasting tastes and textures that prolong our interest in and enjoyment of the food.

So what happens to all the excess food we eat? Food has two basic functions. It provides the energy or fuel we need to keep alive, and it provides the building materials from which our bodies are built.

The thousands of chemical processes constituting 'life' are powered by energy, and this comes from the food we eat. In the process of respiration, oxygen breaks down complex substances obtained from digested food and supplies energy. So there is a simple formula: physical exercise demands extra energy; energy comes from food; the more you exercise, the more you must eat.

Unfortunately, many men ignore the first part of the formula. When physical exertion is insufficient, all the extra energy provided by food is unused. The body solves the problem by storing excess energy as fat, and in doing so creates yet another problem - obesity.

The other reason for eating is to provide the materials from which our bodies are constructed. The need for these materials varies widely throughout life. In childhood and adolescence, our bodies increase in size and complexity, requiring large amounts of food to supply the building materials. Later, however, our bodies need only sufficient building materials to replace those lost through damage or by the body's normal repair and waste removal systems. The *need* for food as a building material steadily decreases thereafter and, in elderly men, may drop sharply.

Digestion starts as soon as food enters the mouth, and continues as it is moved along through the digestive system. At each stage enzymes in the digestive juices break the food down into its various constituent elements, which can be converted into a form the body can use.

1 *The teeth break up the food, the tongue mixes it with enzyme-rich saliva released from three pairs of salivary glands* 2.
3 *The oesophagus is a muscular tube which moves the food down by wave-like muscular peristaltic contractions until it reaches the stomach.*
4 *The stomach churns the food around mixing it with acidic gastric juices and turning it into chyme which is released into the duodenum over the next four hours.*
5 *The duodenum releases hormones into the blood when food arrives from the stomach. This stimulates the pancreas to secrete an alkaline juice rich in enzymes into the duodenum to break down the food.*
6 *The liver secretes a fluid called bile.*
7 *The gall-bladder (concealed by the liver) stores and concentrates bile.*

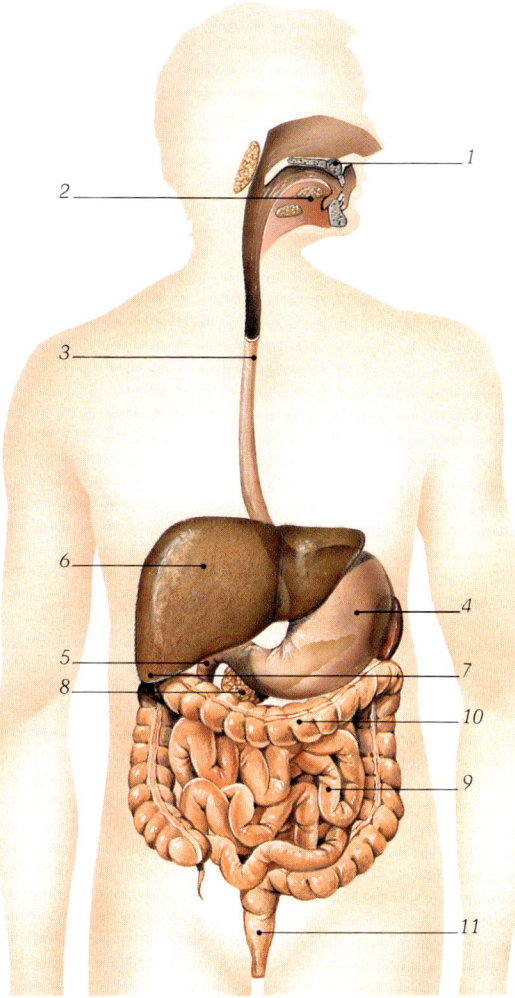

8 *The pancreas also secretes the hormones insulin and glucogen into the blood, to control the level of glucose in the blood once it has been absorbed.*
9 *Small intestine is divided into the duodenum, jejunum and ileum and is the site of both digestion and absorption. Once food has been broken down by digestion it is absorbed into the bloodstream through villi which line the intestinal wall. Proteins are used for the growth and repair of tissue. Surplus is converted into urea by the liver. Carbohydrates are used as energy. Fat is absorbed by lymph vessels. These carry fat to the thoracic duct of the lymphatic system which feeds it into the large vein above the heart. It is then stored in the body.*
10 *The colon plays no part in digestion. It absorbs considerable amounts of water and electrolytes such as sodium.*
11 *The rectum, the second part of the large intestine, is usually empty. As it fills with faeces a reflex triggers its muscles to contract and expel them through the anus.*

THREE BASIC BUILDING BLOCKS

The nutrients we obtain from our food fall into three basic groups: carbohydrates, fats and proteins. It is important to understand the sources and uses of these substances in any discussion of food and diet.

Carbohydrates   A group of substances obtained almost entirely from plant sources and including sugars and starches, carbohydrates are the body's main energy source, for they are eventually broken down to form glucose. Carbohydrates do not contain materials to build body tissues; they simply power the system.

Fats and oils   The only differences between fats and oils is that fats are solid at room temperature. Both are composed of fatty acids and, like carbohydrates, they are a source of energy, although they contain, weight for weight, more than twice as much energy. They are also used for repair and for growth. There are important differences between saturated and unsaturated fats from the point of view of health, and these are discussed more fully later in this chapter.

Proteins   The true building materials of the body, proteins make up much of the solid part of the body (about 12 per cent by weight, compared with 70 per cent water and 15 per cent fat). Proteins form the basis of all living tissue as well as of most of the chemicals produced within our body, such as enzymes. We produce our own proteins, from simpler building blocks called amino acids, a number of which cannot be synthesized within the body and have to be obtained from our food. These are the so-called 'essential' amino acids. Excess proteins are broken down and used as an energy source, although this process is much less efficient than the systems using carbohydrates and fats. We obtain proteins from fish, meat, dairy products and vegetable foods.

WHAT ELSE IS IN FOOD?

As well as carbohydrates, fats and proteins, the body needs small amounts of other substances: minerals, vitamins and fibre.

Minerals   Apart from calcium and iron, minerals are needed in only small amounts. Mineral deficiencies are rare, although they may occur in certain diseases and in areas where iodine or fluoride are absent from drinking water. Calcium is the main constituent of bone, and is only stored in the body in quantity in this form. If there is insufficient calcium in the system for the body's needs, it will be extracted from the bones to compensate which, in the case of some serious diseases, can cause the bones to become spongy. Calcium is also present in large amounts in the teeth, and gives them their hard structure. Calcium is obviously important in giving strength to the bones, but it also takes part in some fundamental chemical reactions in the body, helping the blood to clot after an injury, and assisting in the electrical conduction of signals through the nervous system. The main dietary sources of calcium are dairy products and green vegetables.

Iron is used by the body in large amounts. Its primary use is in haemoglobin, the red pigment in blood cells which carries oxygen around the body, releasing it when needed. Iron is mostly needed to replace the small amounts lost through bleeding. Bleeding can take place in the gut, as in peptic ulcers, or through the over-use of aspirin, at which times there will be an increased need for iron if anaemia is to be avoided. Foods such as kidney, liver, eggs and many vegetables contain large amounts of iron, and any reasonably mixed diet will provide the necessary requirement.

Vitamins   Our bodies require only small amounts of vitamins, usually as catalysts - substances that help to speed up chemical reactions. The idea that the more vitamins we take the healthier we will be is a mistaken one. The vitamins we need can be obtained from a normal diet and, in some cases, an excess of them can be harmful.

Fibre   Although it is a form of carbohydrate, fibre is not, strictly speaking, a nutrient, as it is not digested or absorbed into the body. Fibre is composed largely of cellulose, the material that forms the cell walls of plant tissue. Although apparently inert and without obvious nutritional function, fibre has recently been recognized as being extremely important in a healthy diet.

PRODUCING AND USING ENERGY

Energy is released from the breakdown of nutrients using a complicated chemical called ATP (adenosine triphosphate). Wherever energy is required in the body, ATP is stored.

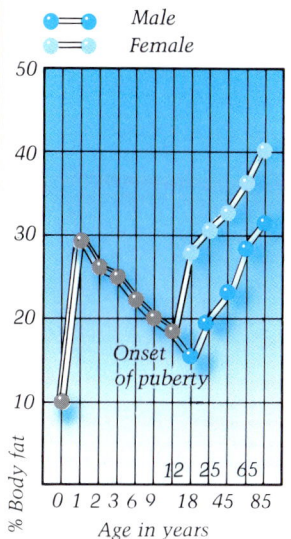

Male
Female

% Body fat — Age in years

Onset of puberty

During the first year of life the fat content of the body increases rapidly, but during childhood it falls. At the onset of puberty the fat content begins to rise again. On average men never lay down the same amount of fat as women but it increases with age in both sexes.

With the aid of oxygen and chemicals, derived from glucose or other food materials, ATP is split into another substance called ADP (adenosine diphosphate) and energy is released, powering the muscles or causing a chemical reaction to take place. The whole process is self-renewing and ensures a continual supply of energy where it is needed. It is called the Krebs cycle and is one of the most important processes of the body.

Oxygen is essential for the process and is the basis of aerobic activity, when food materials provide the energy needed for muscular (or other) activity. Normally, carbohydrates are the primary energy source but, when they are in short supply, as during a diet, fats are broken down instead. Proteins are less useful as an energy source and are used only when nothing else is available, body tissues being broken down to provide energy. When someone is on a particularly severe diet, it is sometimes possible to smell the products of the breakdown of protein on their breath. These substances are called ketones, and they smell rather like nail varnish remover or pear drops; a similar smell may sometimes be detected during diabetic emergencies.

The chemical activity of the body is known as metabolism. The efficiency with which the body uses the energy obtained from food is usually referred to as a basal metabolic rate (BMR), which varies very widely between the sexes, and with age and build. In general, thin men who eat a lot have a higher than normal BMR; overweight men tend to have a low BMR. This means that a thin man disposes of excess energy without storing it away as fat more efficiently than an overweight man. Metabolism is usually an inherited characteristic, and this can lead to the discouraging circumstances of some people claiming that they can eat as much as they want without ever seeming to put on weight.

Men have a higher BMR than women and thus tend to put on weight less readily than women but, at the same time, BMR declines with age, so an older man will put on weight, unless he reduces his food intake as he ages. BMR increases with aerobic exercise because of the changes that occur in the body as fitness improves. When you achieve peak fitness, therefore, you not only need more food to provide energy, but you are better able to dispose of the excess without turning it into flab. Another factor to consider is the genetic predisposition to put on weight, which varies between individuals.

The phrase energy balance is used to decribe the situation that occurs when you use all the energy that is provided by your food. If you take in too much food, you will begin to store the excess as fat; if you take in too little, you begin to break down body tissue to provide energy. To keep the energy balance of your body constant, you need to be aware of the energy value of the food you eat. This value is usually expressed as calories, but this is a misnomer, as the popular term 'calorie' is more actually a kilocalorie, which is 1,000 times greater. However, the standard calorie is likely to be in universal usage for the foreseeable future.

The higher the calorific value of a food, the greater the amount of energy

CALORIE COUNT

Energy is burnt up at different rates depending on the type of exercise that you do. These figures are only a guide because different people have different metabolisms and burn energy at different rates for the same task. To maintain an energy balance, you should consume the same amount of calories as you burn up during exercise and rest.

ACTIVITY	CALORIES PER HOUR	TIME TAKEN TO BURN 500 CALORIES
Sleeping	65	7 hrs 40 mins
Driving, cooking, sitting at desk	100	5 hrs
Walking, dancing, badminton	250	2 hrs
Brisk walking, tennis, skating, cycling, jogging	300	1 hr 40 mins
Football, climbing, gentle running	400	1 hr 15 mins
Swimming, skiing	500	1 hr
Running, squash, weight lifting, competitive swimming	650	45 mins

AGE	LIFESTYLE	CALORIES PER DAY
18—35	inactive active very active	2,500 3,000 3,500
36-70	inactive active very active	2,400 2,800 3,400
70+	inactive active	2,200 2,500

FOODS CONTAINING 500 CALORIES

1 oz butter
3 oz peanuts
3.2 oz potato crisps
4 oz chocolate cake
4 oz cheddar cheese
5 oz French fries
5 oz corn flakes
6 oz tuna fish
7 oz wholemeal bread
7 oz fried fish
7 oz dates
8 oz avocado pear

1lb boiled spaghetti
1½ lbs boiled potatoes
½ lb oysters
5 lbs raw carrot
11 lbs boiled cabbage

that food can provide. As most foods consist of varying mixtures of carbohydrates, fats and proteins, their calorific values also vary widely. Because the BMR differs widely among individual men, it is not possible to make precise recommendations for the daily calorific value of food. However, your average daily calorie intake should be somewhere between 2000 and 3000 calories.

The effect of your daily activity on your energy balance is crucial, and the chart below shows the amount of calories you would use if you did one of the activities for one hour. These figures can be added together and compared with those in the table opposite to see if your calorie intake is in balance with energy needs - or, more probably, how far you have tipped the balance toward excess calorie intake! Remember, your personal BMR will also help tip the energy balance, but in which direction, you are the best judge. If you are slim and active, you can probably cope with an excess intake of calories; if you have a tendency to be overweight, you probably have a low BMR, and your calorie needs may be lower than those shown.

You can use this data in conjunction with the calorie tables for common foods listed in this chapter to develop a sensible diet that will help you to control your weight.

DIET AND DISEASES

Like most men, you are probably confused by the changing view of what constitutes 'healthy' eating. Foods that were once thought to be 'good for you', are now to be avoided, while the potatoes and bread that we were once warned against are now advocated enthusiastically.

It is not surprising that there has been a cynical reaction. The same people who say they have smoked for years and are in perfect health, can now use the same argument against changing their diets. Like diseases caused by smoking, there may be no warning of the diseases caused by a poor diet. You can't argue with a heart attack that strikes down a relatively young and fit man.

But why have the recommendations for a healthy diet changed so much? As we have already seen, it is neither feasible nor ethical to experiment on people in such a way that their health could be adversely affected. Identifying the health risks associated with patterns of eating is possible only by comparing the food, health and life expectancies of different groups of people living in different areas. Using data obtained internationally over many years, nutritionists have concluded that most of us living in the Western world are overfed and badly fed, and that numerous serious health risks are associated with our 'sophisticated' diet.

Opinions about what constitutes a 'good' diet have also been influenced by the change in lifestyle within our own culture. From 1914 until about 1945, wars and economic decline meant that few people were overnourished. Many suffered deprivation, and actual dietary deficiency was common among poor families. High-energy foods such as eggs, dairy produce, meat and sugar were promoted as being essential to health, but the actual quantities consumed were not high. These foods were either not available or they were too expensive for most people. Bread and potatoes were cheap and filling.

Recently, relative affluence has meant that we can eat more or less what we choose, and this has led to a swing toward the more expensive dairy produce, meat and sweets while the cheaper 'fillers' like bread and potatoes are in less demand.

In terms of health this swing to more expensive items has, generally speaking, led to a decline in our health, although the effects can take many years to become apparent. Certainly heart disease and some cancers were much less common in the days when we ate less or simpler foods.

Who says what's healthy?   A vast amount of information about nutrition is readily available to any man who is concerned about his diet and his health. Unfortunately, this information is not being put to good use.

Surveys have shown that most men have heard of the nutrients in the food they eat, but relatively few of them make use of the knowledge to change their diets. This is partly due no doubt to our upbringing, when we are told what is 'good' for us; it is also partly due to the active counter-propaganda put out by the food industry, which has a vested interest in maintaining the *status quo* or, at the very least, in influencing any changes in our food preferences. For example, as soon as public health authorities publicize the potential health problems from eating too much butter or drinking too much milk, counter-campaigns are mounted to extol the traditional virtues of dairy products. This is, of course, exactly what many of us really want to hear: who wants to be told that they have been doing things wrong for most of their lives?

Unfortunately, scientific 'facts' and statistics are notorious for being manipulated to obscure vital issues, and it is difficult to unravel the truth. For that reason, a number of official bodies have issued guidelines on healthy eating. These advisory bodies include the World Health Organization (1982); the National Advisory Committee on Nutrition Education or NACNE (1983); and the Committee on Medical Aspects of Food Policy or COMA (1984).

Many diseases can be directly related to the Western style of eating.

DISEASE ▼	DIETARY FACTOR ▼
Coronary heart disease	*High fat, salt and cholesterol*
High blood pressure	*High salt*
Strokes	*High salt*
Varicose veins	*Low-fibre*
Bowel cancer	*High-fat and low-fibre*
Appendicitis	*Low-fibre*
Irritable colon	*Low-fibre*
Diverticular disease	*Low-fibre*
Constipation	*Low-fibre*
Haemorrhoids	*Low-fibre*
Gallstones	*High fat and cholesterol*
Diabetes	*High fat and sugar intake, low-fibre*
Obesity	*High calorie*
Tooth decay	*High sugar*

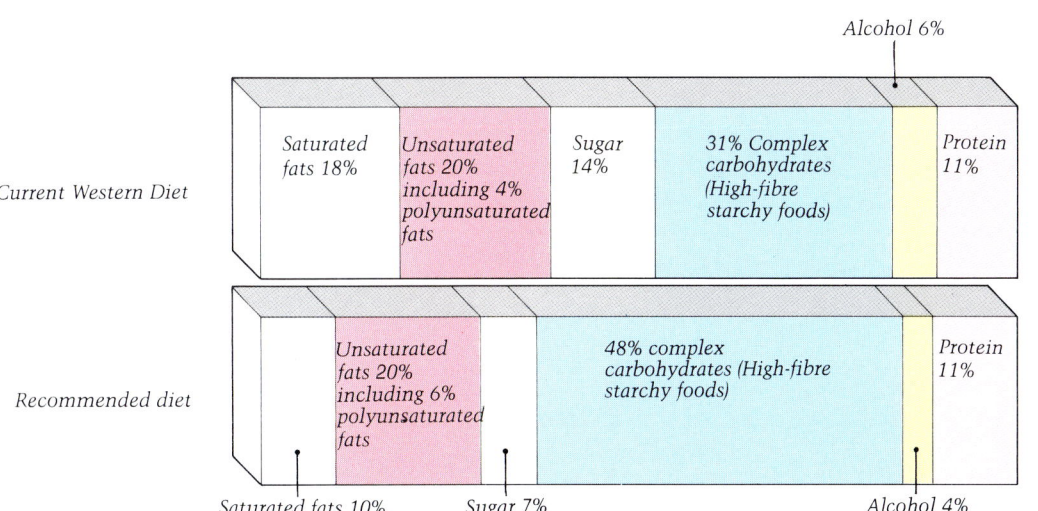

Alcohol 6%

| Current Western Diet | Saturated fats 18% | Unsaturated fats 20% including 4% polyunsaturated fats | Sugar 14% | 31% Complex carbohydrates (High-fibre starchy foods) | | Protein 11% |

| Recommended diet | | Unsaturated fats 20% including 6% polyunsaturated fats | | 48% complex carbohydrates (High-fibre starchy foods) | | Protein 11% |

Saturated fats 10%   Sugar 7%   Alcohol 4%

Both diets give the same amount of calories but the balance of nutrients is different. It is now believed to be more healthy to get the majority of your calories from carbohydrates in the diet.

Although the findings of these bodies vary in detail, there is a remarkable degree of consistency in their recommendations for changes in diet. They and organizations working in countries with similar health problems have concluded that the average person's diet should be modified in the following ways:

● *Eat less fat.* NACNE recommends cutting down the total fat intake by 25 per cent and switching to unsaturated fats where possible.
● *Eat less sugar.* NACNE recommends reducing intake by 50 per cent.
● *Eat less salt.* NACNE recommends cutting down intake by 3 grams a day.
● *Eat more fibre.* NACNE recommends increasing the daily intake by 50 per cent.

The rest of this chapter considers the health reasons for these recommendations and their implications for everyday eating.

FIT WITH LESS FAT

Adopting the recommendations to cut our intake of fat by 25 per cent would involve making radical changes in our diet, but such changes would be worthwhile, for high fat intake is implicated in a number of diseases of the circulatory system.

Fats are an important energy source for the body and a number of substances derived from fat circulate in the blood, ready to be used wherever required. Cholesterol, a fat-like substance that is made in the body, is important in the manufacture of hormones within our bodies, and there are large amounts of cholesterol in the brain and certain other organs, including the kidneys and liver. However, essential as it is, cholesterol seems to be a key factor in the development of certain diseases.

The large blood vessels are lined with a slippery membrane; this reduces friction, allowing the blood to circulate freely, and prevents fluids leaking from the blood vessels into the surrounding tissues until the blood reaches the capillaries. As we age, this slippery lining becomes less 'non-stick', and cholesterol penetrates the surface, building up into rough patches called an atheroma. Once a rough patch is established, blood cells and fibres of a material called fibrin stick to it, making it thicker, larger and tougher. Eventually the calcium may become deposited in the atheroma, making it rigid. If the atheroma is deposited thickly the arteries become narrowed, and the deposits also make the walls of the arteries rigid and unable to expand to allow increased blood flow, so that the system can no longer respond normally to the extra demands put on it during exercise.

Probably 90 per cent of adult men have some degree of damage to their arteries. This 'hardening of the arteries' (atherosclerosis) can cause leg pains during exercise, as the nerve receptors in the muscles warn of inadequate oxygen supply for their normal aerobic activity. Another symptom is that affected limbs become cold, because of inadequate circulation.

Much more serious, however, are the effects of these fatty deposits on the heart. Like any muscle tissue, the heart needs an adequate oxygen supply, and the heart has a separate blood supply to its powerful muscles, the muscular ventricles being supplied with blood through the narrow coronary arteries, which are all too susceptible to silting up with deposits of atheroma.

This atherosclerosis may not cause symptoms at rest, but during exercise the heart speeds up and the damaged coronary arteries may no longer be able to keep up an adequate blood flow. The heart responds with the crushing chest pain called angina pectoris, which at first feels like very severe indigestion. Although the pain goes away quite rapidly on resting, it is a clear warning that the circulatory system is in trouble. Immediate medical attention is needed.

Sometimes a blood clot can be formed very suddenly on a patch of atheroma, causing the blood flow to be blocked off completely. In much of the body, the blood will find an alternative route, but when the clot, or thrombus, occurs in a coronary artery, a coronary thrombosis or heart attack results. The area of heart muscle supplied by the blocked coronary artery dies, and the heart's ability to pump is seriously threatened. The heart may continue to work reasonably well, or it may twitch erratically and fail to pump unless swift medical aid is given.

Similar effects occur when a thrombus on a patch of atheroma blocks the blood supply to the brain. This causes the death of a whole section of brain tissue, resulting in a stroke, which often affects those areas of the brain that control movement.

Three major factors are associated with heart disease: high cholesterol levels, high blood pressure and cigarette smoking. Although only 20 men out of each 1000 are normally at risk from dying as a result of their first heart attack, for men with a high cholesterol level, with high blood pressure and who smoke, the chances of dying from their first heart attack rise to 171 in 1000.

It is known that large amounts of saturated fats in the diet are associated with high levels of cholesterol in the blood, which in turn are related to an increased risk of heart disease. Cholesterol is made by your body as well as being taken in from the food you eat; therefore different men have different levels of blood cholesterol. Some men, for instance, have a genetic tendency to produce high levels of cholesterol, and if they can be identified, their risk of arterial disease may be reduced by careful treatment and a modified diet. Such hereditary tendencies may become apparent when family history is considered.

PROBLEMS WITH FATS

Although the high level of saturated fat in our diet is usually associated with an increased risk of coronary heart disease, it is also blamed for a high level of certain forms of cancer.

A comparison of Japanese men with those in Western countries shows that cancers of the prostate and testes are ten times less common in the West, although among Japanese men who emigrate to the United States and eat a Western diet, the risk soon increases to the same level as for native Americans.

Cancer of the bowel, which is very common in the West, is sometimes ascribed to a high fat diet. This causes the liver to secrete large amounts of bile acids, which assist in the digestion of fat, and it is believed that excess bile acids may be broken down by bacteria in the gut to form substances capable of causing cancer, a theory supported by the observation that people who excrete excess bile are more prone than the average to develop bowel cancer.

The causes of bowel cancer are, however, far from clear. The condition is, for example, less common than average among Seventh Day Adventists, a Christian group whose members abstain from alcohol, meat and smoking and who are of considerable interest to nutritionalists as they have a much lower than usual rate for most of the common diseases.

THE FATS WE EAT

At present, we get about 40 per cent of our energy requirements from fat, and we are told that this figure should be reduced to about 30 per cent of the total with the consequent 10 per cent shortfall in calories being derived from high-fibre starchy carbohydrates. In practice, this need not mean much of a change in your diet, as fat is an effective source of calories and only a small reduction will be needed.

However, improving our health is not just a matter of reducing the level of fat we eat. We must be sure that we eat the right types of fat. All the fats we eat are built up from various types of fatty acids, long chains of carbon atoms, joined together like a necklace by chemical links or bonds. In one type of chain, each carbon atom has a pair of hydrogen atoms attached to it, and the fatty acid is called a *saturated* fatty acid because every available carbon atom has its two hydrogen molecules firmly attached.

The carbon atoms in the fatty acids may be linked with a double bond, which means that only a single hydrogen atom can be attached. This is called an *unsaturated* fatty acid. If there is only one of these double bonds in the chain of carbon atoms, it is *mono*-unsaturated; if there are many, it will be *poly*-unsaturated, and this is the term you will often see on the label of processed foods.

All fats and oils are made up of a mixture of saturated and unsaturated fatty acids, and the relative amounts of each decide if the fat itself is saturated or unsaturated. We know that the saturated fats we eat that derive mainly from animals products (eg, meat and dairy products) are involved in furring up your arteries.

Mono-unsaturated fats do not do this; in fact, their effects on the system seem to be neutral. Olive oil is the only common mono-unsaturated fat in our diet. Poly-unsaturated fats, on the other hand, seem to be positively beneficial in that they may lower the blood cholesterol level, and they may possibly help to 'de-fur' the arteries. Most poly-unsaturates are derived from vegetable sources, such as nuts and seeds. Oils such as corn, sunflower and soya are good sources, but poly-unsaturates are also found in large amounts in mackerel, herring, trout, salmon and similar oily fish.

It is important to emphasize, however, that the belief that animal fats are 'bad' and vegetable fats are 'OK' is a misconception. Some vegetable fats - especially the cheapest types such as coconut and palm oil, which are widely used in processed food - are high in saturated fats.

Processing can change the nature of fats. For example, margarine may be made from sunflower oil, a poly-unsaturated fat that is actually a thin oil. To thicken it, the sunflower oil is put through a process called hydrogenation, which means adding hydrogen atoms and breaking the double bond, so making the fat more saturated and, at the same time, more solid. So, if the label says that the margarine (or any other product) contains

All fats are made of the same atoms, but the factor that makes them different is the order in which these atoms are arranged in a chain. Most saturated fats are hard at room temperature and tend to come from animals but coconut and palm oils are the exceptions. Hydrogenating an oil will make it saturated and hard at room temperature, so even if your margarine is made from vegetable oil, it is no healthier for you if it is hard at room temperature.

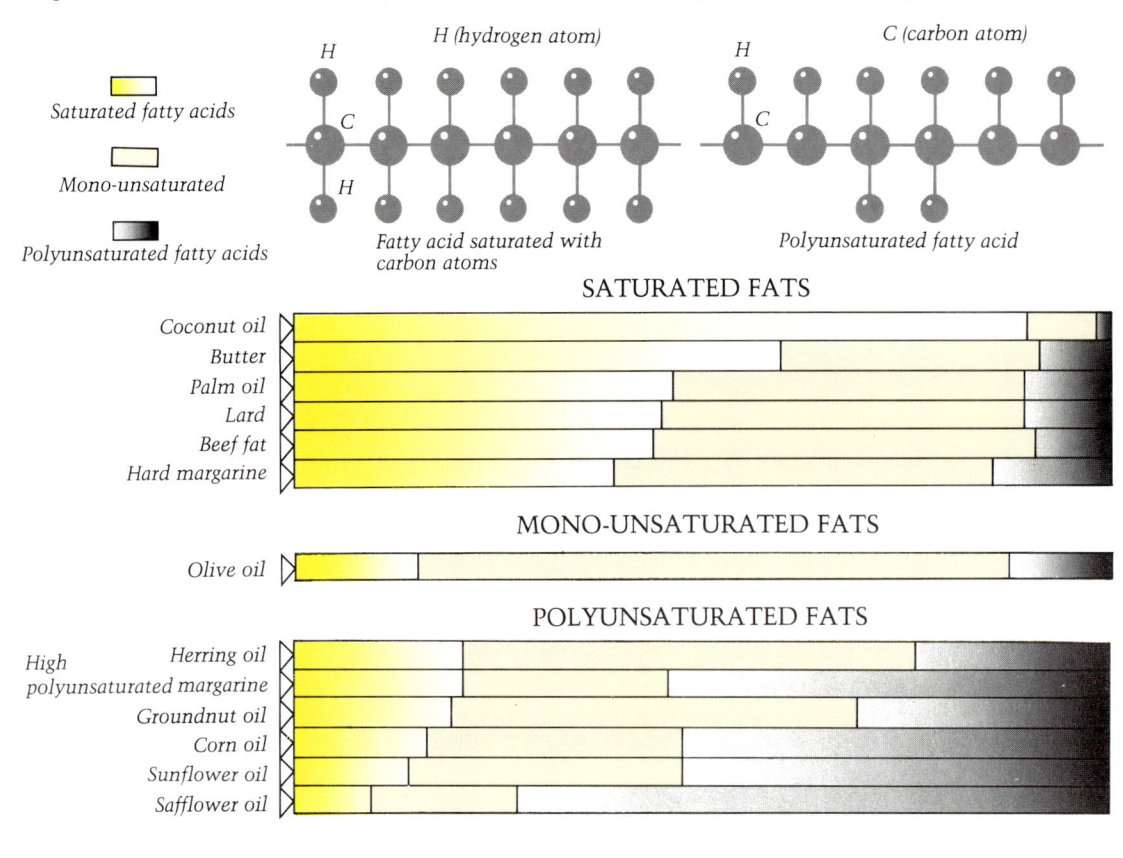

Saturated fatty acids

Mono-unsaturated

Polyunsaturated fatty acids

H (hydrogen atom)   C (carbon atom)

Fatty acid saturated with carbon atoms

Polyunsaturated fatty acid

SATURATED FATS

Coconut oil
Butter
Palm oil
Lard
Beef fat
Hard margarine

MONO-UNSATURATED FATS

Olive oil

POLYUNSATURATED FATS

High polyunsaturated margarine
Herring oil
Groundnut oil
Corn oil
Sunflower oil
Safflower oil

'hydrogenated vegetable oils', this is simply a way of avoiding having to say that it contains high saturated fat.

The evidence linking a diet high in poly-unsaturates to health is not as clear cut as the established risk of a diet high in saturated fat. The NACNE and COMA reports have been cautious in recommending increased levels of poly-unsaturates, but the growing number of products featuring the words 'high in poly-unsaturates' on their labelling is an indication of the rising demand from a public that is becoming increasingly well informed on matters of healthy eating.

SOURCES OF FAT

Our total fat intake comes from a variety of sources. Some can be classed as visible - butter, margarine, cooking oil, the fatty rind on bacon or pork chops, for example - but probably at least half is 'invisible', incorporated into the foods we eat, such as biscuits, pies and eggs.

Dairy products   A third of our daily fat intake comes from dairy products, and on average it is 63 per cent saturated fat, making up no less then 40 per cent of the total saturated fat we consume.

Half the total dairy fat we consume comes from butter, which is almost entirely fat, and highly saturated at that. Cutting down on butter intake is fairly simple: spread it more thinly, and don't pile butter on your vegetables. A switch to poly-unsaturated margarine is beneficial or to the newer low-fat spreads.

Most of the rest of our consumption of dairy fat is from milk, which is a classic example of how traditional 'wisdom' has been proved wrong. The full-cream milk we have been brought up to regard as the best type of milk is extremely high in saturated fat, and even ordinary whole milk is not much better. Semi-skimmed and skimmed milk have much lower fat contents, and although they may tast slightly watery when you first try them, they are generally acceptable in tea, less so in coffee.

Needless to say, cream is 'naughty but nice', being extremely high in both saturated fat *and* calories. But there is no reason not to use cream for the occasional treat. Cream substitutes are usually made from processed vegetable fats, and are therefore no 'healthier' than real cream.

Other visible fats   Margarine has as much fat and as many calories as butter. Unless specifically labelled as 'high in poly-unsaturates', margarine, which is a high-fat product, is likely to have been heavily hydrogenated to give it the proper consistency; it is, therefore, probably highly saturated. The claim 'blended vegetable oils' is no recommendation, as those oils can be highly saturated. Margarine can, in fact, be manufactured from a variety of animal and fish fats and oils, as well as from vegetable oils.

Low-fat spreads resemble margarine, but do not contain sufficient fat to be legally labelled as margarine. They are an acceptable butter substitute for spreading and contain around 50 per cent of the fat found in either margarine or butter, but are not suitable for frying or baking.

Cooking fats and oils contain varied proportions of saturated/unsaturated fats. Lard, dripping and the white solid fats used to make pastry are all high in saturates, as are most of the cooking oils that are

High levels of cholesterol in the blood have been closely linked with the onset of coronary heart disease but medical opinion is still divided as to the exact source of this cholesterol because the body has an ability to manufacture it. However, a diet high in cholesterol inevitably adds to the load with which the body has to deal. Cholesterol does not occur in vegetables, but all animal products contain a proportion of it. Should you wish to keep your daily intake below 300 milligrams, a single egg would supply that quota.

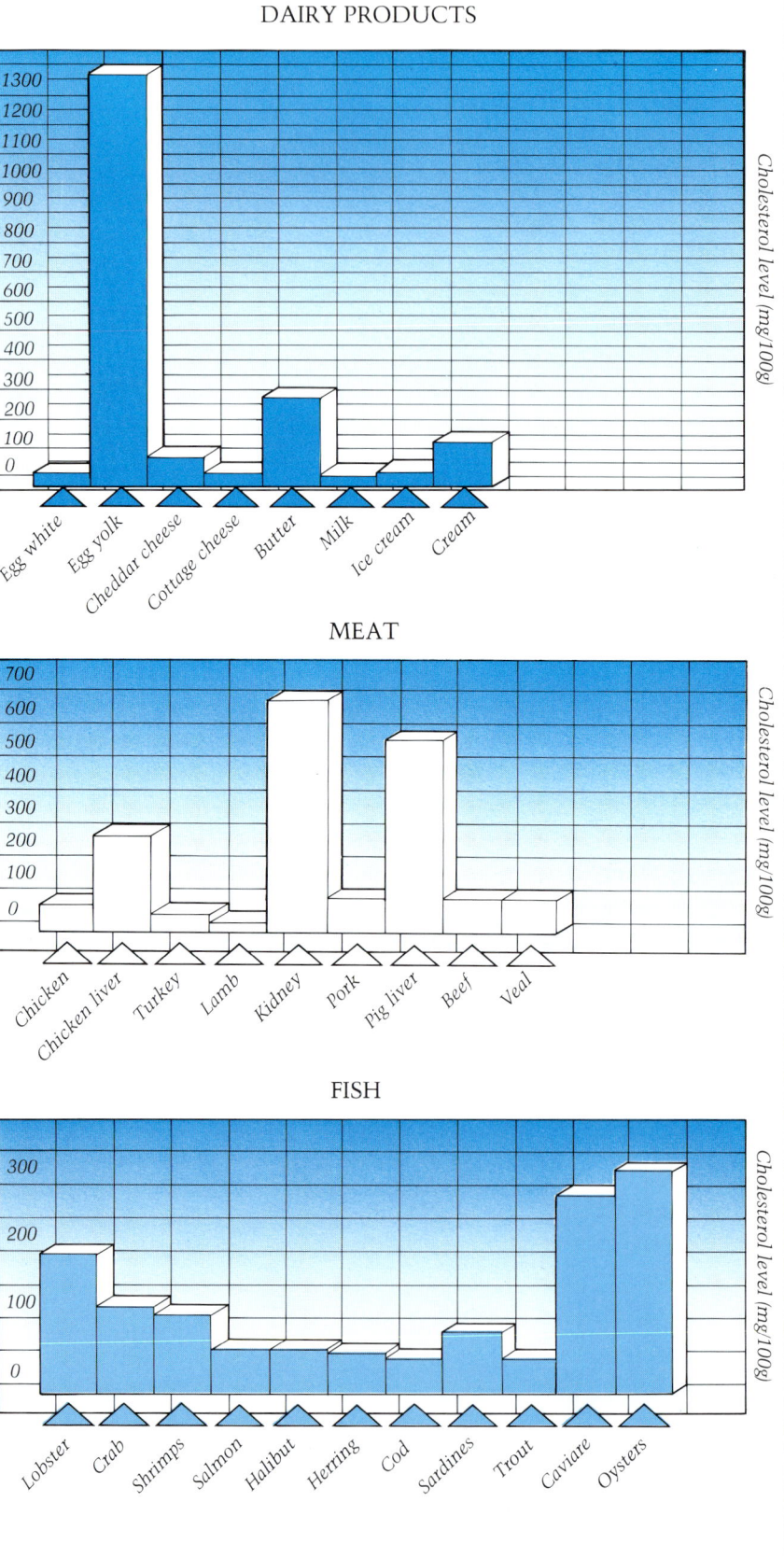

DAIRY PRODUCTS

Cholesterol level (mg/100g)

1300, 1200, 1100, 1000, 900, 800, 700, 600, 500, 400, 300, 200, 100, 0

Egg white, Egg yolk, Cheddar cheese, Cottage cheese, Butter, Milk, Ice cream, Cream

MEAT

Cholesterol level (mg/100g)

700, 600, 500, 400, 300, 200, 100, 0

Chicken, Chicken liver, Turkey, Lamb, Kidney, Pork, Pig liver, Beef, Veal

FISH

Cholesterol level (mg/100g)

300, 200, 100, 0

Lobster, Crab, Shrimps, Salmon, Halibut, Herring, Cod, Sardines, Trout, Caviare, Oysters simply labelled as 'vegetable oil'. However, there are now many satisfactory alternatives, which can be used for cooking, frying (if you must!) and for salads and which are low in saturated fats. Olive, soya, corn, sunflower, peanut and walnut oils contain less than 20 per cent saturated fat.

Pastries, including cakes and biscuits, are well known as rich sources of sugar, but they are probably more of a health risk because of their high content of saturated fats. The fat content usually varies from 5 to 25 per cent, and 'cream' fillings, which are usually based on a mixture of palm oil and coconut oil, can contain as much as 90 per cent saturated fat. Chocolate-covered biscuits also have a very high fat content.

Meat and meat products   All meat, even the leanest cuts, contains fat, as fat forms an integral part of the individual cells that make up the muscle tissue constituting the meat we eat. Usually this 'invisible' fat is of the unsaturated variety and is not, therefore, of great concern for our health. The saturated fat is highly visible: it is the layer of fat around the outside of the meat and may also be seen as yellowish streaks or marbling within the meat. Trim off the fat from the outside of meat, preferably *before* cooking or it will melt and soak into the meat, and avoid meat in which the fat is deposited in marbling or streaks, as this is impossible to remove.

Mince is inevitably made from the cheapest meat, including trimmings that would otherwise be wasted; poor quality mince can contain 50 per cent fat. Use only the best quality, which should have a better meat/fat balance.

Sausages can be even worse than mince in terms of high fat levels, their fat content varying from 30 to 60 per cent. In addition, they contain additives.

Offal is very low in fat; usually 10 per cent or less, with the exception of brains, which contain large amounts of cholesterol. You are unlikely to eat enough brains to endanger your health, but offal such as kidneys and liver can be eaten freely, and they contain large amounts of vitamins A and D, and liver is especially rich in iron.

Convenience foods such as prepared pies, hamburgers and pasties are generally made from low-grade meat and waste materials. Unfortunately the description 'meat' on labels is legally interpreted as meaning almost anything derived from an animal, so the label will not help you to determine fat content.

Fish is the most neglected of foods and its consumption is undeservedly low. The fat content of white fish is *very* low, and what fat is present is usually poly-unsaturated.

DOWN WITH SUGAR!

A recent report by NACNE recommends that we halve the amount of sugar we eat. On average, we each consume around 40kg (over 88lbs) of sugar each year, and about half of this is 'visible' sugar, bought to add to tea or coffee, cook with, or sprinkle on food. The other 50 per cent is 'hidden' in prepared foods - not just in cakes, pastries, biscuits and conserves but in savoury foods such as sauces, pickles and some tinned vegetables.

Continued on page 60

EATING STYLES AROUND THE WORLD

The major cause of death to emerge in the twentieth century in industrialized countries has been heart disease and there is a marked international difference. The same is true of many other diseases associated with diet, and researchers have shown that people migrating from a low-risk country to a high-risk country tend to have risk rates approaching the host country.

GREAT BRITAIN

This is now top of the list of heart disease risk countries. The nation still consumes most of its energy requirement in the form of animal fats and proteins. The average body fat content has increased over the past 40 years by 10%.

USA

Since 1968 the incidence of heart disease has been gradually dropping. One of the reasons for this is a reduction in the amount of animal fats in the national diet, but increasing physical activity and reduction in cigarette smoking are also contributory factors.

AUSTRALIA

The incidence of heart disease rose steadily during post-war affluence when meat production rose, but the incidence is now dropping. Aborigines have the lowest salt intake of any culture in the world, about 2g a day, and hypertension is an unknown disease although ordinary white Australians exhibit the normal risk.

FRANCE

There is a high prevalence of cirrhosis of the liver because the consumption of alcohol per head of population is one of the highest in the world.

ITALY

The consumption of fat in Italy is high but the incidence of coronary heart disease is low. This is because the Italians use olive oil for cooking, and eat food high in starchy carbohydrates but comparatively low in meat.

FINLAND

In 1970 Finland was top of the list of heart disease risk. The diet included high quantities of milk, cheeses, butters and meat. Changes in government agricultural policy and eating trends have reduced this figure dramatically.

SOUTH AFRICA

A study was done on a privileged group of South African whites living in university, compared with a similar group in establishments for the needy. The diet of the latter group contained a higher proportion of fibre and the incidence of appendicitis was substantially lower.

UGANDA

The consumption of sugar is low and so is the incidence of dental caries. In the parts of Africa where unrefined grain forms the basis of the diet, appendicitis, hiatus hernia, constipation, diabetes, varicose veins, piles, diverticular disease and cancer of the bowel are virtually unknown.

INDIA

In places where rice is eaten in its natural state, the incidence of diabetes is very low. However, in the more affluent parts of India where the rice is polished and therefore low in fibre, the incidence of diabetes rises again.

CHINA

The diet here consists mostly of rice, with vegetables and meat added as accompaniments. The incidence of heart disease low, as is dental caries.

JAPAN

The incidence of heart disease in Japan is very low — about 15 in 10,000. The Japanese diet is high in fish and low in meat. However, it is also high in salt, the average Japanese man consuming 25g per day, and hypertension is higher here than anywhere else in the world.

PAKISTAN

The diet contains a high proportion of complex carbohydrates and a small amount of animal proteins. Diabetes has been found to be less common in the areas where wholewheat chapatis are eaten.

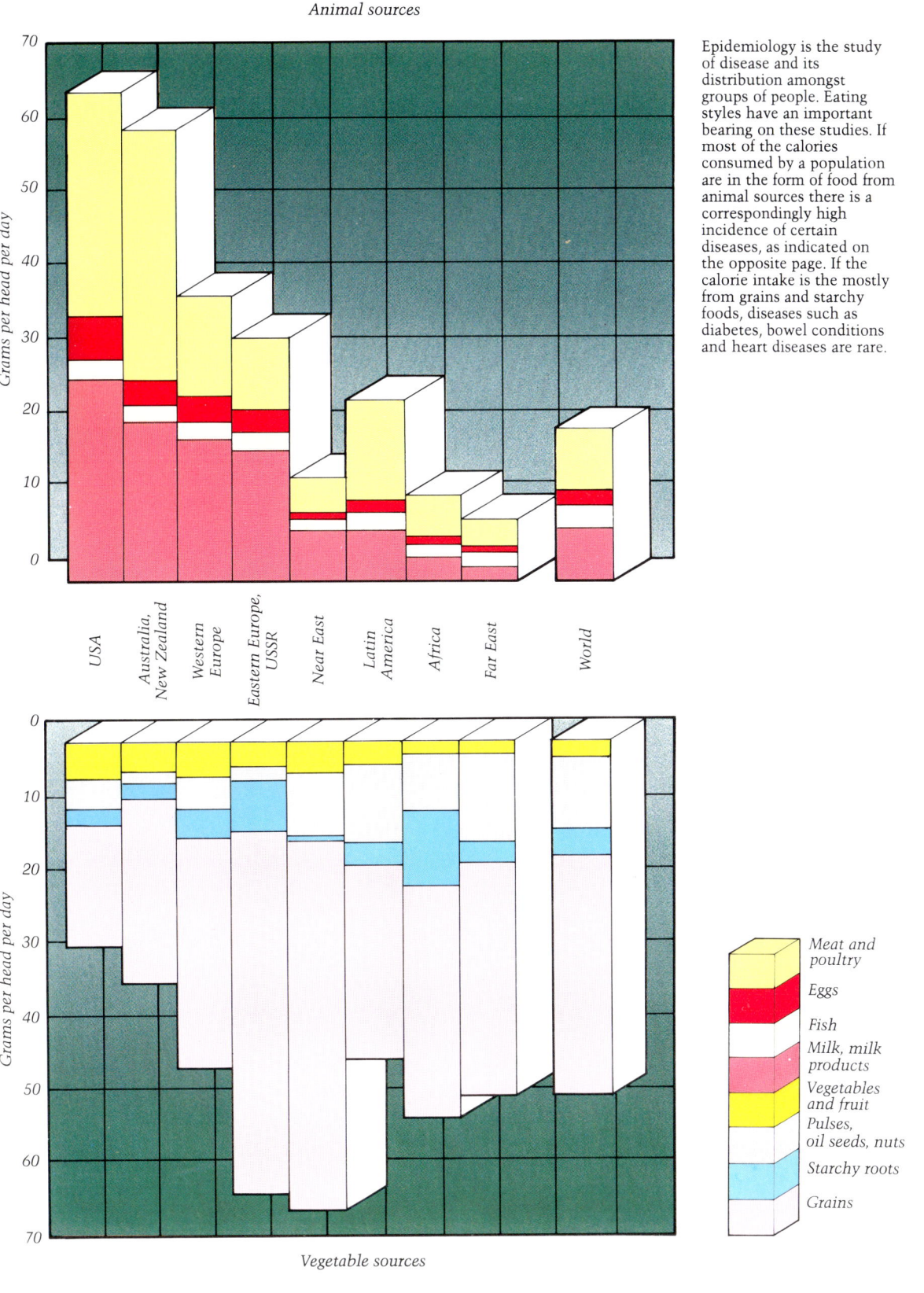

Animal sources

Grams per head per day

USA
Australia, New Zealand
Western Europe
Eastern Europe, USSR
Near East
Latin America
Africa
Far East
World

Epidemiology is the study of disease and its distribution amongst groups of people. Eating styles have an important bearing on these studies. If most of the calories consumed by a population are in the form of food from animal sources there is a correspondingly high incidence of certain diseases, as indicated on the opposite page. If the calorie intake is the mostly from grains and starchy foods, diseases such as diabetes, bowel conditions and heart diseases are rare.

Grams per head per day

Vegetable sources

Meat and poultry
Eggs
Fish
Milk, milk products
Vegetables and fruit
Pulses, oil seeds, nuts
Starchy roots
Grains

Continued from page 57

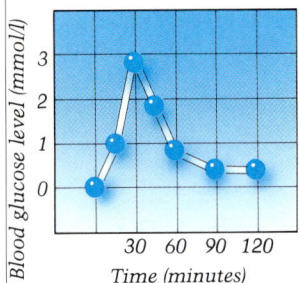

You do not need to eat sugar to supply your body with energy. Any type of high calorie food raises the levels of glucose in the blood. This graph shows that rise after the subject has eaten 50g of wholemeal bread.

The latest recommendations are that we should take only eight teaspoonfuls each day (including 'hidden' sugar). But can we afford to do without this extra sugar and, in any case, why should we? Most men believe that sugar gives them energy, but that is only true in the strict sense of the word 'energy'. Sugar provides energy, meaning calories, but virtually nothing else. It has no nutritional value, although there may some benefit in the other ingredients of sugary foods, and excess energy, in the form of calories, is simply stored away as body fat. Sugar does not give you energy in the sense of vitality or vigour, any more or less than other high-calorie foods.

High levels of blood glucose (sugar) do provide energy for the muscles, but even if you eat neat glucose, blood levels increase only briefly, for the excess is immediately converted to glycogen and stored in the liver and elsewhere until required. On the other hand, your blood glucose level does *drop* after exercise or if you miss a meal, and this causes an internal signal to be produced, switching conversion of stored glycogen into glucose, thus restoring the level. The blood glucose levels are restored rapidly after eating even a small snack.

THE TYPES OF SUGAR

The word 'sugar' covers a variety of related substances. If you look at food labels you may see terms such as fructose, sucrose, lactose, maltose, glucose or dextrose. All are sugars and, for nutritional purposes, they are identical.

The white sugar we sprinkle in tea or coffee, the commonest form of sugar in our diet, is pure sucrose. Syrup is a concentrated solution of sucrose. Honey contains some fructose and minute amounts of minerals, but despite its healthy image does nothing for your diet in terms of nutritional benefit. Brown sugar and other forms of sugar may taste slightly different, but there is absolutely no difference between them in terms of their effect on your health. Some slightly different sweeteners are used for diabetic foods; sorbitol, for example, is absorbed only slowly, so that it does not produce the changes in blood sugar that can be dangerous for diabetics. However, using 'diabetic' foods is not a short cut to weight loss. Diabetic foods are produced for a specific purpose; they should be used only as part of a special, medically controlled diet.

There are several types of artificial sweeteners on the market, which can provide sweetness without calories. Most contain no calories at all, although a few are mixtures of sugar with an artificial sweetener. Saccharin has been around for many years, and is used widely in processed foods and in soft drinks. It is also used by people who are unable to do without their accustomed sweet flavourings in coffee and tea, or in cooking. Saccharin does have a drawback - although it is extremely sweet, it leaves a bitter aftertaste. Some newer artificial sweeteners that are now available do not have this drawback. There have been occasional scares over possible health hazards with artificial sweeteners. It is unlikely that there is any real risk in their use, but it makes sense to cut down on all sweet things, including sugar and artificial substitutes. Re-educating the palate is the best way to get over the sugar craving.

THE DANGERS OF A SWEET TOOTH

Tooth decay is the most obvious hazard from excess sugar. It is not long since it was normal for most men to have lost their teeth by the time they were 35. This was partly due to lack of dental care and partly due to the very high levels of decay caused by sugar in the diet.

Teeth are composed largely of calcium hydroxyapatite, a hard mineral that is easily attacked by acid. Saliva is slightly alkaline, and conditions in the mouth should prevent acid damage to the teeth. But the mouth contains billions of bacteria, in a yellow cheesey film of plaque over the teeth, and these bacteria feed upon sugar and other nutrients in our food. Within a few minutes of our having eaten any sugary substance, they are producing their own waste products, in the form of acid. This acid eats away at the teeth and in time penetrates the hard external layer of enamel. Once a cavity has begun to develop, bacteria enter the tooth and their acid attacks the softer underlying material, enlarging the cavity and eventually causing the destruction of the tooth. (Our saliva neutralizes the acid within about 20 minutes but by then much damage can be done. The real danger is eating or drinking sugary substances throughout the day, especially between meals.)

The same bacteria, nourished by sugar, encourage the deposition of hard scale on the teeth, and this can eventually lead to gum disease and tooth loss.

While tooth decay is the most obvious, obesity is the greatest hazard from excess sugar, although it usually results from an excess of all types of high calorie food, not just sugar alone. Obesity is thought to be implicated in a form of diabetes appearing in maturity (late-onset diabetes), and it has also been associated with high blood pressure and gall bladder problems. Obesity itself, with its association of sugar intake, is also responsible for damage to the hips and knee joints, which are not able to cope with the increased load they must bear.

Dental caries occurs when bacteria in the pits of the teeth erode the hard enamel covering of the tooth, creating a cavity. Decay spreads rapidly into the soft dentine and eventually infects the pulp at the heart of the tooth.

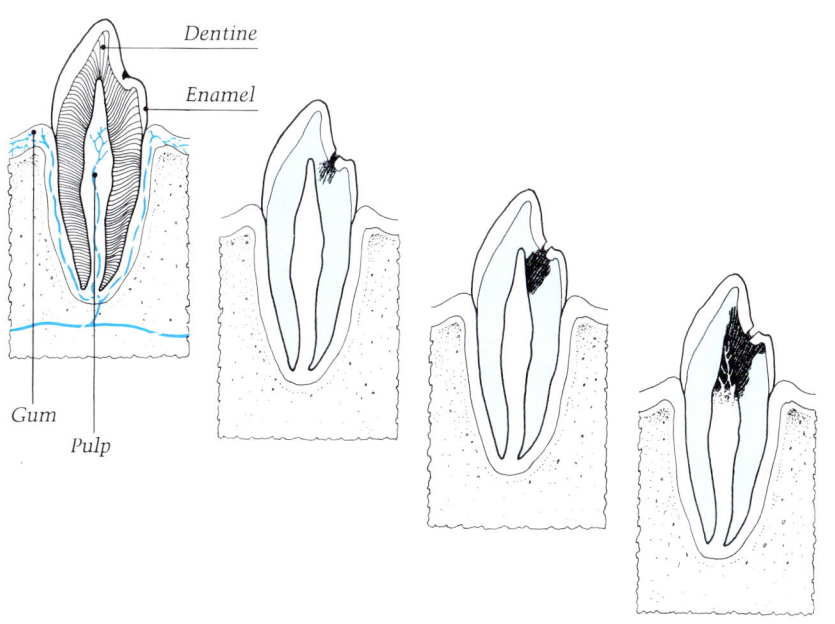

Dentine

Enamel

Gum

Pulp

SALT – THE UNPALATABLE TRUTH

Why do we crave so much salt in our food? It is true that in some parts of the world there are remote land-locked tribes who have difficulty getting sufficient salt for a healthy diet. It is also true that salt is one of the most abundant substances in our blood, and we do need to top up our salt balance regularly if we are to remain healthy. But to remain healthy, we need only a half to one gram of salt each day - we actually consume nine to twelve grams a day. (This figure is an average for both sexes, but men actually consume more salt than women, probably because of their taste for fried food and larger meals, usually eaten with more salt.)

If we enjoy the flavour of salt *and* it is necessary, why should we be advised to cut down our intake? The medical view is that if we cut our salt intake by about three grams a day or by up to one-third of our normal intake, the risk of developing hypertension, or high blood pressure, and its associated disorders like coronary heart disease and strokes, will be greatly reduced. These diseases are the main killers and salt, or rather its constituent sodium, has a very important part in controlling blood pressure. Sodium controls the flow of water in and out of the body's cells, and it is important that the correct sodium balance is maintained. When we take in too much sodium, the kidneys dispose of the excess in the urine; in some people, this process of eliminating excess sodium seems to lead to high blood pressure. The mechanism for this is not known but one theory is that sodium passes into the walls of the tiny capillaries carrying blood through the tissue. This causes the cells forming the capillary walls to swell, narrowing the tubular blood vessel and restricting the amount of blood flowing. Blood pressure rises, as the heart attempts to force blood through the restricted capillaries. The causes of hypertension are by no means as simple as this, however, and several other factors are involved.

Up to ten per cent of people who suffer from hypertension have a specific cause of the condition; in the other 90 per cent there is no known cause. There is an inherited tendency to developing hypertension, but there is no way of detecting this until you already have high blood pressure!

A proportion of the population - perhaps over one person in every four - is salt-sensitive in regard to blood pressure, and these may be the people who are at risk from hypertension through eating our current high-salt diet. The theory is that cutting down moderately on salt may help protect those at risk, and will not do any harm to non-salt-sensitive people.

The evidence for yet another recommendation to change our diet lies in a comparison of the eating habits of contrasting populations. In countries where salt intake is low there is little or no hypertension and blood pressure does not rise significantly with age. Studies in California have demonstrated that when salt intake is reduced, the average blood pressure in the community falls.

Controlling or avoiding hypertension is certainly worthwhile, especially when the results of untreated high blood pressure are known: seven times greater risk of strokes, four times greater risk of heart failure and three times greater risk of heart attacks; and atherosclerosis, or hardening of the arteries, is much more common in blood vessels damaged by the effects of high blood pressure.

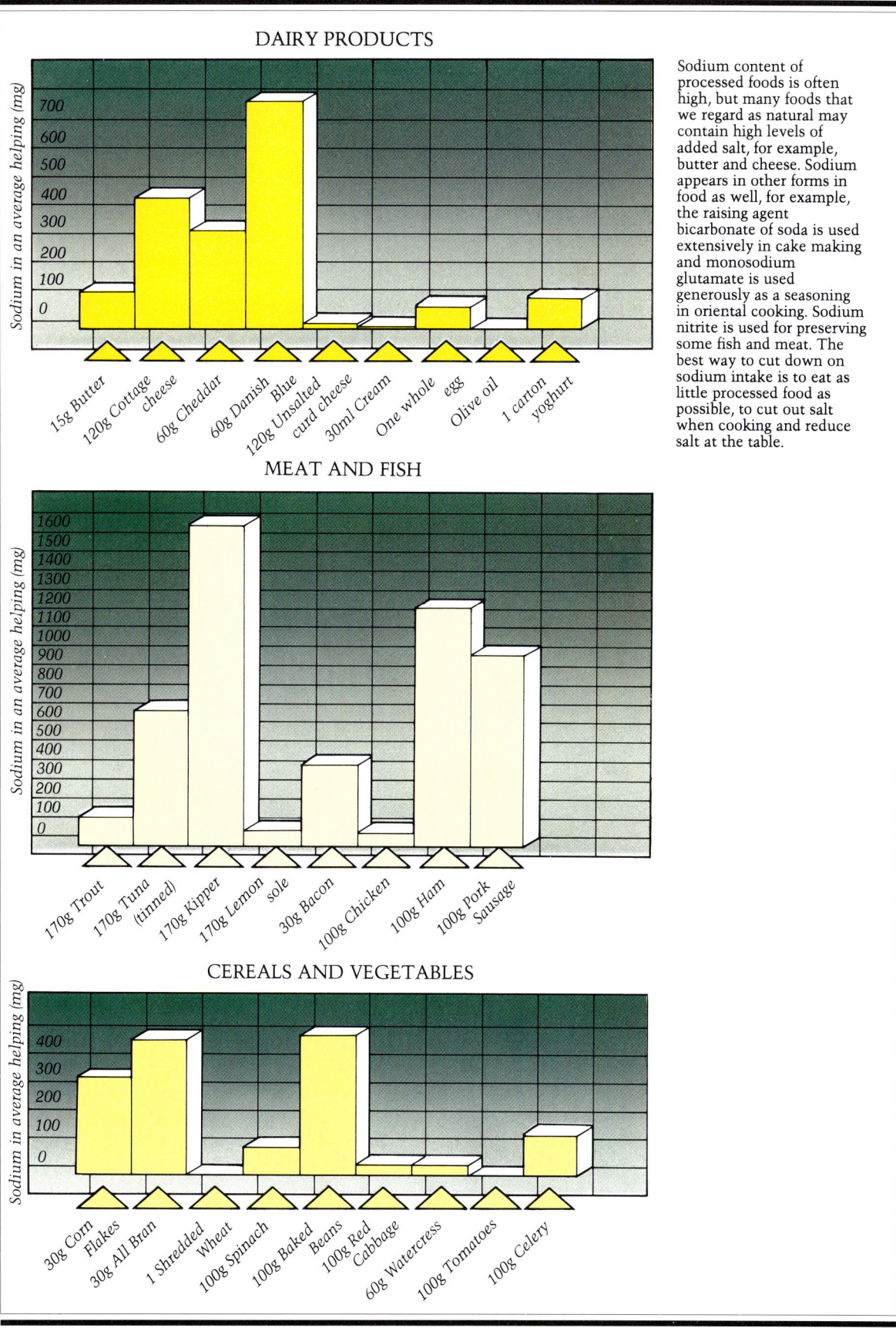

DAIRY PRODUCTS

Sodium in an average helping (mg)

700, 600, 500, 400, 300, 200, 100, 0

15g Butter, 120g Cottage cheese, 60g Cheddar, 60g Danish Blue, 120g Unsalted curd cheese, 30ml Cream, One whole egg, Olive oil, 1 carton yoghurt

Sodium content of processed foods is often high, but many foods that we regard as natural may contain high levels of added salt, for example, butter and cheese. Sodium appears in other forms in food as well, for example, the raising agent bicarbonate of soda is used extensively in cake making and monosodium glutamate is used generously as a seasoning in oriental cooking. Sodium nitrite is used for preserving some fish and meat. The best way to cut down on sodium intake is to eat as little processed food as possible, to cut out salt when cooking and reduce salt at the table.

MEAT AND FISH

Sodium in an average helping (mg)

1600, 1500, 1400, 1300, 1200, 1100, 1000, 900, 800, 700, 600, 500, 400, 300, 200, 100, 0

170g Trout, 170g Tuna (tinned), 170g Kipper, 170g Lemon sole, 30g Bacon, 100g Chicken, 100g Ham, 100g Pork Sausage

CEREALS AND VEGETABLES

Sodium in average helping (mg)

400, 300, 200, 100, 0

30g Corn Flakes, 30g All Bran, 1 Shredded Wheat, 100g Spinach, 100g Baked Beans, 100g Red Cabbage, 60g Watercress, 100g Tomatoes, 100g Celery

CUTTING DOWN ON SALT

As many as 60 per cent of us sprinkle salt on our food, and of these a quarter of us don't taste the food first. In the same way, most people add salt to vegetables or other food they are preparing without tasting to see if it is necessary. This 'visible' salt is easy to control.

You can make a conscious effort to reduce the amount you sprinkle on your food or that you use in cooking. By gradually cutting down on added salt you can train your taste-buds to become less salt-dependent in about two to three weeks. Once you've done that, you'll actually prefer food that is less salty.

Avoiding a rather bland flavour is possible if you use more spices, herbs and lemon juice in cooking. It is also possible to use commercial salt substitutes. These are usually based on potassium chloride, rather than the sodium chloride of ordinary table salt, and some contain a mixture of sodium and potassium chloride. Salt substitutes certainly taste salty, but most are also bitter and need to be used in moderation. There is some evidence that the balance between sodium and potassium in the body can affect blood pressure, so increased potassium intake *may* be beneficial, provided it is combined with a reduction in sodium intake. An increased potassium intake is better than the use of salt substitutes, and most fruits and vegetables are rich in potassium. But remember, boiling reduces potassium content drastically.

If you have any sort of kidney or heart problem, you must check with your doctor before regularly using a salt substitute as it could interfere with your medication.

Some people have switched to sea salt or rock salt, which are widely promoted as being more 'healthy'. The effects of sea salt on the body are exactly the same as ordinary table salt. Sea salt does, however, contain other 'trace' elements and has a slightly different taste. Use it by all means, in moderation, especially if it helps you to be more conscious of the amount of salt you are using.

About 70 per cent of the salt we eat is already added to food when we buy it. Manufacturers claim that the public demands high salt levels, but it has been argued that, because salt enhances flavour to some extent, manufacturers can make economies in more expensive ingredients. It may be quite difficult to estimate the amount of salt present in any manufactured food, even when the constituents are listed on the pack or can.

The chart on page 63 shows the salt content of some common foods. Processed foods are always high in salt, but some 'natural' foods like butter and cheese can also contain added salt. It is worth noting that certain breakfast cereals, pickles, cheeses and smoked meat and fish contain very high levels of salt.

Try to remember the worst offenders so that you will know what to avoid, although it will be very difficult to cut down if you use a lot of prepared or manufactured foods. But you can substitute foods with a low salt content for more commonly used ones.

In addition, sodium, but not sodium chloride, can be added to the food in the form of monosodium glutamate (a flavour enhancer), sodium bicarbonate (self-raising agent for dough), sodium benzoate and nitrate (preservatives), as well as in many other forms.

Always read the label to see if salt or anything containing sodium is listed among the ingredients; if possible, buy a sodium-free substitute. Health-food stores now stock salt-free foods, and even some of the large supermarkets are stocking tinned foods without added salt. So the salt story is yet another reason for sticking to fresh or home-prepared foods as much as possible.

THE FIBRE FACTOR

One other important dietary recommendation that has been generally accepted is that we should eat more fibre and increase our intake from an average of about 20g a day to 30g a day. Such an increase is relatively easy without drastically altering the traditional diet. In fact, much can be taken in by eating more of the foods we were traditionally taught were 'good for us' such as fruit and vegetables, wholegrain cereals and wholemeal baking.

To most people, fibre means bran, the relatively unpalatable, and certainly uninteresting, material that is discarded during the processing of cereals. And many men have come to believe that a high-fibre diet means endlessly chewing mouthfuls of boring bran. Bran is high in fibre, but very little of the fibre in food is actually bran.

Fibre, or roughage as it used to be known, is not necessarily either fibrous or rough in texture. It is actually the remains of plant material in our food, which pass through the digestive system without being changed or absorbed. Instead it soaks up water in the intestine and forms a soft, smooth mass; indeed, 'smoothage' would be a better term for it. In simplified terms, its general effects are to keep the intestines well filled, and to produce a larger, softer bulk of stools or faeces, thus keeping the bowel contents moving and preventing constipation.

We know that fibre is good for our health, by examining the diet and health statistics of other cultures. In general, cultures with high-fibre diets eat proportionately less fat (and vice versa), which can make it difficult to distinguish the effects of high-fibre from low-fat, but the diseases of Western civilization that have been linked to our existing over-refined, low-fibre diet are constipation, obesity, diverticular disease, cancer of the bowel, piles, varicose veins, appendicitis, hiatus hernia, gallstones, diabetes and coronary heart disease.

The modern move toward increasing our fibre intake came in the 1950s and 1960s, when the diseases listed above were described as 'diseases of affluence' and linked to over-refining of our diet, a process that effectively removes most of the fibre from flour. It was found that while we tend to eat only 15-20g of fibre a day, people in Third World countries in Africa and Asia consumed around 40-60g a day, most of which was from cereal sources. People from these countries tend to suffer very many serious health problems but they do not generally suffer from 'diseases of affluence' to any significant extent.

Although fibre is not affected by digestion, it seems to have a beneficial effect on the whole digestive process. The effects start in the mouth, when foods containing fibre are more work to chew. Wholemeal bread, for example, takes longer to chew than an equivalent slice of white bread. And it is obviously more work to eat an orange, complete with fibre, than to drink a glass of orange juice. Chewing food for a long time encourages the flow of saliva, which is beneficial for dental health, and also provides enzymes to help digestion. It also helps to deter over-eating!

Once swallowed, food passes down the oesophagus to the stomach, where it mixes with digestive juices, and digestion begins in earnest. Food low in fibre is runny when mixed with digestive juice, and leaves the stomach quickly; food that is rich in fibre is thicker and remains in the stomach for two hours or more. Digestion is then more complete, and the stomach *feels* fuller, so you will not feel hungry again so quickly.

Part-digested food moves along into the small intestine. Here again the benefits of high-fibre food are apparent. The food mixture is thicker and stickier, and sugar is released into the walls of the intestine more slowly than with a low-fibre diet, helping to avoid a sudden rise in the blood sugar level.

Fibre is also thought to reduce the amounts of fat available for absorption, and a high-fibre diet is associated particularly with a lower level of cholesterol in the blood. This could be a significant factor in the development of coronary heart disease.

Once the nutrients have been digested and absorbed in the intestine, the indigestible remains move on to the large intestine or colon. Waste is moved along the colon (and the rest of the gut) by wavelike muscular contractions (peristalsis), which move the faeces with them. If the faeces are bulky, because of the presence of fibre, the contractions can move them with relative ease. Fibre has another valuable function here: it clears away various chemical wastes before they can be absorbed into the body.

The presence of large amounts of fibre in the food is critical in avoiding some all too familiar, and some serious, health problems. Most dangerous of all these is bowel cancer, a fairly common condition among men in Western nations. It is, however, rare in Third World countries, where people eat high-fibre diets. Bowel cancer is thought to be caused by irritant substances - produced by the billions of bacteria that normally live in the large intestine or colon - which feed on the waste from the process of digestion. In fact, a large proportion of the faeces consists of these bacteria. It is thought that if the remains of the food linger in the gut, the bacteria are more likely to produce these cancer-forming toxins (or carcinogens). It is beneficial, therefore, to move the faeces through the gut more rapidly. The best way to achieve rapid transit time is *not* to use laxatives, which are mostly harmful irritants and should only be used if recommended by the doctor, but to eat a high-fibre diet, which will provide a completely natural stimulus to the actions of the gut.

SOURCES OF FIBRE

Most men in Britain have inadequate fibre intakes, largely because they consume considerable amounts of processed or refined food, which are mostly based on low-fibre, white flour.

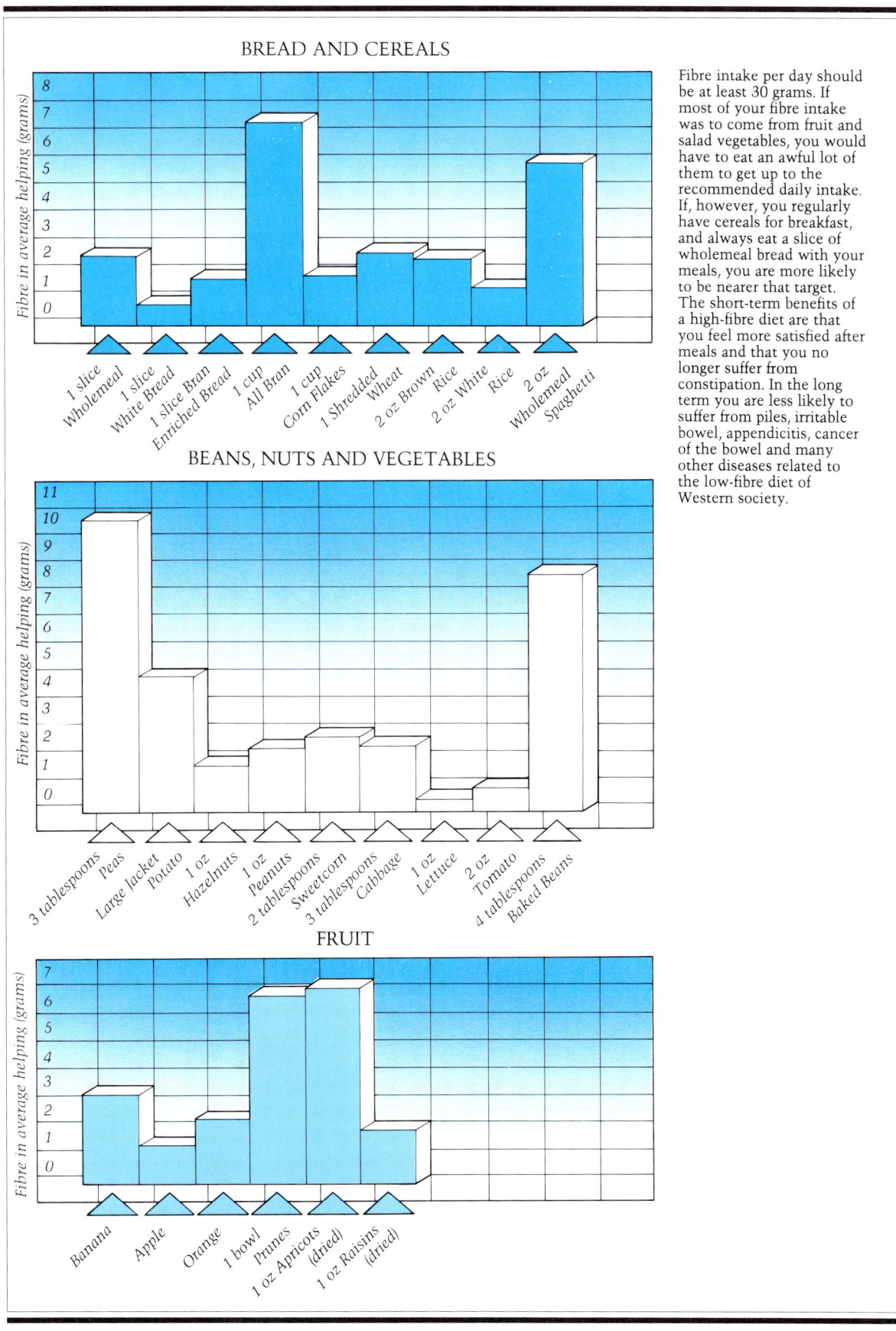

BREAD AND CEREALS

Fibre in average helping (grams)

1 slice Wholemeal
1 slice White Bread
1 slice Bran Enriched Bread
1 cup All Bran
1 cup Corn Flakes
1 Shredded Wheat
2 oz Brown Rice
2 oz White Rice
2 oz Wholemeal Spaghetti

BEANS, NUTS AND VEGETABLES

Fibre in average helping (grams)

3 tablespoons Peas
Large Jacket Potato
1 oz Hazelnuts
1 oz Peanuts
2 tablespoons Sweetcorn
3 tablespoons Cabbage
1 oz Lettuce
2 oz Tomato
4 tablespoons Baked Beans

FRUIT

Fibre in average helping (grams)

Banana
Apple
Orange
1 bowl Prunes
1 oz Apricots (dried)
1 oz Raisins (dried)

Fibre intake per day should be at least 30 grams. If most of your fibre intake was to come from fruit and salad vegetables, you would have to eat an awful lot of them to get up to the recommended daily intake. If, however, you regularly have cereals for breakfast, and always eat a slice of wholemeal bread with your meals, you are more likely to be nearer that target. The short-term benefits of a high-fibre diet are that you feel more satisfied after meals and that you no longer suffer from constipation. In the long term you are less likely to suffer from piles, irritable bowel, appendicitis, cancer of the bowel and many other diseases related to the low-fibre diet of Western society.

The relative merits of some common types of bread

•100g wholemeal
Fibre: 8.5g
Calories (Kcal): 216

•100g white
Fibre: 2.7g
Calories (Kcal): 233

Very high levels of fibre intake can at first lead to a feeling of being bloated and also to the production of large amounts of wind or flatus, but this discomfort eases after a week or two. You should obtain your extra fibre from a mixture of all the various sources. Fibre from bread and cereals is thought to be particularly beneficial for the bowels because it is more effective in increasing faecal weight than fruit or vegetable fibre.

The easiest way to increase your intake of fibre is to eat more bread, particularly bread made from wholemeal flour, despite what we have been taught about the 'evils' of bread in causing obesity. In fact, wholemeal bread is much more filling than ordinary white bread, and it contains around three times more fibre for each portion, so you will not want to eat so much at a time. There are pitfalls, however, for not all brown-coloured bread is wholemeal - it may be white flour with added colouring, or an admixture of wholemeal flour. Other types of bread, such as granary, wheatmeal and wheatgerm, contain varying amounts of fibre, and it is not easy to determine how much fibre you will be getting from them. A further pitfall with *all* forms of bread is that the manufacturers include unnecessarily large amounts of salt; increasing your bread intake will also increase your salt intake: a further reason to cut down on the table salt while increasing your fibre intake.

Because fibre is not digested, eating wholemeal bread is a convenient way to cut down on your calorie intake. And don't forget, white bread is 'good' for you but wholemeal bread is a whole lot better!

Breakfast cereals are another convenient way of getting extra fibre, but check to make sure that they are actually made from the whole grain, as many are made from refined grains. Avoid too those cereals with added salt and sugar.

Pasta, especially if it is made from wholemeal flour, is another good source of cereal fibre, as is brown rice. Fibre from pulses (eg, beans, peas and lentils) and fruit and vegetables is thought to be particularly beneficial in helping to control blood sugar and cholesterol. Pulses contain very large amounts of fibre, and there are reasonable amounts in leaf vegetables such as cabbage and brussels sprouts. Nuts and dried fruits too are very high in fibre. Fresh fruit is a palatable but not so rich source of fibre as it contains so much water.

It is not easy to determine your fibre intake; vegetables such as celery and other salad stuffs, for instance, contain little fibre, while beans and peas contain a great deal. The table below shows the fibre content of a range of common foods and will help you determine if you are getting near the recommended 30g a day.

WHO NEEDS VITAMINS?

The general view of vitamins is that they are good for us and that we need as much as possible of all of them, and this belief has received enthusiastic support from certain 'experts' on health and nutrition.

Vitamins are essential to health and life for they are required by the body to assist in the manufacture of enzymes and other vital substances. The body cannot make vitamins, so they must be obtained from the food we eat, but

VITAMIN ROUND-UP

VITAMIN	BEST SOURCES	ROLE	RECOMMENDED INTAKE
Vitamin A (retinol)	Liver, milk, eggs, green and yellow fruit and vegetables	Healthy eye retina, lung and digestive system lining	1mg
Thiamin (Vitamin B1)	Pork, whole grains, nuts, pulses, enriched flour and cereals	Efficient calorie burning	1.0—1.4mg
Riboflavin (Vitamin B2)	Milk, cheese, eggs, liver, poultry	Repair and energy release in cells	1.2—1.7mg
Nicotinic acid	Whole grains, liver, poultry, lean meat	Needed by all cells	13—19mg
Pyridoxine (Vitamin B6)	Liver, meat, grains, milk, eggs	Needed by red blood cells	2mg
Pantothenic acid	Egg yolk, meat, nuts	Energy production	4—7mg
Biotin	Liver, kidney, egg yolk, nuts, vegetables	Skin and circulatory system	100—200 micrograms
Vitamin B12	Eggs, meat, dairy products	Red blood cell production, nervous system	3 micrograms
Folic acid	Vegetables, fish, poultry	Red blood cell production	400 micrograms
Vitamin C	Citrus fruits, cabbage, potatoes, tomatoes	Bone, teeth and tissue repair	60mg
Vitamin D	Oily fish, eggs, dairy products, sun	Blood calcium levels and bone growth	5—10 micrograms
Vitamin E	Vegetable oils and many other foods	Cell membrane production, fat metabolism	8—10mg
Vitamin K	Leafy vegetables	Blood clotting	70—140 micrograms

Vitamins are needed by the body to help the metabolic processes. Our Western diet usually provides us with an adequate supply of these vitamins, but vitamins are sensitive chemicals and can be destroyed if the food is handled incorrectly. Cooking, storing and processing food can lead to vitamin loss, for example, exposure to high temperatures inactivates vitamin C. The B vitamins can wash out of food and be discarded with the cooking liquid. Your daily diet should include as many raw, fresh vegetables and fruits as possible. It is not necessary to supplement your diet with vitamin tablets, and vitamins A and D taken in excess can cause disease.

with one or two exceptions, our daily requirement of most vitamins is about one milligram (one thousandth of a gram) - about as much as one grain of sugar.

The vitamins that are required in the smallest amounts are those that are stored in body fat. Water-soluble vitamins are needed in larger amounts, as they are lost from the body in the urine. The table on page 69 shows the daily requirements of vitamins for healthy men; more may be needed by growing adolescents.

Vitamin deficiency can lead to serious diseases of the kind that are common in Third World countries. Their effects are especially crippling in children and can lead to blindness or rickets. Even in Western countries, vitamin deficiency can occur, but only in people who eat what most would consider to be an inadequate diet. For example, some old people, particularly widowers, may not have the strength or the will to shop and cook for themselves and may be missing out on various vitamins.

Anyone eating a varied range of foodstuffs including plenty of fresh fruit and vegetables is unlikely to suffer from vitamin deficiency. Taking a multi-vitamin tablet won't do you any harm, but it is unlikely to do you any good. Because of the way in which the body uses vitamins, larger amounts than the minimum requirement of water-soluble vitamins are simply disposed of in the urine. Fat-soluble vitamins can actually be harmful if they are taken in large amounts, because they are stored in our bodies.

The use of vitamin pills is promoted on the basis that, if vitamins are good for you, more of them must be better; but this is not true. Our traditional diet, even without the improvements recommended in this book, provides more than enough vitamins for almost everyone. There are only a few medical reasons for taking vitamin supplements; such as after a debilitating virus illness like influenza, when they *may* help you get over the after-effects, or in pregnant women, who may need a particular type of vitamin.

HEALTH FOODS

It should be clear by now that there is no such thing as a 'health food'. All foods are healthy - if eaten as part of a balanced diet. But some foods have more place in a sensible balanced diet than others, which, when consumed in excess, have been shown to have harmful long-term effects.

The growing interest in healthy eating has led to an enormous increase in the number of specialist health-food outlets. More and more supermarkets and chemists stock health foods, and there has been a significant growth in the number of specialist health-food shops. Such shops sell a wide range of foods and herbal preparations, as well as food supplements such as vitamin and mineral tablets. This is something of an admission of failure, for as these substances are unnecessary for a person eating our ordinary 'unhealthy' diet, they should be doubly unnecessary for the diet-conscious customers of the health-food shop.

Most of the food sold in health shops is valuable to healthy eating and is often especially rich in fibre. Health food shops (and wholefood shops) tend to specialize in wholegrain cereals and flour and in pulses: dried peas, lentils and beans. Nuts, dried fruit and cooking oils are also available, and nearly all of these are free from colourings and additives.

Organically grown foods, produced without the use of fertilizers or pesticides, may also be sold. Opinions differ as to whether there is any difference in the taste or quality of this food compared to crops produced by more orthodox farming techniques, and it is true that the organically grown crops tend to be more expensive, because of the more labour-intensive methods of farming and reduced yields.

PROCESSED FOODS – ARE THEY 'HEALTHY'?

Many people would consider processed foods to be the absolute opposite of the type of food supplied by health-food shops and to be nutritionally inferior. But the term 'processed food' actually covers a wide range of foodstuffs that may have been 'processed' for a variety of reasons.

Preserving food by treating it with chemicals or by other means such as refrigeration means that wastage is reduced and that seasonal foods can be obtained all year round. Safer food results from the elimination of dangerous organisms, including those causing food poisoning, and the control of the toxins produced by organisms growing on the food. Adding colourings and flavourings and altering the texture gives food more 'eye appeal', while the production of convenience foods, minimizing preparation time, has revolutionized family eating over the past 20 years or so. Finally, in addition to extending the shelf life of food, processing has reduced production costs which has led to lower prices.

These alterations have been made to increase the foods' appeal to the consumer, but does processing affect the nutritional value of food?

Drying, one form of processing, has been used for thousands of years to preserve meat and fruit. The dried fruit sold in health food shops has been subjected to the process and even the freshest of fresh fruit has probably been stored for weeks or even months, after having been kept in an atmosphere laden with an inert gas to delay ripening, or with a different type of gas to speed ripening when they are needed at market.

Processing can also mean the cooking of food, which causes some loss of nutrients. Vitamin C, folate, lysine and thiamine are destroyed by prolonged cooking, and water-soluble vitamins and minerals are flushed out of food during boiling. This happens whether food is cooked in a huge processing plant or at home, but in some processed foods, unstable substances like vitamins are replaced or added later in the processing. In contrast to processed foods, home cooking allows you to use better quality ingredients, to avoid overcooking, to avoid too much salt, sugar and other additives and cut down on fat.

In general, the nutritional value of processed food need not be inferior to that of home-cooked foods. In practice, however, the techniques used in food processing may allow the manufacturer to use inferior produce, or to use bland materials to bulk out a small amount of food. And, of course, large amounts of cheap ingredients like salt and sugar may be added to suit the 'taste' of the consumer, not to mention other additives. It is these points that are increasingly worrying people concerned about what they are eating. In response to this new consumer demand the food manufacturers are beginning to produce processed foods without sugar or with reduced salt levels or additive-free. Always read the small print on the label.

THE ADDITIVE CONTROVERSY

Large manufacturers have begun to accept, albeit reluctantly, the recent recommendations to cut down on fat, sugar and salt, and increase fibre levels in our diets. Yet market research studies have shown that the public is more concerned with chemical additives to food than with the balance of nutrients in our food.

Although it seems sensible to avoid unnecessary additives, don't develop a phobia about foods with additive numbers on the label. Some are wholly innocuous, natural substances that are highly unlikely to cause problems.

•**Numbers allocated to food additives fall into the following groups:**
100s colouring agents
200s preservatives
300s anti-oxidants
400s emulsifiers, gelling agents, stabilizers etc.

Chemicals are added to food for a variety of reasons. They may be flavourings, colourings, flavour enhancers, emulsifiers (which stop fat globules from settling on it), anti-oxidants (to prevent rancid tastes developing), preservatives or others. Not all are synthetic chemicals with unknown effects on the body. Some are natural extracts or 'nature-identical' analogues. The most widely used preservatives are salt and sugar, and many substances added to food as pure chemicals are naturally occurring.

There are reckoned to be about 6,000 additives in use today, about 95 per cent of which are flavourings. It has been estimated that we consume an average of about 4.5kg (10lb) of additives per head per annum (excluding salt and sugar). In the United Kingdom, only about 300 additives are regulated and these must be identified on the label of foodstuffs. They are given a number to denote the chemical substance, which may be prefixed by the letter 'E', which indicates that the additive has been approved by the European Economic Commission. When there is no 'E', the substance has either been rejected or has not yet been approved by the EEC. Some of these additives have been around for many years. Nitrates and the similar nitrites have been used for centuries to preserve ham, bacon and similar 'cured' meat products. It has long been known that the nitrates break down to nitrites, and it is these that have the 'curing' properties. Recently it has been found that the bactericidal nitrite can combine with amines, which are found both in food and in our bodies, to produce nitrosamines, a process that may be helped by gut bacteria. Nitrosamines are known to be potential carcinogens, or cancer-inducing agents. The problem has been played down by various governments and vested interests, but nitrite levels have been gradually reduced, although eliminating them completely would carry the risk of food-poisoning organisms developing in certain meat products.

It has been estimated that, while 35 per cent of all cancer deaths may be attributable to our diet, only 1 per cent can be attributed to food additives. This is not, however, a view shared by many other workers in this field, who are particularly suspicious of the dyes and colourings added to processed foods, often for no good reason. Food manufacturers decided that raspberry jam should be bright pink for example, and, until recently, a popular brand of blackcurrant juice had added colouring; this in a

Additives were originally given a letter E to put the public's mind at rest. The E signifies that the additive has been approved by the EEC as being safe for consumption. However, the public is still concerned by the quantities of chemicals that are added to processed foods such as packet soup, pork sausages or instant dessert (right).

Colours: E150 is caramel and E160(a) is an extract of natural plant pigment. E122 is a synthetic dye and can produce allergic reactions in some people.

Emusifiers: Many are safe and natural, and these two have no known adverse effects. E322 is made from soya beans.

Ingredients: Sugar, Modified starch, Hydrogenated vegetable oil, Emulsifiers: E477, E322; Gelling agents: E339, E450(a); Fat-reduced cocoa, Caseinate, Lactose, Colours: E150, E122, E160(a); Whey powder, Flavourings, Antioxidant: E320.

Anti-oxidant: E320 is prepared synthetically to stop food going rancid. This additive is not allowed to be used in foods intended for young children and babies.

Gelling agents: Substances that form a jelly. Neither of these E additives has any known adverse effects.

substance which is naturally strongly coloured!

Several food colourings are based on synthetic azo-dyes, or coal tar-compounds, and are related to substances known to be hazardous to health, in some cases causing cancer. Those dyes used as additives, however, have been thoroughly and expensively tested, and are regarded by government and the food industry as quite safe for long-term use. However, there is strong evidence that at least one widely used yellow dye, tartrazine (E102), can cause severe hyperactivity in susceptible children, and several other food additives are suspected of causing allergic reactions, and may be a contributory factor in stress-related illnesses in adults.

Some major supermarket chains are now reducing or eliminating unnecessary additives from their own-label ranges of foods, and some independent food manufacturers are introducing 'additive-free' ranges. This sometimes means that we have to eat foods that are now the usual colour or that have shorter shelf-lives than usual; inevitably, it might also mean that we have to pay more.

THE VEGETARIAN DIET – FAD OR FITNESS?

Interest in vegetarian diets is increasing rapidly, and they are no longer regarded as 'cranky'. Indeed, many restaurants now offer some vegetarian dishes.

People become vegetarians for a variety of reasons. Religious or spiritual beliefs influence many, and several religions teach that it is wrong to take the life of animals to provide food; many non-religious people are concerned about the exploitation and possibly inhumane treatment of animals. Others become vegetarian for health reasons or because they dislike the taste of meat.

VITAMIN ROUND-UP

VITAMIN	BEST SOURCES	ROLE	RECOMMENDED INTAKE
Calcium	*Dairy products, green vegetables*	*Blood clotting, bone and tooth structure, nerve function*	*800mg*
Phosphorus	*Meat, dairy products, pulses, cereals*	*Cell energy store*	*800mg*
Potassium	*Avocados, bananas, apricots, potatoes*	*Fluid balance cell metabolism*	*3g*
Magnesium	*Pulses, nuts, cereals, leafy vegetables*	*Electrical activity of nerves and muscles*	*500mg*
Iodine	*Seafood, liver, meat, eggs*	*Thyroid gland function, manufacture of haemoglobin in blood*	*0.1—15mg*
Iron	*Red meat and offal, also shellfish, cereal products, fruit and vegetables*	*An essential component of haemoglobin, which carries oxygen in the blood. Deficiency causes anaemia.*	*10mg*
Fluorine	*Tap water (in certain areas), toothpaste*	*Helps prevent tooth decay*	*Trace*
Copper	*Liver, seafood, meat*	*Oxygen metabolism*	*1.5mg*
Zinc	*Seafood, meat, pulses, wholewheat, nuts*	*Cell enzyme structure*	*15mg*
Chromium	*Trace element in many foods*	*Minor roles in body chemistry*	*Trace*

Minerals are 'metallic' elements required by the human body. Many other elements, such as gold, silver, barium, bromine and rubidium appear in the body but as yet their significance has not been discovered. Mineral deficiency diseases are rare in Western society. A diet low in zinc has been shown to retard growth in some children, and areas where levels of fluorine in the water supply are low show an increase in the levels of dental caries. However, too much fluorine in the diet eventually weakens the enamel and results in chalky white patches on the teeth which may eventually become pitted and discoloured. In severe cases the bones may also be affected. Other trace elements are toxic if consumed in excess over time. Cadmium accumulates in the body and much of it comes from cigarette smoking. The concentration may be especially high in the kidneys and contribute to high blood pressure in later life.

●For discussion of sodium, see pages 62-5

Many vegetarians eat eggs and milk products as well as vegetable foods. A minority of vegetarians eat no food of animal origin whatsoever, eve cutting out eggs, butter and milk. This is a vegan diet, which is exclusively based on fruit, vegetables, cereals, nuts and other materials of plant origin. The macrobiotic diet is more extreme; its exponents eat only those foods derived from plants in season.

In general, the more austere the vegetarian diet, the less fat it contains, and vegetarians generally consume less of this calorie source. This makes the vegetarian diet a good slimming aid. It is possible to overcompensate for the absence of meat, however, by taking large amounts of cheese and eggs, causing an overconsumption of saturated fats.

There are good and bad points about a vegetarian diet. The diet may be inconvenient, especially if you are dining with friends who must produce special dishes for you. It need not be monotonous, however, and there are many highly flavoured and attractive vegetarian dishes that are easily prepared and palatable. It is, on the whole, a cheap diet, as plant foods are an economical source of protein and other nutrients. And above all, the vegetarian diet is healthy, probably because of its low-fat, high-fibre nature. Vegetarians are much less prone to coronary heart disease, strokes, constipation and diverticulitis, as well as the many diseases related to obesity.

It is a myth that you need meat for protein. Equally spurious is the claim that red meat is essential for strength and muscle bulk. Many athletes - champion weightlifters among them - are vegetarian. Vegetarian diets demonstrate that you don't need to eat meat to be healthy, and it has been shown that vegetarians on a properly balanced diet tend to live longer than people on a diet that includes meat. Some authorities recommend eating at least two or three vegetarian main meals each week, provided that they do not contain more dairy products.

JUST PLUMP, OR OBESE?

As you have seen, excess energy obtained from eating too much calorie-rich food is stored away in the form of fat. Normally, 10-20 per cent of your body weight is in the form of fat; much more than this, and you could soon be in trouble.

Fat is laid down in many parts of the body. It is stored in bulk inside the abdomen and packed around the internal organs, and it is this excess fat that contributes to the pot-belly characteristics of the over-weight middle-aged man. Fat is also stored in a layer beneath the skin, but in obese men this subcutaneous layer is usually thinner than it is in obese women. Men tend to put on weight around their neck, shoulders and abdomen. (Women tend to put on weight around their breasts, buttocks and thighs.) Where fat appears is determined entirely by your genes.

It is not possible to measure fat accurately without special equipment, but you can make a rough check by pinching the back of your arm, between the elbow and shoulder, with your thumb and forefinger. If you can pinch up more than 2.5cm (1in) of tissue, you are too fat. Another test is to get someone else to pinch the skinfold below your shoulder blade; here too there should be no more than 2.5cm (1in) thickness. This is a very rough

Continued on page 78

FOOD AND THE WORKING MAN

All this good advice about your diet is all very well, but it may not be so easy to put into practice. If you eat in a factory cateteria or have to snatch a pub lunch, you may not always have a good enough choice of food from which to get a healthy, balanced meal. And that is even more likely with motorway snacks and business lunches.

The factory cafeteria or motorway restaurant are in many cases the worst places to eat from the point of view of your health. Chips, almost certainly fried in cheap and saturated cooking oil, are served with everything. You should avoid most of the other cafeteria standbys — sausages, fried eggs, fatty bacon and so on. Of course, you *may* be lucky. You may be offered wholemeal bread rolls, salads or pasta, and you can always concentrate on grilled foods for the main dish. It is up to you to use the guidelines provided here to help you choose your food wisely.

Business lunches are more of a problem. Just as when you are entertaining at home, the occasional 'binge' won't do any harm, especially if you follow all the commonsense rules outlined in this book. But if you eat out frequently, your figure and your health are likely to suffer. Check the menus carefully and select the most sensible combination of courses. Avocado for a starter and fresh fruit for dessert are much better than prawn cocktail laden with mayonnaise and a gateau or rich cheese. For your main course, you could choose a lean grilled fillet steak with plenty of vegetables instead of meat cooked in a rich sauce laden with saturated fats.

If you really want to control your diet, you will probably have to rely on a packed lunch, which

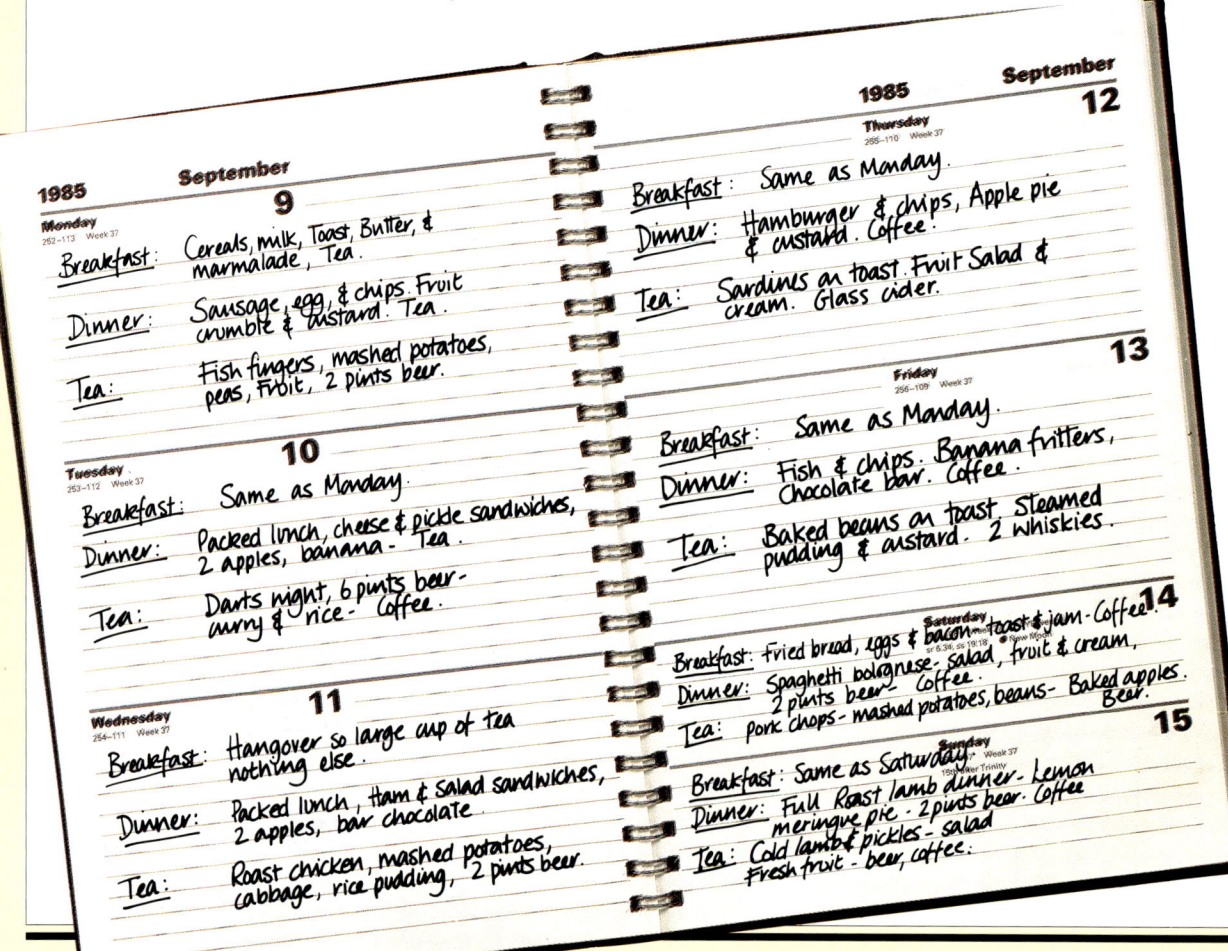

need not be sandwiches, although they can be an excellent way of getting the right balance, especially if you have thick-cut wholemeal bread, little butter or margarine and plenty of low-fat nutritional fillings.

Many other convenient (not 'convenience') foods can be added to your lunch: wholemeal crackers, dried fruits, or, if you want some meat, try a leg of chicken (grilled or roast, of course). Take some fresh fruit, too, such as apples or grapes, or munch a raw carrot or a stick of celery.

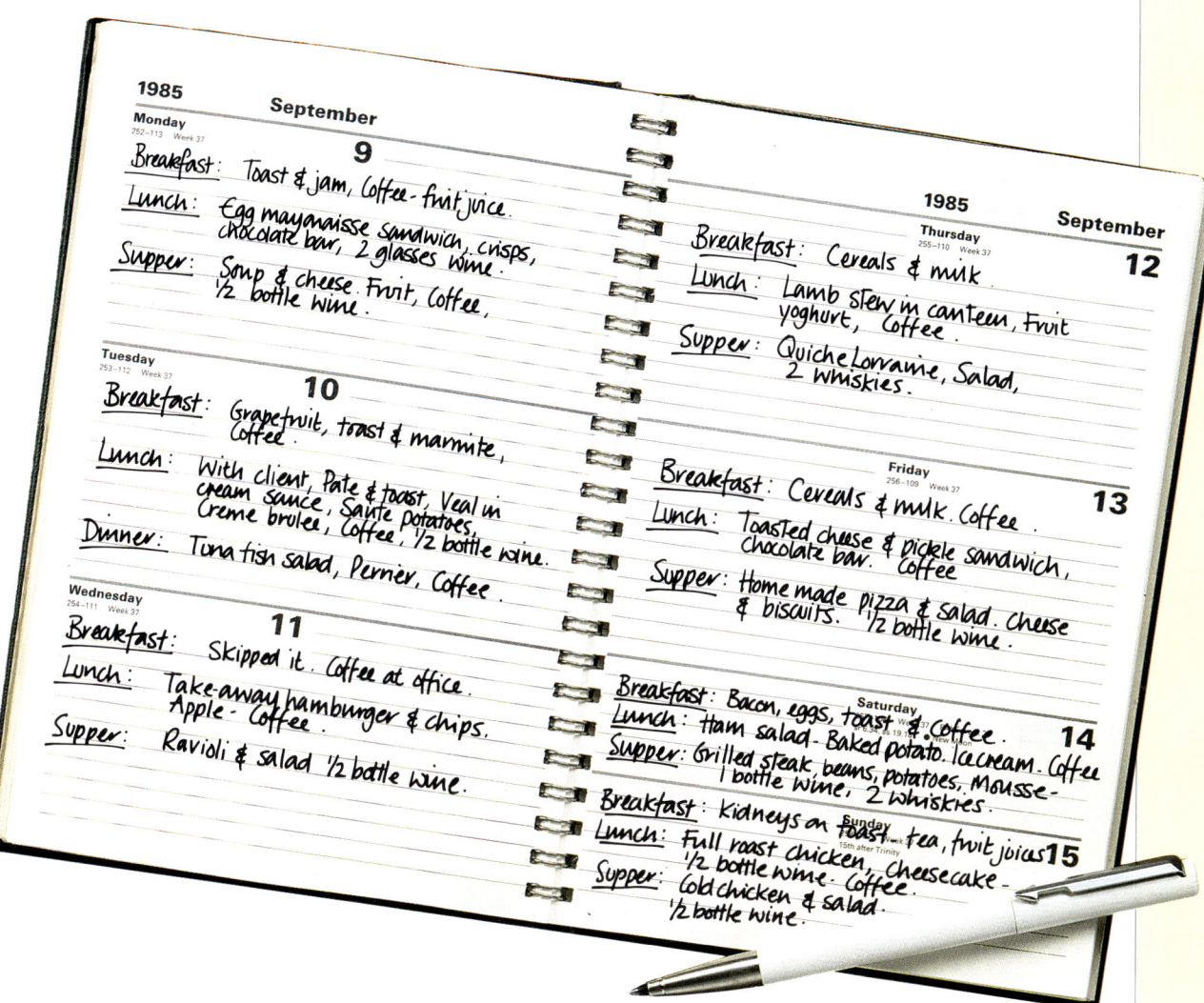

A healthy diet is something that you maintain over a space of time. The diet of the manual worker (*left*) is good in some aspects — he does not drink as much alcohol as the white collar worker, and breakfast tends to consist of a healthy fibre cereal, but his diet is fairly high in fat due to canteen meals. His sugar intake is also rather high. He would be better off taking a packed lunch like Tuesday. The white collar worker is eating a lot of fresh fruit and salads, but needs to cut down on alcohol and coffee. The high fat weekend breakfast is acceptable occasionally, as is the business lunch. Both men need to modify their diets but neither has to cut out any one food completely.

Continued from page 75

measurement of your subcutaneous fat, but to decide how much you have stored away in your abdomen, you will have to check yourself against a standard chart that has been based on studies of very large numbers of men.

The band in the middle of the graph represents men with a healthy weight. It is broad enough to allow for adjustment for stocky, muscular build or for less muscular men, and you must decide for yourself where you fit on the chart. If you weight is above the coloured band, you are under-weight. If you want, you can indulge yourself in more high-calorie food, but you're probably better off as you are.

If you are below the coloured band, you are overweight. The further below the band, the more overweight you are and the more at risk of ill-health. The chart shown was compiled by life insurance companies, after studying large numbers of their clients, and the coloured band represents the weights where fewest men died prematurely.

We all know that being fat is no longer fashionable. You know how you appear when you look in a mirror, and if you are too fat, you are probably acutely aware of it. But appearance is not the main problem with the overweight male. There are some simple and brutal truths to be faced if you are overweight: insurance statistics show that the fatter you are, the more likely you are to die prematurely. Being overweight means that you are more likely to become ill, particularly with hypertension or diseases of the heart and blood vessels. Diabetes is much more common in fat people too. The extra weight also puts more strain on joints, so fat people are more likely to get joint disorders and back problems.

People run extra risks from being grossly overweight or obese — and if you are 20 per cent or more above the normal weight limit for your height, you are obese.

If you are obese, you will already know about it: you will feel unfit and breathless, and you will be subject to all sorts of unconscious, but cruel, prejudices from other people. If you are really fat, you should be receiving treatment from your doctor; losing weight is an urgent medical problem.

Fortunately, however, most men are not grossly overweight, but you may be one of the many who need to shed a few pounds. If you are, you will be looking for sensible ways to lose weight.

CALORIE-CONTROLLED WEIGHT LOSS

You are probably bored stiff by having people nag you to lose weight and by reading magazine articles about dieting. Some people have made a lot of money out of advising others how to lose weight, usually by the most involved systems or by persuading them to attend slimming clubs. But like most men, you probably don't want to be bothered by all that.

The secret of successful dieting is that there isn't a secret at all. If you are taking in more calories than your body burns up, you will store them away as fat. If you take in fewer than you need, then you burn up the stored fat and lose weight. It's as easy as that!

The usual way to lose weight is to count calories and, after having established your normal daily calorie usage, to cut down so there is a

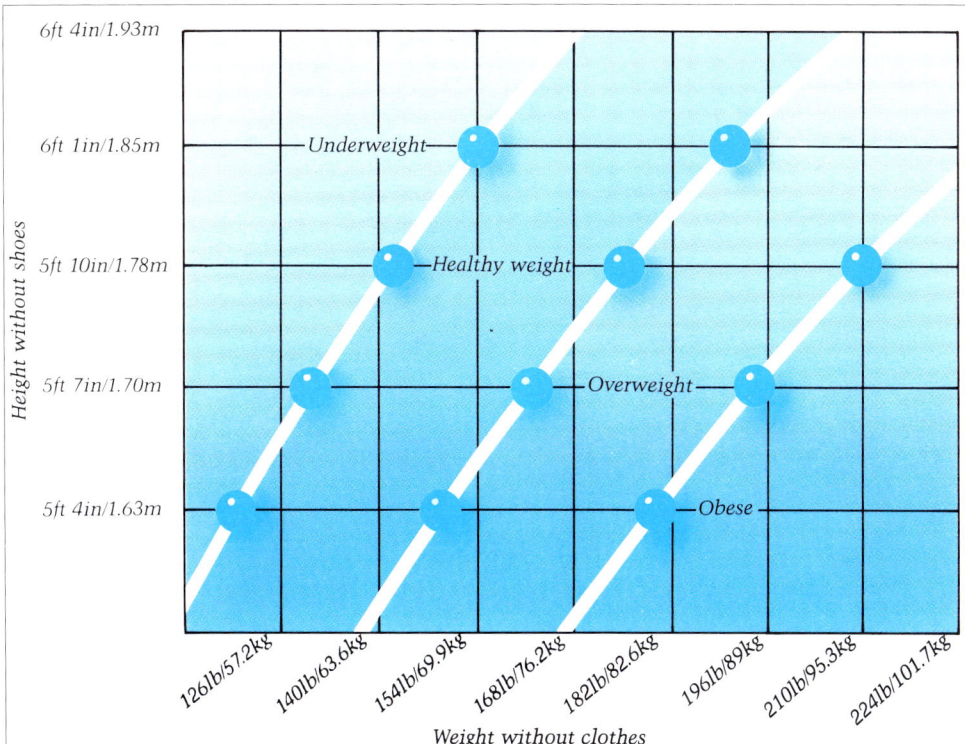

Height without shoes

6ft 4in/1.93m

6ft 1in/1.85m — *Underweight*

5ft 10in/1.78m — *Healthy weight*

5ft 7in/1.70m — *Overweight*

5ft 4in/1.63m — *Obese*

126lb/57.2kg 140lb/63.6kg 154lb/69.9kg 168lb/76.2kg 181lb/82.6kg 196lb/89kg 210lb/95.3kg 224lb/101.7kg

Weight without clothes

Ideal weight charts are worked out by life insurance companies on death rate statistics. If you are within the range of weights for your particular height you are more likely to reach old age than if you are either under or overweight. Once you move into the obese section of the chart, you **are more likely to suffer from a range of disorders throughout life as well as shorten your life expectancy.**

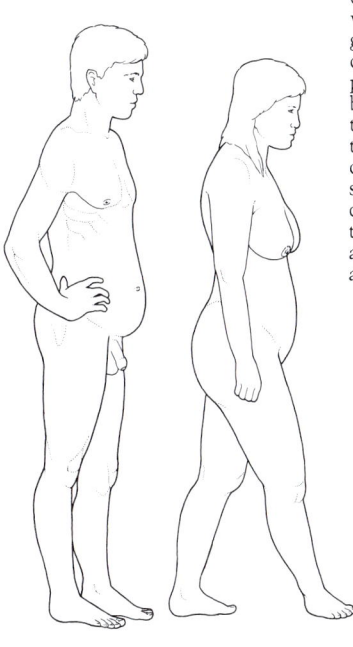

Men and women lay fat down in different ways. A woman has more body fat generally and it is laid down as surface fat, particularly around the bosom, buttocks, legs, thighs and knees. Men, on the other hand, lay fat down on the inside of their stomach wall, giving the characteristic belly shape of the middle-aged man accompanied by thin arms and legs.

●How many calories do you need? See chart, page 48

'calorie gap' of around 750 calories per day. As you can see, the first week or so produces the greatest weight drop, because the first energy stores to be broken down are the easily accessible glycogen stores in the muscles. Later, as you start to burn off fat, the process is much slower.

To carry out a calorie-controlled diet properly, you must weigh and

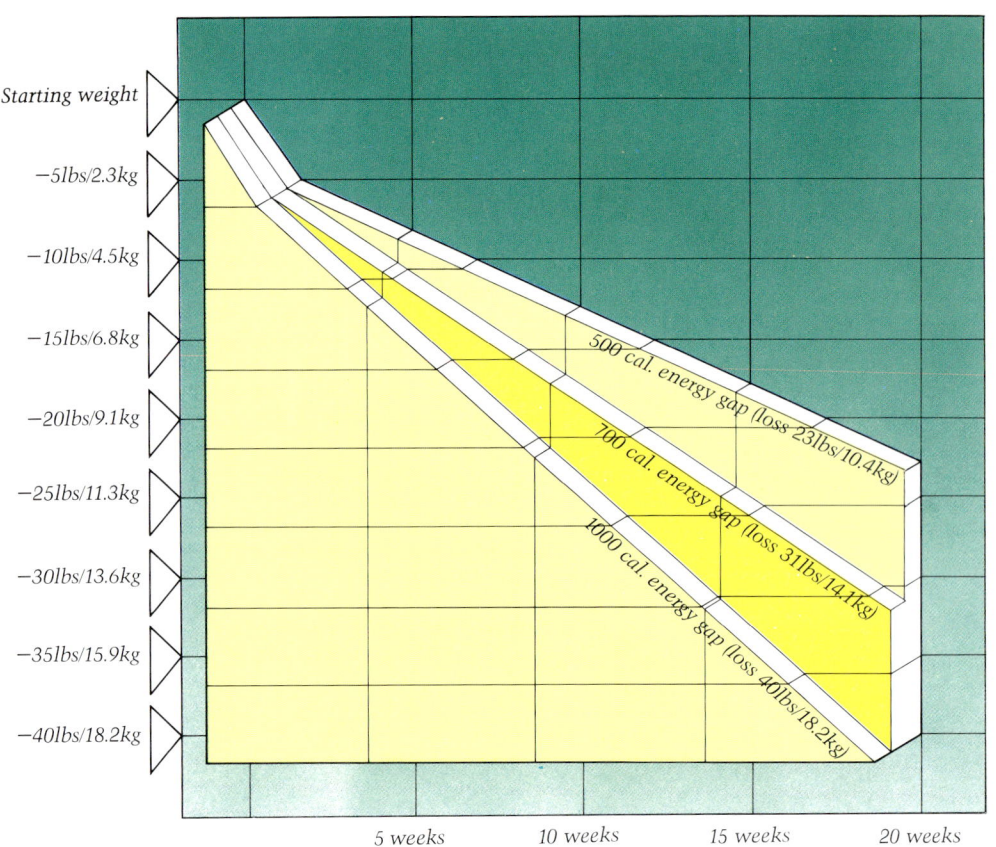

Starting weight

−5lbs/2.3kg

−10lbs/4.5kg

−15lbs/6.8kg

−20lbs/9.1kg

−25lbs/11.3kg

−30lbs/13.6kg

−35lbs/15.9kg

−40lbs/18.2kg

500 cal. energy gap (loss 23lbs/10.4kg)

700 cal. energy gap (loss 31lbs/14.1kg)

1000 cal. energy gap (loss 40lbs/18.2kg)

5 weeks   10 weeks   15 weeks   20 weeks

Weight loss speed depends on the difference in energy input (food and drink) and energy output (exercise and metabolism). If your exercise regime is very energetic and your food intake low, your weight loss will be swift. However, it is probably better to maintain a slower weight loss by reducing the energy gap because the regime will be easier to maintain after you have achieved your goal weight. Whatever the energy gap, inital weight loss is fast for the first week before levelling out into a more gradual loss.

measure every portion you eat and drink, and keep this up for weeks until you gain a rough idea of the calorie values of different foods. Remember, individual calorie needs vary widely among individuals (because of variations in basal metabolic rate), so you will have to establish your daily calorie target very carefully.

Some diets are just plain silly; others are potentially dangerous. For example, a crash diet that produces a calorific deficiency of 1000 to 1500 calories a day is likely to make you feel very ill and weak. And the popular all-fruit diet, like all extreme diets, can be particularly dangerous. Some diets consist almost entirely of fibre, others are almost all protein, but with all these diets, and with artificial meal replacements too, you will not be receiving the proper balance of nutrients for health.

With almost any calorie-controlled diet, there is evidence that your basal metabolic rate adjusts itself to the lower availability of calories, so you no longer use so much energy to power muscles and internal organs. Because your body no longer needs so much energy, having adjusted itself to a lower calorie intake, once you come off the diet and start eating normally again, you will put on weight much faster than before.

It is easy to get into a cycle of over-eating, dieting then over-eating again and, although an awareness of high calorie foods is obviously sensible so that you will know what foods to avoid, this is the great danger of all forms of calorie-controlled diet.

WEIGHT LOSS BY HEALTHY EATING

By now, you have probably realized that a sensible diet for the sake of your health will also benefit your weight. You are recommended to eat less fat, eat less sugar, eat less salt and eat more dietary fibre.

The effect of this is to cut down on high-calorie fat and sugar, so if you adopt the new diet you are automatically reducing your calorie intake. By eating fibre-rich low calorie foods you will feel more full up, so your total food intake will be less than normal. You should be taking more exercise too, so this will help burn off a few more calories, and it will also help you set your basal metabolic rate a bit higher, to burn calories off even faster.

So do not cut down on the total *amount* you eat, just alter the *types* of food you eat. This way you can control your weight readily without bothering to count calories. If your scales tell you that your weight is creeping up, just cut down a little more on the fats and sugars.

Don't expect any single part of this advice to change your life, for token efforts here and there will not suffice. It is what you eat day after day, week after week, year after year that is important - the adage 'You are what you eat' is not an old wives' tale. Your body can cope with the occasional bout of over-indulgence so long as you redress the balance by cutting down at other times. Moderation, balance and variety in your eating habits are what matter. When you eat, you are eating for life - literally.

HEALTHY AND HAPPY

Well-being demands not only a sensible approach to the physical aspects of life· - diet, exercise, sex - but also finding satisfactory ways of coping psychologically with the stresses and strains of life.

Stress is a word that is used widely and rather loosely. We need to distinguish between events in our lives which may stress us and our reactions to those events. These will be referred to here as stress and strain respectively. The same event may cause a severe strain or be enjoyed as an interesting experience, according to how we deal with it. As individuals, men differ in the way they deal with stress; the things that one man finds easy to cope with may put another under strain. Our abilities and propensities to deal with stress are not, however, fixed. By studying ourselves and the way stress affects us, we can find ways of dealing with it more effectively and increasing our enjoyment of life.

THE STRESSES OF LIFE

Two psychological concepts are helpful in thinking about stress. These are the need to maintain an optimum level of arousal and the need to cope successfully with loss.

Arousal   We need change and stimulation in order to remain healthy. Experiments on sensory deprivation, when men have been kept in darkened rooms or suspended in tanks of warm water, have shown that they become confused and disoriented, eventually beginning to have hallucinations and delusions. On a more everyday level, we are all familiar with the lethargy that comes with boredom and little activity. Conversely, if we are over-stimulated, over-stretched and too many demands are made upon us, we function less well and are 'distressed'. Either situation, if it persists, can lead to physical, psychological or social malfunction. To function adequately men need to have an optimum level of stimulation and of demands placed upon them. If too little is demanded, boredom, lethargy and depression follow. If too much, anxiety, physical and mental illness and eventually breakdown will occur. What the optimum level is not only varies from individual to individual, but will also vary in the same individual at different times.

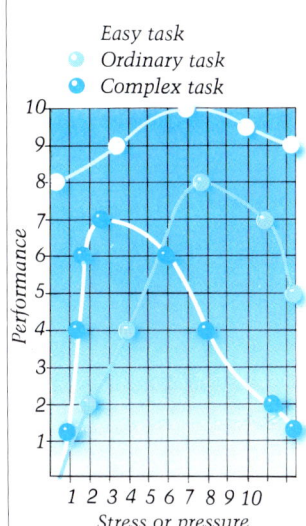

Easy task
Ordinary task
Complex task

Yerkes-Dodson curve alters according to the type of task but in each case stress initially stimulates performance, but if the stress increases, performance begins to drop. During an easy task the stress has little effect on performance. An ordinary task shows the classic curve, but the performance of a complex task is greatly increased by stress at first, but efficiency drops off more rapidly.

This cycle does not merely apply to well-being; our performance is affected in a similar way. Thus, if you are working extremely hard you may *feel* that you are being very virtuous and achieving more than everyone else, but you may not in fact be *doing* so.

Each of us has his own arousal-performance curve, which is sometimes referred to as the 'Yerkes-Dodson' curve. Although arousal is a psychological concept and does not necessarily refer to anything physical, it is probably closely associated with the degree of activity in certain parts of the brain. Up to a certain point, as arousal increases so performance improves. Beyond that point, however, a further increase in arousal leads not to an increase in performance but to a decrease. Not only does performance then become less efficient, it may disintegrate completely. It is not hard to think of everyday instances of this: it is good to be keyed up for an interview, an examination or a sporting competition, for example. If we are too relaxed, the motivation to perform well is lacking, and we miss that extra 'edge' that gives us an advantage, or we make silly mistakes through over-confidence. However, if we are too nervous, we stumble and fail to think clearly, often making errors of judgement and failing to perform as well as we can.

If we are carrying out tedious or repetitive tasks, checking figures, driving on the motorway, working in a factory assembly line or monitoring equipment, for example, we may find our arousal level falling too low. Listening to the radio, moving to a different environment or taking a stimulant such as coffee are actions that we often use to keep our minds functioning effectively while we complete a boring job. On the other hand, if an activity generates a lot of arousal, the reverse is necessary; we should make a deliberate attempt to relax and so reduce our level of arousal. Difficult interviews, conflicts at work or at home, or driving in heavy traffic are circumstances when this often applies.

Arousal is determined partly by external events - the amount and complexity of stimulation coming in from around you - but is also modified by the way you respond to events. There are techniques that can be used as filters to reduce the arousal produced by external events, and other ways in which arousal can be increased at will. Some of these will be discussed later in this chapter.

Loss   Our self-confidence, our security and the satisfaction we get from life depend on a whole range of things outside us. Our relatives, our friends, our job and our possessions give us pleasure and contribute to our image of what we are.

Much psychological stress comes from adjusting to the loss of these things, whether it is a small possession, such as a wallet or a watch, or a major loss such as the death of a parent or spouse. Disappointment, which is the loss of something hoped for, is another common stress. The anger and sorrow associated with such losses are an inevitable part of life, but our attitude to these losses can help us deal with them or allow them to overwhelm us.

St Ignatius advised that we should 'not prefer health to sickness, riches to poverty, honour to dishonour, a long life to a short one'. Such equanimity is a goal few of us are likely to achieve, but having a balanced view of life and a positive view of ourselves will help us to cope with such losses more effectively.

TYPES OF STRESSOR

Anything that happens to a man can act as a stress, although some experiences are usually stressful while others are rarely so. Stress can arise in any area of life - at work, in family relationships, financial affairs, sexual relationships or in one's relationship with oneself.

Work In a period of social and technological change, some men find themselves under pressure because of the great demands of their jobs; others suffer equally because there is no longer a need for their skills. His work role, be it manual or mental, as a boss or a worker, is central to a man's identity and self-confidence. Men have been brought up to think of themselves as the breadwinner, and to expect that their principal activity and satisfaction will come from their job, whereas women have been conditioned to get their major satisfaction from running the home and caring for children. Men have not been led to see that as their role, although an increasing number are taking on all or part of this work, and doing so very successfully.

Because of the emphasis that tends to be placed on the man as a worker, men often find unemployment difficult to cope with. Time hangs heavily on their hands, and they become bored and lacking in energy. This lack of mental stimulation and social contact predisposes them to depression. As well as the loss of purposeful activity that employment can bring, the lack of a job produces a fall in self-esteem. Even though it may be clear that unemployment is not due to individual inadequacy but to social factors

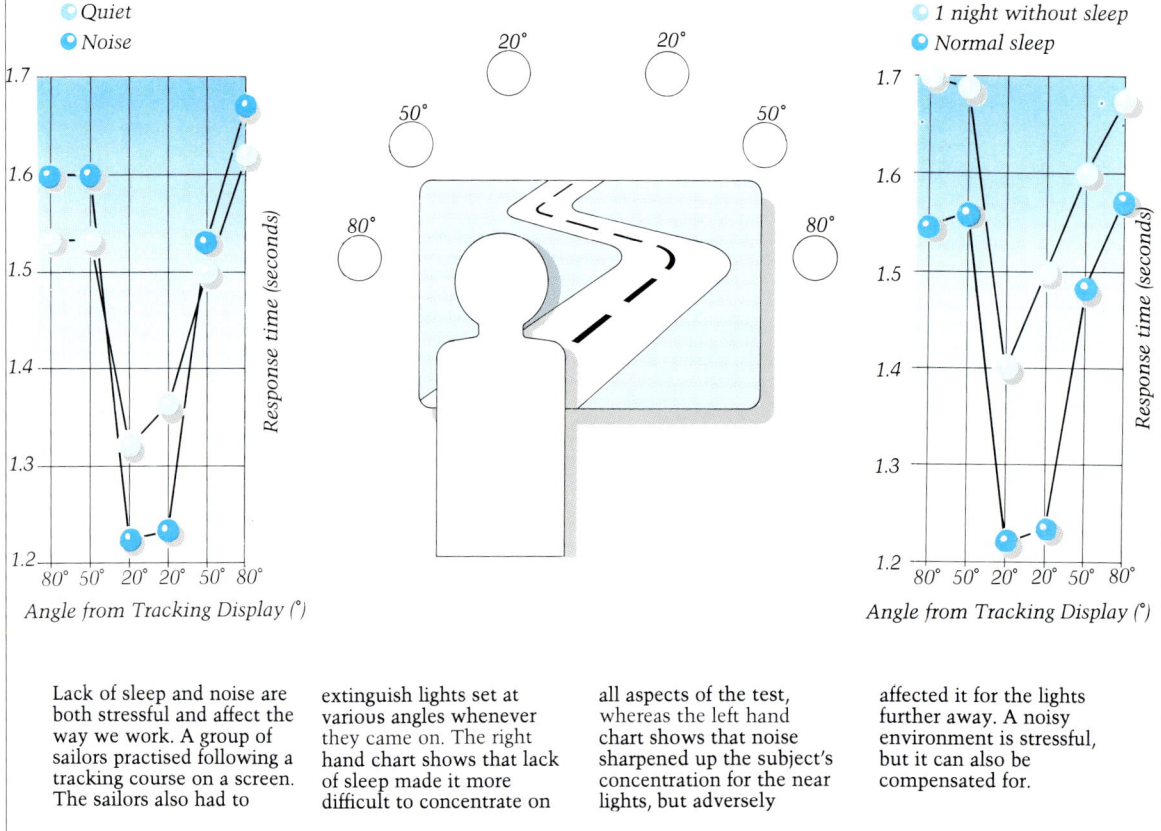

Lack of sleep and noise are both stressful and affect the way we work. A group of sailors practised following a tracking course on a screen. The sailors also had to extinguish lights set at various angles whenever they came on. The right hand chart shows that lack of sleep made it more difficult to concentrate on all aspects of the test, whereas the left hand chart shows that noise sharpened up the subject's concentration for the near lights, but adversely affected it for the lights further away. A noisy environment is stressful, but it can also be compensated for.

(such as when the major employer in an area closes), a man's role as a worker is so central to his self-image that it is difficult for most men to remain happy without this and depression frequently creeps in. The financial difficulties associated with unemployment, of course, often add to the problem, while unemployment that results from illness also frequently causes depression and hopelessness.

Relationship stresses   The second major cause of stress in most men's lives is their personal relationships. The first important relationship a man has is usually with his parents. As he grows up and leaves home the nature of this relationship changes. Young men frequently have conflicts with parents over choice of job, sexual partner or sexual orientation, sometimes even after they have achieved adulthood and left home. The struggle to sustain a good relationship while maintaining a degree of autonomy can be a difficult one later in life; as parents become older and frail, the stress becomes that of being the supporter in financial and/or psychological terms, and this often happens at a time when a man has many other responsibilities as well.

The stress generated by sexual relationships within and outside marriage is endlessly talked about and provides the principal theme of most European literature. The anxiety generated by 'does she/he love me?' or 'she/he does love me but I don't reciprocate', and the conflict of 'which shall I choose?' is well documented. Less widely discussed are the social pressures that are put on a man to succeed in this as in other areas, and the strains such pressures produce. Even more than being a success at work, men are supposed to be great lovers. These expectations come in different ways from both men and women. By his peers a man is expected to be able to have a girl, or, if he is gay, a boy, to show off. The ability to attract girls is part of the demands of a macho image. Once he has achieved a sexual relationship, the pressures from women, while not the same, are equal. A man is expected to give sexual satisfaction, but also to be tender, loving and kind. The women's movement and the greater equality they have achieved have, in a way, increased the strain on men, for not only are women's expectations higher than they used to be, but men are being asked to behave in ways that are different from those they were brought up to expect. Women's attitudes and expectations differ, too, some wanting an old-fashioned 'gentleman', others wanting to be treated as equals. In times of social change even addressing an envelope becomes a dilemma!

Although most men find fatherhood a pleasure, it brings about a major change in the relationship with their partner. Formerly, they were two people relating to each other; now there is a third, taking much of the attention that was formerly theirs, and disturbing sleep and sexual relationships. Not surprisingly, many men feel that their noses have been put out of joint, a feeling that is not helped by the fact that the happy father is not allowed to express this jealousy. This may need recognizing by both partners if it is to be successfully dealt with.

Sexuality can create stress in many other ways - coming out as gay, experiencing problems with sexual performance and dealing with infertility are just some examples. Many of these will be discussed in subsequent chapters.

Life event stress   We tend to think of stress in terms of unpleasant events, but it seems that change *per se*, whether it is in the long term for the better,

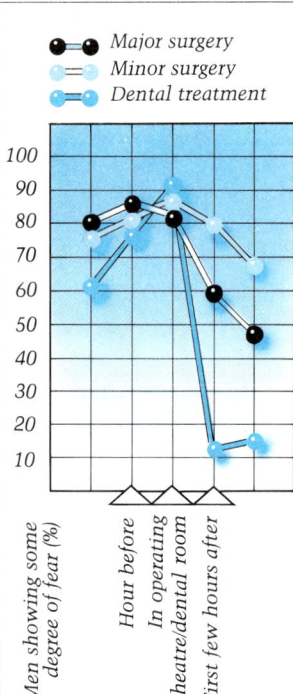

Major surgery
Minor surgery
Dental treatment

100
90
80
70
60
50
40
30
20
10

Men showing some
degree of fear (%)

Hour before

In operating
theatre/dental room

First few hours after

Dental treatment causes
the maximum amount of
short-term stress, which
disperses the moment the
treatment is complete.
Minor surgery is highly
stressful in anticipation,
probably because the
procedures are usually
done under local
anaesthetic, but once the
treatment begins stress
lessens. Major surgery,
however, continues to
cause high levels of stress
even after the operation.

the worse or merely different, can be stressful. It has been shown that all major changes in life such as starting a new job, moving house, getting married or being bereaved are associated with an increased risk of both physical and mental illness.

The strain of such events can be minimized by forward planning. Try to avoid too many changes at once where possible; for example, it would be sensible not to get married, change your job and move house all at the same time. Some changes can be planned for; many men now go on pre-retirement courses to help them cope successfully with that change, for instance. Ensuring that you are well rested and relaxed prior to a major upheaval such as moving or changing jobs will make the change easier.

Bereavement and loss   Perhaps one of the greatest stressors is the death of a parent, a partner or close relative or friend. The death of a parent is a common but particularly stressful event, since it is the loss of something that one has never before been without, even if the relationship has not always been close or amicable. At the other extreme, the loss of a son or daughter, whether as a child or as an adult, often causes profound distress. Bereavement (and other losses) are dealt with psychologically in three stages.

The first response is numbness. The truth of what has happened cannot be accepted: the bereaved person may not be able to grasp that the loved one is really dead and constantly thinks that it must be a mistake. Or, although it may be accepted apparently calmly and reasonably, the person may feel nothing at all. This accounts for the self-possession and apparent indifference often exhibited by close relatives at funerals.

The second stage is one of realization and grief. This is a very emotional period, full of strong feelings and confusing ideas. Men often feel guilty at this time; they believe that they have failed to do something for the departed or that they did not say what they should have said. Conversely, they often blame others and become angry with doctors, nurses or others involved in the caring in the final illness, particularly if, as may be the case, care has not been 100 per cent perfect. The minor errors or omissions of human frailty may assume great importance during this period.

Because of the taboo against men expressing their grief by crying in public and their conditioning to respond with aggression, this sort of anger is particularly likely in bereaved men, although individual differences in personality are probably more important. This stage is particularly difficult for men who have been taught since early childhood that 'big boys don't cry'. Although one might not wish to see men (or women for that matter) bursting into tears at every minor loss or frustration, as children of both sexes do, crying is a natural expression of human emotion, and it is a right and appropriate way to deal with the emotions at times such as a major bereavement. Men are embarrassed and disconcerted by tears in themselves and in others, and they try to hide them or bottle them up. In fact, if you feel like crying then there is usually a good reason for it, and the best way to deal with it is to let it happen until you feel like stopping. Then dry your eyes, wash your face and carry on.

If a man or woman cries in your presence, above all don't be embarrassed and don't try to stop them or run away; make yourself useful and find a handkerchief; sit quietly and let it take its course. A gentle hand on the shoulder is often appreciated and will not be thought of as an

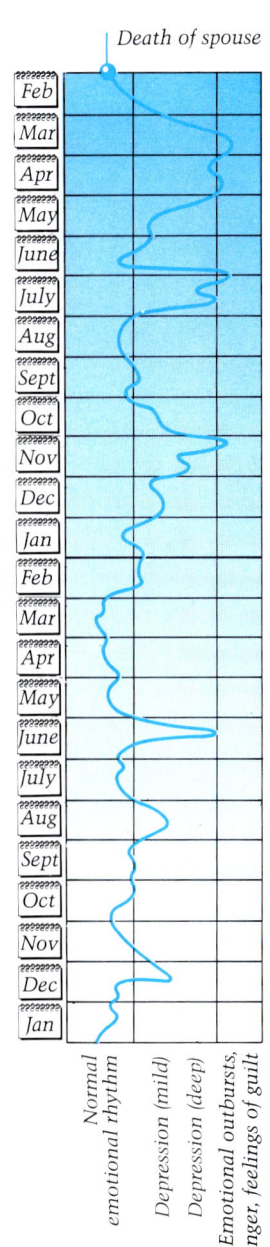

Death of spouse

Normal emotional rhythm — Depression (mild) — Depression (deep) — Emotional outbursts, anger, feelings of guilt

Bereavement is followed by at least two years of grief before a normal emotional rhythm is established again.

intrusion.

The third stage of bereavement is acceptance of loss and reconstruction of life without the person who has died. The negative emotion passes and the enjoyment of life again becomes possible. Although usefully thought of as three different stages, these responses do not necessarily follow one after the other in clearly separated shapes. Men frequently appear to have accepted their loss, but then may go back to a period of anger or grief. The whole process takes much longer than is usually expected in our society, which tries to ignore death. For someone not very close the emotion, though real, may be quite short lived; for a close relative or friend two years or more is not uncommon.

Anniversaries, both of the death itself and of events such as birthdays and wedding anniversaries that would have been celebrated if the person had lived, are often particularly difficult times. They can be easier to cope with if a definite act of memorial is planned - a visit to the grave or to a favourite spot - rather than by trying to ignore them.

Although death is the most obvious way in which a person can be bereaved, the effect of other major losses by separation or the break-up of a relationship or a marriage is very similar. The same stages of numbness, grieving, guilt and anger, and resignation may occur, and in the same way these emotions are part of the re-adjustment process and cannot be avoided.

Facing death   Perhaps the most difficult stress that most of us face is the knowledge of our own imminent death. Whatever we believe about life beyond death, the recognition that we are dying is hard to face. The same resources that enable men to live successfully - a positive image of themselves, the ability to face anxiety and depression without being absorbed by it, and to cope with feelings without being overwhelmed by them - help them to die well too.

Minor stressors   So far we have considered the major stresses of life in work, personal and social life. Much of the avoidable stress and strain occurs not because of major events, however, but because of the minor irritations of everyday life. Each of us has our own list of these, but common ones are losing small but vital objects such as keys and cheque books; struggling to remember everyday jobs; and being constantly interrupted by the telephone or callers while trying to get on with a job. Transport provides a whole set of minor irritations, which cause many men enormous strain; getting stuck in traffic jams, and the irrational and selfish behaviour of every other driver on the road plague those who travel by car. The delays and impatience felt while waiting for buses and trains affect those who use public transport. For everyone, the pressure of being late causes stress.

Other people's irritating habits or incompetence can cause strain out of all proportion to their importance and raise your general level of arousal. Telephonists who make wrong connections, waiters who get the order wrong and shopkeepers who are surly or unhelpful are examples of situations in which, while a complaint might be justifiable, the anger and heat (and therefore the strain) generated are out of all proportion to their importance. Other strains are totally irrational: the colleague whose accent, whistling or way of answering the phone irritates beyond endurance, is an example of this.

STRAIN – NOT COPING WITH STRESS

The effects of stress may be mainly physical, mainly psychological, or a combination of both. The exact pattern of response will vary from individual to individual; from time to time certain common patterns of strain, however, occur and can be recognized.

Flight or fight? The body's response to an acutely stressful situation is often referred to as the 'flight or fight' response. Various changes, transmitted through the sympathetic nervous system, prepare the body for 'instant action'.

•**Sympathetic system build-up**
Pupils, bronchi and blood vessels to muscles dilate
Heart races
Bladder relaxes
Digestion is inhibited

•**Parasympathetic system cool-down**
Pupils and bronchi constrict
Heart beat slows
Bladder contracts
Digestion normal

Flight or fight? Our bodies and intuitive psychological responses developed for life in a very different world from that in which we live. For all but the last few thousand of the million or so years man has lived on earth, man developed as a hunter/gatherer in an environment where the appropriate response to most types of threat was physical. This environment has determined our nervous systems (and our digestions!)

The body's response to an acutely stressful situation is often referred to as the 'flight or fight' response. A set of nerves, known as the sympathetic nervous system, increases its activity, leading to various changes that prepare the body for 'instant action'. The heart beats more rapidly and also more forcefully; blood is directed away from the digestive system and kidneys towards muscles; muscles become tense; and the rate and depth of breathing increases. These changes prepare the muscles for rapid movement towards, or away from, the threat by providing the oxygen and the fuel, carried by the blood stream, needed for exertion.

Other changes also occur. The pupils dilate so that vision is improved. Sweating increases, partly no doubt to prepare to lose heat by vigorous exertion, and perhaps also because being sweaty and slippery is useful in a fight. Sympathetic nerves work by releasing chemical messengers, adrenalin and noradrenalin. In situations of acute stress these substances are also released into the blood stream by glands near the kidneys - the adrenal glands - so that their effects may be felt throughout the body. Mental alertness also increases.

These responses, while useful in the environment in which they developed, are of little value in today's world. Few of our challenges are best met by running away and even fewer by physical violence. Instead they require considered responses involving little physical exertion but much thought. The anticipated effort is never made, and the physical changes made in preparation for it instead lead to distress and illness.

Anxiety Many of the symptoms of anxiety can be regarded as the inappropriate functioning of the 'flight or fight' response. The acute experience of a churning stomach and racing pulse are familiar to most people who have had a near miss or car accident or have made a potentially serious mistake. If the feelings are only transient, they are of little significance. Sometimes, however, these physical responses get out of hand. They may be interpreted not as normal physical reactions but as symptoms of a serious illness, or they may act in other ways to increase fear. This in turn makes the physical responses increase, leading to a vicious circle or 'positive feedback loop'. If this happens quickly a 'panic attack' may occur. In particular, if the increase in rate and depth of breathing is not accompanied by vigorous exercise, it may lead to a variety of frightening physical symptoms - tingling in the fingers, pounding of the heart, thumping in the head and a tightness in the chest. Even spasms of the fingers may occur. Those experiencing these symptoms and those observing them often fear a life-threatening attack is taking place, thus increasing everyone's anxiety.

More often, however, strain manifests itself as a chronic state of over-arousal. The symptoms are similar to those of a 'flight or fight' response, but rather than being short lived they become a way of life. We all recognize the state of being jumpy, responding too quickly and without thought to stimuli and talking too much and too rapidly. Muscular tension is a common feature of such chronic over-arousal and can lead to headaches - indeed it is their commonest cause - and to neck and back pain. It can also cause a general feeling of exhaustion. If you are continually over-aroused, it is often difficult to rest in spite of being tired. The brain has difficulty in 'switching off', and sleep is slow to come or is broken and fitful. This exacerbates tiredness and worsens the situation.

Coronary prone behaviour   The type of response to stress that includes being hostile, having a feeling of being pressed for time and talking very rapidly with many violent gestures is known as 'type A' behaviour. 'type B' responses, on the other hand, are placid, unconcerned with time and altogether more sedate. It has been shown that people who display a lot of 'type A' behaviour in a given situation are more prone to heart attacks than those who deal with stress in a 'type B' way.

Depression   The second major psychological response associated with stress is depression. Whereas anxiety is often associated with uncertainty or with the anticipation of problems, depression more commonly occurs when there is loss or failure. However, both anxiety and depression can occur in the same situation, and men often suffer from a mixture of the two, particularly in their milder forms. Often depression is easily recognized: you feel miserable, everything seems to be too much trouble and nothing seems worthwhile. You feel a failure.

Sometimes, however, a man can be depressed without recognizing it. He may feel tired all the time, yet sleep badly and wake up feeling awful early in the morning. He may lose his appetite or he may be unable to stop eating. Constipation is a feature of severe depression. Many men think they are physically ill, when in fact they are depressed. Conversely, physical illness or tiredness can make you feel depressed. Depression is particularly common after viral illnesses such as influenza, glandular fever or hepatitis.

Almost everyone suffers from 'black days' when everything goes badly and life seems a fairly pointless exercise, and these mild degrees of 'fed-upness' and even short periods of really quite severe depression are fairly common experiences, frequently passing without any specific therapy. But it is always worthwhile looking for the cause of your depression and trying, if possible, to change that aspect of your life, whether it is physical, psychological or social. This can help to prevent the problem recurring. If depression becomes established then it can become self-perpetuating. When this happens, physical or psychological treatment may be needed to break the circle and to allow mental life to resume as normal. One of the problems with depression is that the condition itself makes any action, including that of seeking help, difficult. Men suffering from depression believe that they are worthless and not worth helping, or they cannot be bothered to look for support. This feeling, allied to the conditioned male fear of being seen not to be coping and the general stigma attached to any form of mental illness, leads to much unnecessary suffering.

DEPRESSION

Depression is an extremely variable condition. It can range from a slight downheartedness to abject despair, and from a simple change of mood to a syndrome affecting the whole body.

Psychiatrists have argued for decades about the various types of depression. Some say that its intensity and form simply depend on the personality of the sufferer and the circumstances prevailing at the time. But most regard depression as falling into two main types:
- Reactive depression — much the commonest, a reaction to adverse events or conditions. This is the type linked to stress.
- Endogenous depression — literally 'coming from within'. No apparent external trigger, but often a metabolic, hormonal or chemical cause.

REACTIVE DEPRESSION

- Accounts for about 8 out of 10 cases of depression
- Usually less severe
- Sometimes called 'neurotic depression' or 'anxiety depression'
- Often set off by the loss of someone or something loved or cherished
- Linked to stress
- Commoner in those with obsessive-compulsive personalities
- Focuses overwhelmingly on causative factor
- Self-esteem usually retained
- Family and friends usually supportive

ENDOGENOUS DEPRESSION

- Usually no triggering loss or disaster
- Cause is often biochemical, 'coming from within'
- Especially common after accidents, infections, surgery, certain medications
- Sometimes alternates with periods of mania (manic depression)
- More likely in older men
- Family and friends less supportive

SYMPTOMS

- Sadness, worsening as day wears on
- Sleep disturbance: difficulty getting to sleep, restlessness
- Appetite disturbance: over-indulgence
- Loss of libido
- Agitation and anxiety
- Increased tendency to cry

TREATMENT

Kindness, understanding and wise counsel
- Distraction from morbid obsession
- May require minor tranquillizer for anxiety element
- Antidepressant drugs and electroconvulsive therapy (ECT) usually ineffective

SYMPTOMS

Sadness, worse in mornings, improving throughout the day.
- Increased tendency to cry
- Sleep disturbance: early morning waking
- Loss of appetite
- Loss of libido
- Slowness of thought. Poor memory. Lack of concentration
- Inability to make decisions
- Loss of confidence. Self neglect
- Guilt complex
- Tiredness
- Irritability
- Hopelessness
- Morbid fears
- Delusions
- Suicidal thoughts

TREATMENT

- Usually not helped by counselling.
- But usually responds well to antidepressant drugs and ECT.
- May also be helped by vigorous exercise.

Psychosomatic or stress related illnesses   Several other physical illnesses may be caused by, or exacerbated by, stress. Indigestion may be a symptom of stress, and some, although not all, forms of stomach ulcer may be partly caused by stress. Eczema, asthma, psoriasis, and migraine are just some of the more common diseases in which stress has been thought to play a part. The mechanism involved is unclear, and in each case stress is only part (possibly a small part) of the cause. If, however, you have one of these illnesses, it may be worth considering whether it is worsened by stress and to see if you can improve it by attempting to change your response to the stress, using one of the methods discussed in the following section. If, however, you can't see the link, don't worry; for many people it is minimal or unclear.

When it is suggested that an illness may be wholly or partly caused by the psychological factors, many men think that this means that 'it's all in the mind', and that they are making a fuss or imagining the symptoms. This is totally false. Symptoms caused by psychological distress are every bit as real as those caused by physical injury. The brain is, after all, the organ that feels pain, whether the pain is caused by a broken leg or a broken love affair, and both are equally real and equally worth taking seriously.

Depression, anxiety and physical illness are described separately as effects of stress. In reality, however, few men have just one or the other. Most experience a combination of these effects and exhibit features together or alternately, perhaps with headaches and other physical symptoms as well.

Acute psychotic breakdown   One of the most extreme responses to stress is the acute psychotic breakdown, in which an individual's mental functioning breaks down completely, and he loses touch with a painful reality. Bizarre, grandiose or paranoid ideas are expressed, and speech becomes disorganized and difficult to understand. He may be immobile and unresponsive (catatonia) and/or have furious violent outbursts. In Western countries such psychotic breakdowns most often occur in a comparatively small number of psychologically vulnerable people, who unfortunately often suffer repeated episodes not necessarily triggered by extreme stress. However, in many cultures such a breakdown is a not uncommon response to a major life stress, and does not imply particular vulnerability.

Phobias   Many men have disabling fears or phobias of some sort, although most prefer not to admit to them since they do not fit in with the image they project to the world at large. For most men, these phobias are comparatively trivial, causing only a minor inconvenience. For some, however, they can become major obstacles to happy and successful living. Common phobias are those of height, enclosed spaces, crowds, spiders, snakes and thunderstorms, but any object or experience can be the focus for irrational fears.

Psychologists believe that phobias arise through a process of conditioning. A man learns to associate fear with a certain situation, either because he has had a traumatic experience of being extremely frightened in that situation, or because he has learnt from others that the situation is frightening. Some stimuli are more likely to become frightening than others - snakes and spiders, for example, present biological dangers. Once such a fear is established, approaching the situation or even thinking about

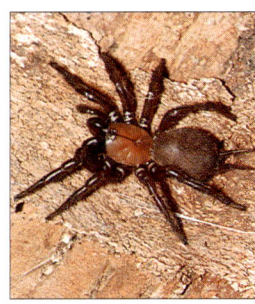

Phobias do not need to be treated with drugs. In the vast majority of cases a person can overcome a phobia using simple, behavioural psychotherapeutic treatment alone. Cures can be achieved in less than five hours and may last a lifetime. The patient is gradually given increasing degrees of exposure to the subject of his phobia. In this instance it is a spider. The patient may be asked to watch the spider in a bottle, then to hold the bottle. Eventually the patient will be able to hold the spider. This exposure treatment can be applied to other phobias such as flying or crowds. By facing the problem in a controlled situation the patient can overcome it.

it provokes an anxiety that is reduced by avoiding the object or situation concerned. This avoidance perpetuates the fear. Many phobias can be overcome by breaking this avoidance cycle, which is usually achieved in one of two ways. The first is to work through a series of progressively more frightening situations, so that the fear felt at each stage may be overcome by relaxation or other methods; this is known as systematic desensitization. Alternatively, the person is put suddenly into the feared situation and given no possibility of avoidance until the fear diminishes; this method is known as flooding.

COPING WITH STRESS

Many of the ways men have of coping with stress, though they make things seem better temporarily, are harmful in the long run. Smoking tobacco or drinking too much alcohol may be used as a means of overcoming stress. Food is another powerful comforter, and many men will eat a chocolate bar or a sandwich for this reason.

Aggression is a typically male way of coping with stress. Although expressing yourself forcefully can sometimes both help the situation and make you feel better, it can be destructive. Coping with stress successfully does not mean being a wimp, but physical violence is rarely helpful, and even verbal aggression is better used sparingly as a deliberate way of influencing a situation, rather than just a way of blowing off steam. Far better than the negative, or 'maladaptive', strategies outlined above are 'adaptive' methods of coping.

Self-awareness and self-analysis   The first stage in coping with stress more effectively is to understand how you function, how things go wrong and why. Are you prone to anxiety, to depression or to irrational fears? Is it at work or at home that things are likely to get you 'uptight'? Are you having difficulties with the major crises of life, or do you cope with these effortlessly and then lose your temper because there is no sugar in your tea? Sitting down and thinking about your reactions to a variety of situations may reveal that you know a lot about yourself already. If, each time you get anxious, angry or depressed, you analyse the cause and try afterwards to think why you felt as you did, you will learn a lot more.

When the stresses and strains that you experience have been identified, your next step is to find a suitable way of dealing with them. Two strategies are possible: either try to control the things that happen to you so that stress is reduced, or change your own reactions to the stress so that you experience less strain.

Organizational approaches to stress   You may find that many stresses can be 'organized out' of your life by setting up systems to prevent them. If you are always losing your car keys, install a hook near the door and get into the habit of putting them on it as you come in. If you can never find the papers you want, try replacing your open brief case with a portable file box or compartmentalized bag. Keeping up-to-date address books and books of telephone numbers can save time and reduce stress. Appointment books and lists of tasks can reduce the stress of trying to remember what you are supposed to be doing. If you have a job to do for which you need to be undisturbed then move out of the office where you are constantly interrupted and find a quiet corner to get on with it.

Organizing your life on a more major scale is also important if you want to avoid stress. Many men find themselves pressurized into doing too much. If you are successful, you are probably flattered to be asked to do things; if you are not, the fear of failure and even redundancy may spur you on. Often you are made to feel you are not a proper man if you cannot cope. Male competitiveness, therefore, may lead you to overdo things, particularly if you have a job with no fixed hours and flexible duties. It is important that you set limits to what you are able and prepared to do, and you must learn to say 'no' to requests, no matter how flattering or attractive they may be, that push you beyond those limits. Even if your hours of work are fixed, you may be forced against your will to work overtime, a combination of the attractions of the money and the fear of the consequences of saying no leading to overwork and exhaustion.

Precisely the same problems can arise outside your work - in clubs, voluntary organizations and even among your friends and relatives. Of course, being involved in the community can be enjoyable and useful, but you must ensure that it does not become a burden instead of a pleasure, otherwise illness and 'burn-out' can easily follow.

Conversely, however, a life that does not have enough variety is inflexible when things change. The most usual example of this is the man whose only real interest is work, who loses his job through redundancy, illness or retirement, and who finds he has no interests left. Active recreation is a useful part of life, and every man must learn what suits him, finding a balance to maintain an optimum level of functioning.

Holidays, evenings and weekends off need to be planned with this in mind. Such times provide a contrast to everyday life and should be spaced to provide a break when it is needed. Taking an annual holiday in the last week of July and the first week of August is rarely sufficient, and perhaps contributes to the high rates of absenteeism seen in men who are forced into this rigid routine.

It is important, too, for everyone to have some time to himself, which can be difficult for a busy man with a job, a wife and a family. Much strain in retirement is caused by devoted couples who do not balance the time they spend together with their time apart. Even a single man may find it difficult to set aside times when he is alone because he is afraid that such times will become large gaps and lead to loneliness. Although working out how best to arrange these periods of solitude is a matter for the individual, they are a necessary part of healthy living.

Altering your response to stress   Some stresses are unavoidable, but it is possible to change your response to them. Carrying a novel to read while you are waiting for a train or listening to music while you are stuck in a traffic jam, can change a source of frustration into a welcome oasis in the day. Even if you are unavoidably held up and cannot use the time usefully, no purpose is served by becoming agitated, which will only make things worse. Relaxation exercises or a 'spot check' technique can help you to stop getting tense.

Relaxation — spot checks   The 'red spot' technique is a simple, but effective, way of monitoring and optimizing your arousal level through the

Continued on page 98

STRESS

Anything that happens to a man can act as a stress, although some experiences are usually stressful while others are rarely so. Stress can arise in any area of life - at work, in family relationships, financial affairs, sexual relationships or in one's relationship with oneself.

Work   Too much work, long hours and overtime, whether compulsory or voluntary, can lead to exhaustion, both physical and mental. Fear of failure drives men to strive for goals, deadlines or targets, so adding more pressure. In a time of economic recession particularly, companies demand more of their employees, and employees know that failure to reach required standards may jeopardize promotion prospects or even continued employment. Inter-personal conflicts at work can be as stressful as those at home.

Repetitive work can become dull and boring, and the most interesting job can, at times, become dull through habit. A certain amount of change - in the work itself or in our attitudes to it - is essential if it is to remain interesting. Again the arousal-performance curve holds, and the correct balance between too much change and too little novelty needs to be sought.

If you experience emotions that you do not understand, you may find it helpful to keep a diary in which you note where you were and what you were doing before, during and after the unwanted feeling of stress occurs; it is also useful to record who was around at the time. Often writing down the details of these occasions allows a pattern to emerge, and once you are able to identify the problem, you are halfway to solving it.

Fear of failure drives men to strive for goals, deadlines and targets and adds to pressure and stress. The man who filled in this questionnaire is a Type A personality and is heading for trouble. Type As are three times more likely to suffer from coronary heart disease. They react to stress with hostility and always feel pressed for time. Type Bs, on the other hand, are placid and more sedate. If you think you may be a Type A, try to modify your behaviour in some aspects to be more like a Type B.

TYPE A	TYPE B
☑ *Are you always punctual?*	☐ *Are you casual about appointments?*
☑ *Are you very competitive?*	☐ *Are you non-competitive?*
☐ *Do you often interrupt?*	☐ *Are you a good listener?*
☑ *Are you always rushed?*	☑ *Are you seldom rushed?*
☑ *Are you impatient?*	☐ *Do you wait patiently?*
☐ *Do you tend to hide your feelings?*	☑ *Do you say what you feel?*
☑ *Do you try to do lots of things at once?*	☐ *Do you take one thing at a time?*
☑ *Are you hard driving?*	☐ *Are you easy going?*

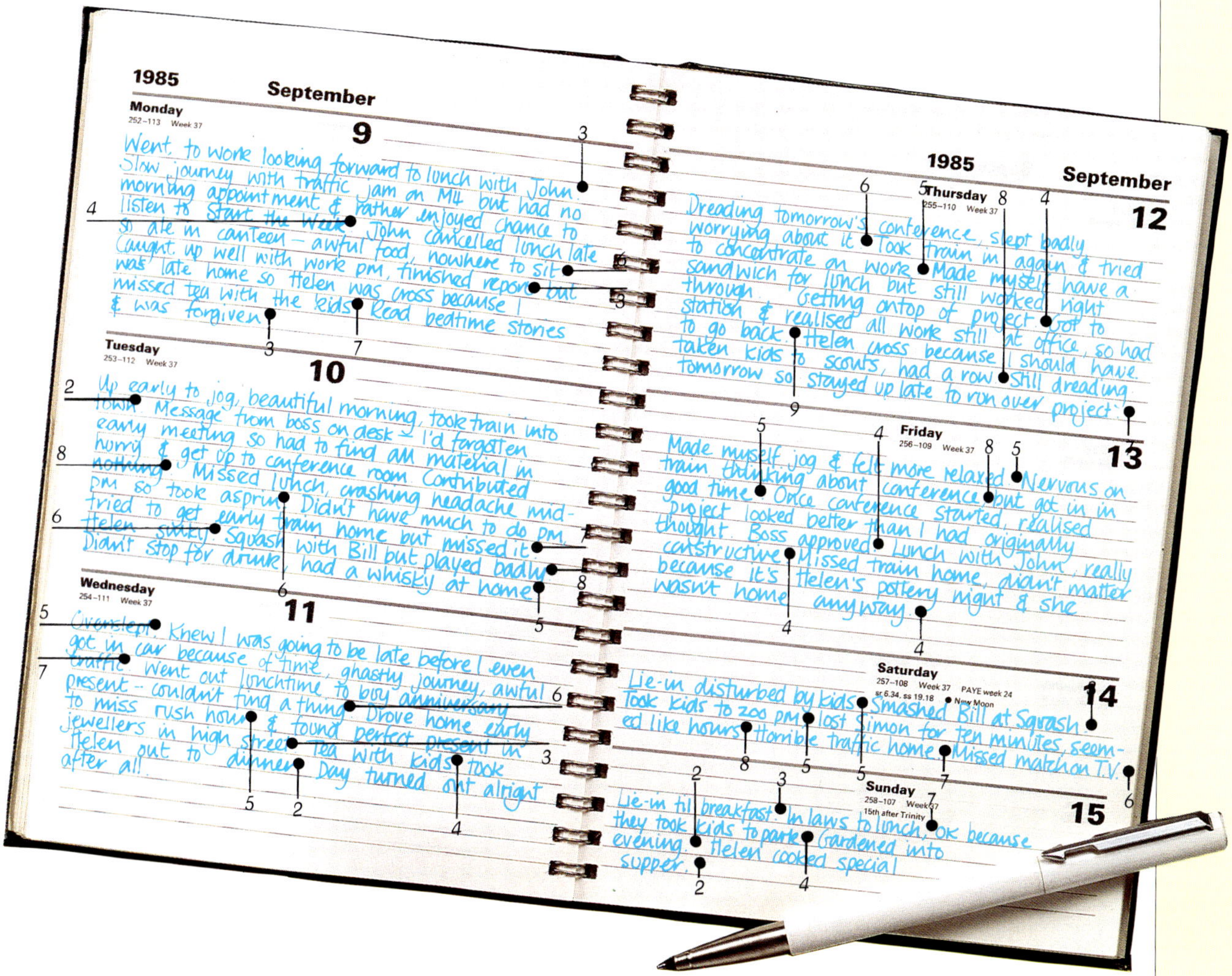

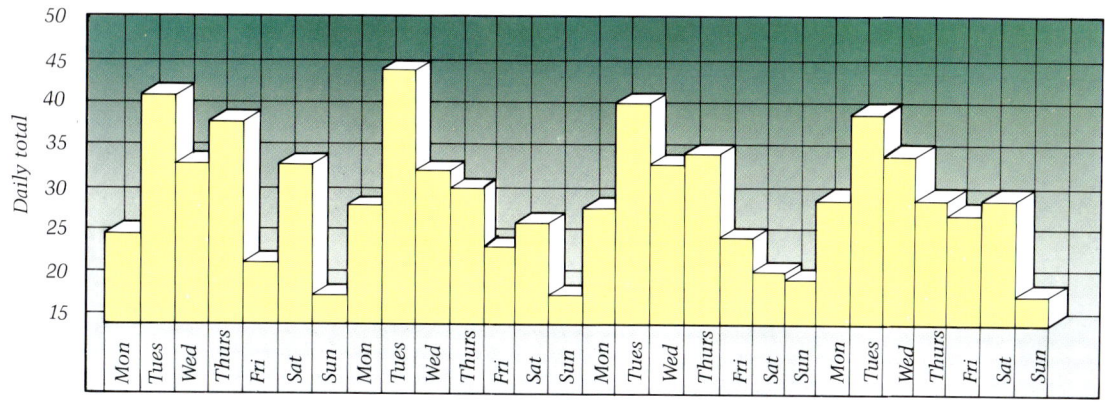

1985 September

Monday 9 — 252–113 Week 37

Went to work looking forward to lunch with John. Slow journey with traffic jam on M11 but had no morning appointment & rather enjoyed chance to listen to start the week. John cancelled lunch late so ate in canteen – awful food, nowhere to sit. Caught up well with work pm, finished report but was late home so Helen was cross because I missed tea with the kids. Read bedtime stories & was forgiven.

Tuesday 10 — 253–112 Week 37

Up early to jog, beautiful morning, took train into town. Message from boss on desk – I'd forgotten early meeting so had to find all material in hurry & get up to conference room. Contributed nothing. Missed lunch, crashing headache mid-pm so took aspirin. Didn't have much to do pm, tried to get early train home but missed it. Helen sulky. Squash with Bill but played badly. Didn't stop for drink, had a whisky at home.

Wednesday 11 — 254–111 Week 37

Overslept, knew I was going to be late before I even got in car because of time, ghastly journey, awful traffic. Went out lunchtime to buy anniversary present – couldn't find a thing. Drove home early to miss rush hour & found perfect present in jewellers in high street. Tea with kids, took Helen out to dinner. Day turned out alright after all.

1985 September

Thursday 12 — 255–110 Week 37

Dreading tomorrow's conference, slept badly worrying about it. Took train in again & tried to concentrate on work. Made myself have a sandwich for lunch but still worked right through. Getting ontop of project, got to station & realised all work still at office, so had to go back. Helen cross because I should have taken kids to scouts, had a row & still dreading tomorrow so stayed up late to run over project.

Friday 13 — 256–109 Week 37

Made myself jog & felt more relaxed. Nervous on train thinking about conference but got in in good time. Once conference started, realised project looked better than I had originally thought. Boss approved. Lunch with John, really constructive. Missed train home, didn't matter because it's Helen's pottery night & she wasn't home anyway.

Saturday 14 — 257–108 Week 37 PAYE week 24 sr 6.34. ss 19.18 New Moon

Lie-in disturbed by kids. Smashed Bill at squash. Took kids to zoo pm. Lost Simon for ten minutes, seemed like hours. Horrible traffic home. Missed match on T.V.

Sunday 15 — 258–107 Week 37 15th after Trinity

Lie-in til breakfast. In laws to lunch, took because they took kids to park. Gardened into evening. Helen cooked special supper.

Daily total (chart y-axis: 15, 20, 25, 30, 35, 40, 45, 50; x-axis: Mon, Tues, Wed, Thurs, Fri, Sat, Sun repeated)

It is not always simple to work out which parts of your life are the most stressful. An incident that is stressful under one set of circumstances (for instance, if it results in failure) may be stimulating under another (when the results are successful). Take a quiet ten minutes at the end of the day to make a note of your day, scoring each stress from 1 to 10. Over the space of a month you may find that stress peaks and causes typical symptoms on one particular day of the week. Here the cause is probably the Tuesday board meeting which makes the subject miss lunch and results in a cyclical stress headache.

RELAXATION

Probably the most valuable way of coping with stress is some form of relaxation training. This term is used here to cover a wide variety of techniques: progressive muscular relaxation, autogenic training or t'ai chi are all methods that emphasize the use of muscular relaxation or regular repetivie movement or breathing to achieve calm.

Various schools of meditation, such as transcendental or Buddhist meditation, emphasize mental techniques of obtaining stillness. In practice, all of these combine physical and mental quietening, and it is not possible to demonstrate clearly the superiority of one method over another. What they probably all have in common is that they are ways of decreasing the overall level of arousal and producing a calm but alert state. Some methods include other elements, such as autosuggestion or positive self-talk, and some are associated with a wider religious or philosophical belief system. The choice of technique is not crucial and is a matter for your individual preference. For those who wish to use it, a simple technique, free from any particular religious or philosophical assumptions, is

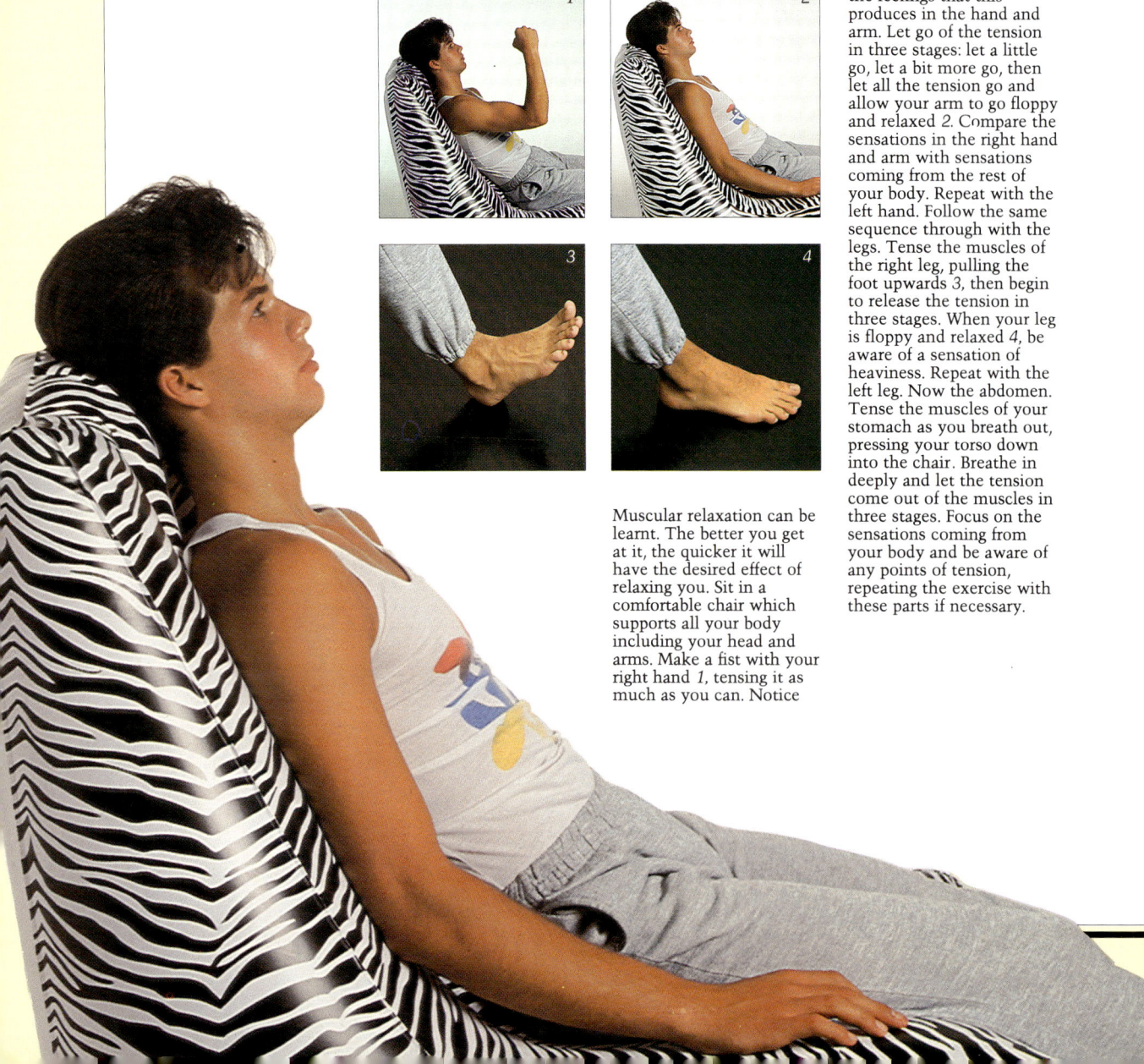

Muscular relaxation can be learnt. The better you get at it, the quicker it will have the desired effect of relaxing you. Sit in a comfortable chair which supports all your body including your head and arms. Make a fist with your right hand 1, tensing it as much as you can. Notice the feelings that this produces in the hand and arm. Let go of the tension in three stages: let a little go, let a bit more go, then let all the tension go and allow your arm to go floppy and relaxed 2. Compare the sensations in the right hand and arm with sensations coming from the rest of your body. Repeat with the left hand. Follow the same sequence through with the legs. Tense the muscles of the right leg, pulling the foot upwards 3, then begin to release the tension in three stages. When your leg is floppy and relaxed 4, be aware of a sensation of heaviness. Repeat with the left leg. Now the abdomen. Tense the muscles of your stomach as you breath out, pressing your torso down into the chair. Breathe in deeply and let the tension come out of the muscles in three stages. Focus on the sensations coming from your body and be aware of any points of tension, repeating the exercise with these parts if necessary.

shown on the opposite page below.

Many men say, 'I can't relax, I'm not that sort of person'. This is not true, however, for relaxation is not a personality trait but a skill like squash or golf or playing the piano. Of course, some people have more natural aptitude than others, but anyone can learn to relax given practice. Nevertheless, it does take time, and many men abandon the effort before they have practised for long enough to benefit. You wouldn't expect to enter the Open the day after you bought your first set of golf clubs; nor should you expect instant results from any system of relaxation. If you practise regularly for a few weeks, the benefits will accrue. At first you will find it difficult to relax at all, but after a few days you will begin to feel less tense at the end of your period of relaxation. However, the moment you encounter aggravation or frustration, you will feel 'uptight' and anxious again. Gradually, perhaps over months or even years, your relaxation will 'generalize', and you will be able to relax at will in any situation in which you begin to feel tense.

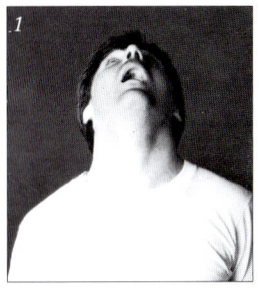
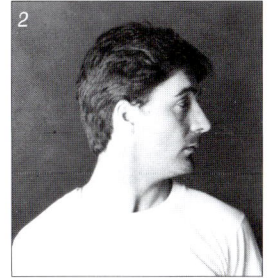
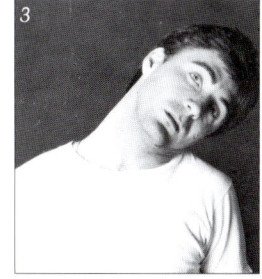
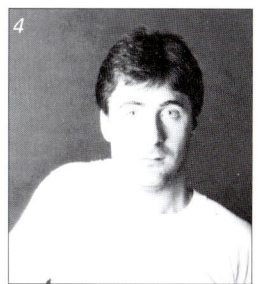

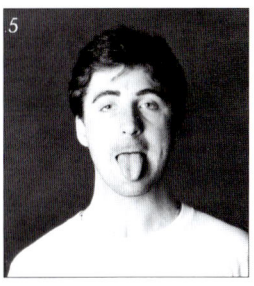
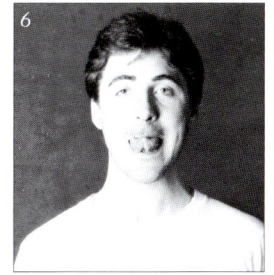
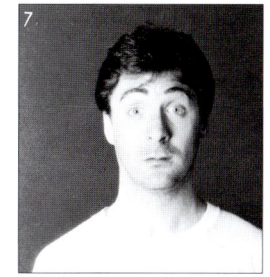
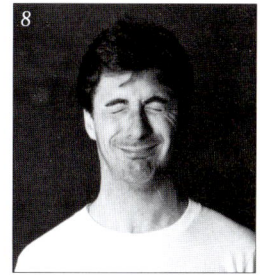

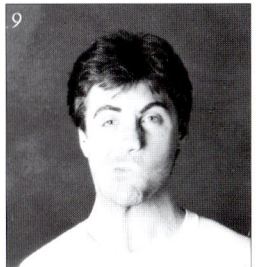

Relax the neck and shoulder muscles by hanging your head forwards then back *1*, letting your mouth drop open. Turn your head left, then right *2*. Face forward and let your head drop to the left shoulder, then the right *3*. Finally lift one shoulder, rotate forward then back *4*. Repeat with the other shoulder. Use the muscles of your face. Stick your tongue out towards your chin *5*, then force it up towards the tip of your nose *6*. Raise and lower your eyebrows *7*. Screw up your face *8* and stretch the skin *9*. Finally massage the skin with the palms of your hands, pushing the skin over the bone structure *10*.

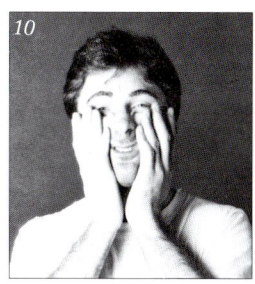

BREATHING

Breathing exercises are very relaxing. Adopt a comfortable position lying or sitting down. Place your hands on your rib cage and begin to breathe in within a count of 8 seconds. Feel your rib cage rise as the inhalation reaches every part of your chest. Start to exhale to count of 8 seconds, pushing the very last bit of air out of the lungs with a sigh. Rest fully exhaled for a couple of seconds, then begin the long, slow and deep inhalation again.

Continued from page 93 day. Buy some adhesive red dots and put them in all the places you are likely to look in tense moments. Your watch, the clock, the telephone and the car dashboard are the usual places, but you can put one anywhere. Then train yourself to do a 'spot check' every time you notice a red dot: check your arousal level - are you anxious or over-aroused? If you are, practise your relaxation method and take a few deliberate breaths, or relax a few muscle groups and use positive self-talk.

Move the red spots every week or so, otherwise you get used to them and stop noticing them. After a while, you can generalize your red dots as you wish. Traffic lights, the brake lights of the car in front or red neon signs - in fact, anything red can become a signal for you to check if you are over- or under-aroused and to take appropriate action.

Exercise   Many men find regular physical exercise helps them cope with stress. Whether this is merely because exercise is an excellent distractor, occupying the mind as well as the body and so helping to turn off stressful thoughts, or whether it has a more specific metabolic effect, is as yet unclear. The type of exercise you take also makes a difference. Difficult and highly competitive sports, such as squash or golf, may add to your stress by being yet another area where there is pressure to succeed. If you are vulnerable to this sort of feeling, non-competitive exercise, such as swimming, running or weight training, may be more appropriate. Immediately after exercise is a particularly good time to practise your relaxation or meditation techniques.

COPING WITH DEPRESSION

So far the methods suggested have been designed to help you deal with anxiety, but equally important is the ability to deal with depression. When someone is depressed he stops doing the things he normally enjoys because he cannot be bothered. Negative thoughts and feelings come more easily to mind, and there is a grey miserable tinge to everything. Experiences that might normally be enjoyed are ignored or interpreted in a negative way. This increased sensitivity to gloom fuels depression and keeps it going, forming a vicious circle.

It is possible to treat this cycle by deliberately acting as though you are ignoring miserable experiences and ideas. A form of psychological treatment known as cognitive therapy is based on this concept, but the principle can help anyone who is depressed, even if not badly enough to need specialist help.

Positive self-talk   An important influence on what we feel is what we think (and vice versa). Thus, if we have depressing thoughts - 'life is meaningless; I'm a failure; I can't do anything' - we feel miserable; if we have anxious thoughts - 'I wonder if I will get that job; will someone break into my house? Will I be able to do this?' - we become anxious. A useful way of reversing this process is 'positive self-talk'. When you catch yourself having one of these negative thoughts, counteract it by talking to yourself positively. For example, if you find yourself thinking 'I'm a failure', say to yourself, 'No, I am not; I've got a good job, a nice flat and some good friends. Everyone makes mistakes from time to time and it is natural and human.

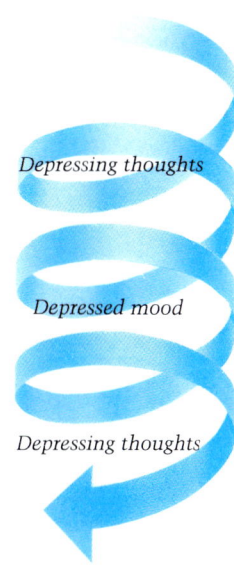

Depressing thoughts

Depressed mood

Depressing thoughts

Depression is a vicious downward spiral. At any one time there are factors in life which are bad and factors which are good but once locked in a spiral, it is impossible to turn the mind onto the positive factors. Depression is often accompanied by insomnia, loss of energy and interest in life, a poor appetite and a drop in body weight. Libido decreases and impotence may be a problem.

Why should I be different?'

This technique is also useful when you are feeling anxious. Counteract anxious thoughts with confident ones. For example, instead of saying to yourself, 'I might not be able to do that job,' say, 'I will; I've done jobs like that before. I've succeeded in the past, and I'll cope again. Keep calm, relax.' Far from being the first sign of madness, talking to yourself in this way may be a major step in helping you to retain your sanity.

Confidants   An important way of helping to solve any problem is to talk it over with someone else. A detached observer often has a perspective on the issues that someone deeply involved in them cannot achieve and so can give valuable advice. The mere act of explaining a problem to someone else also helps to clarify the issues and options in your own mind.

Many women have a 'confidant' - someone to whom they can confide private matters and discuss personal problems - and it has been shown that women who have such a close relationship are less prone to depression than those who do not. Men often find it hard to talk openly, even to a close friend or relative, about matters that are troubling them, and they often feel the need to put a brave face on things. Nevertheless, if a trustworthy person who will respect your confidentiality is available, talking your problems over will often help to resolve them.

Positive self-image   Many of the techniques discussed in this chapter have the same aim - to make you feel better about yourself. A common feature of all failure to cope with stress is the negative view that the person has of himself. A lack of confidence leads to anxiety; not liking yourself leads to depression; guilt leads to over-work and a feeling of responsibility for everyone else's problems. We all use destructive bluster, anger and self-justification to conceal uncertainty and lack of belief in ourselves.

Much of our self-image inevitably comes from things outside us. When, as always happens, these things go wrong, we are prone to a strain reaction. The less easily shaken your self-image is by external events, the more you can continue to have faith in yourself in spite of set-backs, the less strain there will be in your life and the more you will enjoy it.

BODY BASICS

Much of this book is about staying healthy. Sensible eating, relaxation, proper exercise and a well-balanced lifestyle all help to keep a man healthy and active. But we live in a hazardous world. Accidents, environmental disasters and infection by microscopic organisms can beset even the healthiest man, and our own bodies can let us down, producing disease by failing to work properly. So good health is not our automatic right, although we can do much to improve our chances of enjoying and maintaining it.

The World Health Organization has as its target: 'Health for all by the year 2000.' In this context health means more than the absence of disease - or rather, a relative absence. It means 'well being' - physical, mental and social. It is difficult to compare accurately how healthy we are today with earlier periods. Disease patterns vary with the way we live. Many years ago, people died early, as infectious diseases and malnutrition combined with bad working conditions and poor housing to shorten life. Now we have controlled many of the diseases that were killers, and our life span has increased greatly. The result is that we are instead presented with entirely different diseases such as arthritis and some cancers, which tend to develop in older people; formerly they did not show up so frequently because people died earlier. And now we have the biggest killer of all: diseases of the heart and circulatory system, to which the biggest contributory factor is the over-rich diet we eat. This diet is thought also to contribute to the yearly toll of cancer.

So what can you do to help protect yourself from disease? To avoid diseases? Or even to treat yourself. Medical care and advice are available to all, and you should always be able to see a doctor about any medical problem you may have. Your doctor's main concern is dealing with problems once they have developed, so it is up to you to consult him or her and follow the advice you are given. To this extent, your health is in your own hands.

Neither this book nor any other is a substitute for proper medical advice, and to give this, your doctor usually has to examine you. What this book can do is to explain some common medical conditions, and how your doctor may treat them. It also highlights some of the symptoms of disease, which should alert you so that you can consult your doctor promptly.

As with all matters concerned with your health, self-assessment requires common sense. There is little point in rushing to the doctor with a simple headache, sore throat or hangover - provided, that is, these are the only problems. You have to decide if a minor health problem has been going on for too long or if it is getting worse.

IMMUNIZATION

The body develops immunity to infectious diseases after being exposed to the organisms that cause them. Sometimes we become immune spontaneously, without ever developing the symptoms of the disease. Usually, however, we develop immunity after an attack of disease. Most adults have been infected with the common diseases like chickenpox, mumps and measles quite early in childhood, and they are completely immune in later life. For some other diseases, the immunity is brief or incomplete, and these diseases recur (for example, the common cold or influenza), although usually not in quite the same form.

The lymphatic system is crucial to the defence of the body against disease. It consists of a network of vessels which link together the spleen, tonsils, thymus gland and hundreds of lymph nodes which vary in size from that of a pin-head to that of a pea. The lymph vessels feed lymph into the node where foreign particles and bacteria are removed, thus filtering the body's tissue fluid and returning it to the blood. Lymphatic tissue also makes lymphocytes and antibodies.

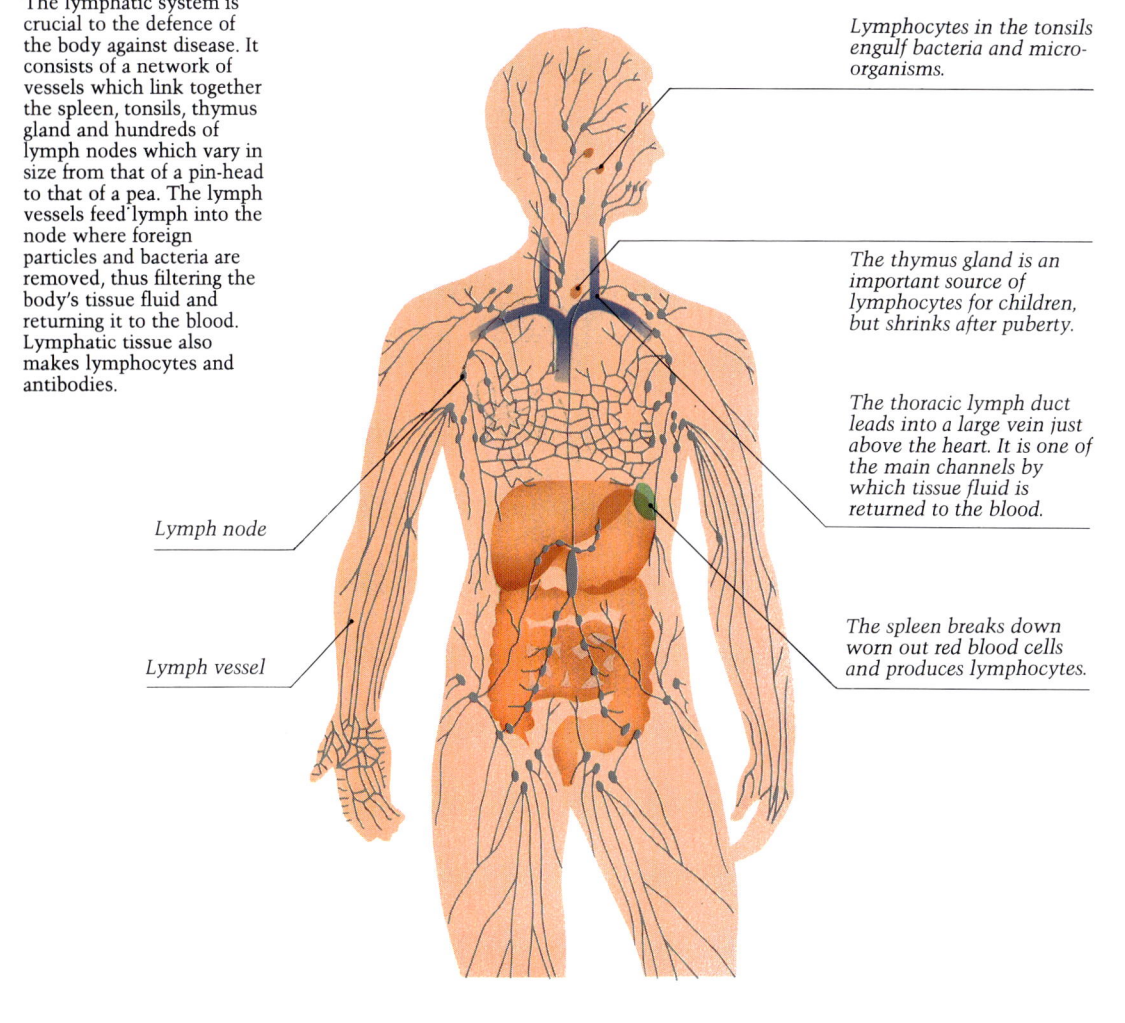

Lymphocytes in the tonsils engulf bacteria and micro-organisms.

The thymus gland is an important source of lymphocytes for children, but shrinks after puberty.

The thoracic lymph duct leads into a large vein just above the heart. It is one of the main channels by which tissue fluid is returned to the blood.

The spleen breaks down worn out red blood cells and produces lymphocytes.

Lymph node

Lymph vessel

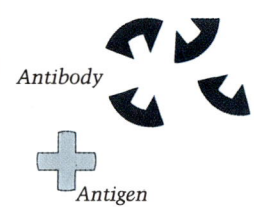

Antibody

Antigen

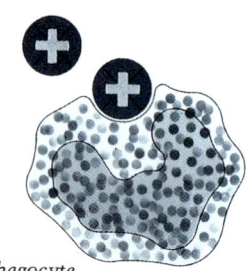

Phagocyte

One type of antibody mirrors the structure of the antigen which is isolated by antibodies that fit themselves around it to form a chemical jigsaw puzzle. Phagocytes then eat it.

Antigen

Antibody

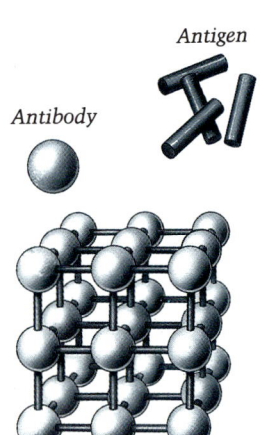

Another type of antibody links together numbers of antigens and neutralizes their poisonous effects. The phagocytes then engulf the lattice and destroy it.

Immunization is the artificial stimulation of the immune response, so that the body can resist disease organisms it has never before encountered. Its success is one of the triumphs of modern medicine and has led to the effective control of several potentially lethal diseases, prevention of many less dangerous diseases and the total eradication of the organism causing smallpox.

In many respects, immunization is an ideal form of medicine. It pre-empts disease and, when a large proportion of the population has been effectively immunized, the disease organism finds it difficult to spread to another host and may die out or persist in only very small amounts. Despite the undoubted success of immunization in preventing infectious diseases, it has not been solely responsible for the dramatic drop in deaths from such diseases witnessed this century. The incidence of killer diseases like scarlet fever and diphtheria had dropped dramatically even before immunization was widely practised, probably because of better sanitation, nutrition, and less crowded living conditions.

Immunization works by persuading your body's immune system that it is being attacked by invading viruses or bacteria. Your body reacts by producing the appropriate antibodies, substances that in turn attack the invading organisms. Having once learned to combat these disease-producing organisms, your body can quickly summon up the same immune response next time it encounters the same invaders.

Foreign substances and invading organisms carry on their surface molecules called antigens, which may be recognized by special cells called lymphocytes. The lymphocytes produce the antibody, a substance that kills or inactivates the invader by latching on to the antigen. Other types of cell assist in destroying the immobilized or damaged attacker.

When you are immunized, antigens with the characteristics of disease organisms are introduced into your body in a vaccine consisting of the bacteria or viruses, either in a weakened or harmless state, or killed, or even an extract from the organisms that contains the characteristic antigens. Depending on how violent a response from your immune system is provoked by the vaccine, the immunity produced is either temporary or life-long. If the vaccine is live and produces a low level of actual disease, it generally provokes a very powerful response and long-lasting immunity. This is the case with the vaccines for tuberculosis, polio and smallpox. The smallpox vaccine in fact contains the related cowpox virus, which is close enough to smallpox to give good immunity.

On the other hand, vaccines that contain dead organisms generally do not give permanent immunity. The vaccines usually given for influenza, typhoid and tetanus, among others, are of this type and need 'topping up' with booster injections periodically.

The other form of immunization is usually reserved for the emergency treatment of people who are at special risk because of an existing health problem. Such people receive injections of gamma globulin, or immunoglobulins, extracted from the blood of a person who has already recovered from the disease. Unlike other vaccines, these immunoglobulins are able to stop an infection in its tracks, but their effects are brief, and they are usually followed by vaccination with the normal types of vaccine once the emergency is past. Extracting the immunoglobulin required for these vaccinations is an expensive process.

The best and strongest immunity is that acquired after natural infection in childhood. Many diseases such as mumps, chickenpox and rubella (or German measles) confer life-long immunity when contracted in childhood. Indeed, it can be said that it is wise to catch these illnesses in childhood and get them out of the way safely. In later life, they can cause serious problems.

DO YOU NEED TO BE VACCINATED?

As an adult male, you certainly won't need to worry about being vaccinated against the common childhood infections. Even if you have not already had them, you may have been exposed to the organisms causing them but not developed symptoms and thus been given life-long immunity.

The diseases you should be vaccinated against are those which can attack people at any age. A few, notably poliomyelitis (polio), tuberculosis (TB) and tetanus, are always a potential health threat; vaccinations against others such as typhoid and paratyphoid, hepatitis A and cholera may also be advisable if you are travelling abroad.

Poliomyelitis   Until an effective vaccine was introduced in 1958, polio was a scourge. It is now quite rare, bu its effects can be so damaging and the vaccination is so easy and without side effects, that it seems foolish not to check with your doctor whether you have been vaccinated against it. If you have not, get vaccinated without delay, especially if you are travelling abroad. Polio is a virus disease that attacks the nervous system, leaving a proportion of its victims paralysed. The virus causing polio lives in the gut and elsewhere and may not cause any disease symptoms. However, it is shed in the faeces, and poor hygiene or inadequate sewage disposal can lead to the infection of others. The vaccine could not be simpler: a drop of live, but harmless, polio organism is taken by mouth, usually on a lump of sugar. This produces very rapid immunity, which lasts for about three years, when a 'booster' is required. Unlike many vaccinations, this gives protection almost immediately, so can be given just before you go on holiday.

Tuberculosis (TB)   In most developed countries tuberculosis rarely appears. However, the rarer such a disease becomes, the more susceptible the population becomes, as individuals are never naturally exposed to the bacterium and do not develop any immunity. So it is important to check with your doctor to see if you have been vaccinated, especially if you are travelling abroad.

Tuberculosis is caused by bacteria that attack the lungs and, sometimes, other parts of the body. The bacteria are usually spread by coughing but can also be caught from infected cattle, and the risk of TB is the primary reason for the pasteurization or heat treatment of milk, which kills any bacteria present. Unlike infections caused by viruses, bacterial infections like TB can be treated with antibiotics, but by the time the symptoms have developed, serious and possibly permanent damage may have been caused to the lungs or other organs. So it is sensible to be vaccinated. A live but weakened bacterium called BCG is given by pricking the skin, which develops to form a small inflamed spot, producing immunity within a few

Continued on page 106

HEALTHCARE FOR THE TRAVELLER

It is common sense to check that you have adequate protection against polio, TB and tetanus, even if you have no intention of travelling abroad. Your doctor receives regular notification of the type of vaccination recommended (and in some cases demanded by law) for travel to any part of the world, and he will be able to advise you what is required and when. Some vaccinations need to be given separately from others and may take a while to confer immunity, so you should consult your doctor at least six weeks before departure. But remember, because conditions and regulations change, the required vaccinations may vary from one year to the next.

Malaria can be a dangerous threat if you are travelling to many warm countries. You *cannot* be immunized against it yet, and you must ask your doctor for a special course of treatment.

Specialist medical advisory services offer detailed personal advice for travellers abroad on immunization, prevention of malaria, and other medical requirements. Computer technology allows these services access to data on the latest health risks worldwide, and they are much used by businessmen.

DISEASES	AREA WHERE ENDEMIC	HOW INFECTION IS CAUGHT
Cholera	*Africa Asia Middle East, particularly in conditions of poor hygiene*	*Contaminated food or water*
Infective Hepatitis	*Most parts of the world, particularly in conditions of poor hygiene*	*Contaminated food or water. Contact with infected person*
Malaria	*Africa Asia Central and South America*	*Bite from infected mosquito*
Polio	*All areas (except Europe, North America, Australia and New Zealand)*	*Direct contact with infected person. Contaminated food or water (rare).*
Rabies	*Many areas of the world*	*Bite or scratch from infected animal*
Tetanus	*Areas where medical facilities not readily available*	*Open injury*
Typhoid	*All areas (except Europe, North America, Australia and New Zealand) in conditions of poor hygiene*	*Contaminated food, water or milk*
Yellow Fever	*Africa South America*	*Bite from infected mosquito*

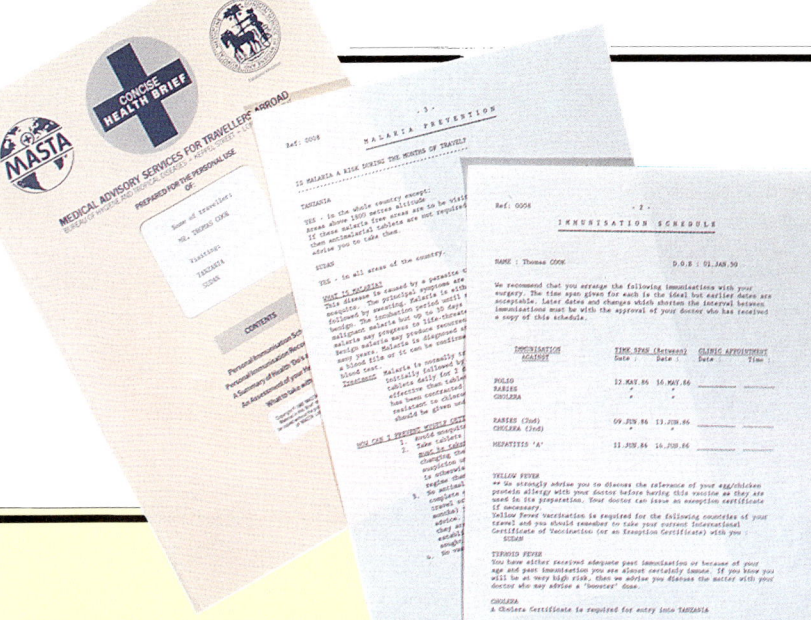

Water Unless you know the water to be safe, sterilize all drinking water, either by boiling it or by using sterilization tablets. Milk should be boiled before use unless it is already sterilized or pasteurized.
Food Foods that can be contaminated include raw vegetables, unpeeled fruit, raw shellfish, cream, ice cream, ice cubes,

VACCINATION	REVACCINATION	VACCINATION CERTIFICATE REQUIRED?	OTHER PRECAUTIONS
Usually 2 injections by your doctor	*Every 6 months while abroad*	*Some countries require evidence of vaccination. Check before you travel.*	*Vaccination does not guarantee full protection. Take scrupulous care over food and drink.*
Seek advice from your doctor		*No*	*Take scrupulous care over hygiene, food and drink*
			Anti-malarial tablets. Avoid mosquito bites.
Drops administered by your doctor; 3 doses taken at 4-8 week intervals	*May be needed after 10 years. Consult your doctor.*	*No*	*Take scrupulous care over food and drink*
		No	*Antiserum given after bite, followed by course of injections*
Seek advice from your doctor		*No*	*Wash all wounds thoroughly*
2 injections by your doctor, usually at an interval of 4-6 weeks	*Usually after 3 years*	*No*	*Take scrupulous care over food and drink*
1 injection at a special centre, at least 10 days before travelling	*After 10 years*	*Some countries require evidence of vaccination. Check before you travel*	*Avoid mosquito bites*

CHECK LIST FOR TRAVELLING ABROAD

underdone meat and fish. Generally, any food that is uncooked, cold or reheated can be contaminated; freshly cooked foods are far safer.
Personal hygiene Be careful to wash your hands before eating or handling food, particularly if you are camping.
Sun burn The sun is often far more powerful than you

think and can burn surprisingly quickly. If you have pale skin, allow only 15 minutes direct exposure to the sun for the first day: thereafter, you can allow a little more sun each day to develop your tan.
Heat exhaustion It is unwise to exert yourself too much in a hot climate; your body will lose too much fluid and salt,

causing headaches, dizziness and nausea. These problems can be avoided by taking extra salt, drinking plenty of fluids, and wearing loose, lightweight clothing (cotton and natural fibres are best).
Sexually transmitted diseases Sexually transmitted diseases are a serious problem throughout the world. If you think you

may have been infected obtain medical advice and treatment immediately.

Small first aid kit You never know when you might need first aid so it is always handy to pack a small kit. Adhesive dressings, insect-repellant and antiseptic cream take up little space and could prove invaluable.

Continued from page 103

weeks. This vaccination cannot, therefore, be given just before your holiday. Your doctor can carry out a simple scratch test to see if you already have antibodies to the TB organism.

Tetanus Sometimes called lockjaw, tetanus is caused by bacteria that live in the soil and may enter the body through a wound. The bacteria are anaerobic, thriving only in the absence of oxygen, and they can therefore only grow in damaged tissue where the blood supply is not effective and oxygen is lacking. Typically, tetanus can occur after deep penetrating wounds, such as cuts received while gardening or handling sharp metal. The tetanus bacterium grows rapidly in the damaged tissue, producing a poison or toxin which causes strong and painful muscle spasms; these can be fatal.

If you suffer any deep wound, especially if it is obviously dirty, it is important that you receive an anti-tetanus vaccination or course of injections. The vaccination needs to be topped up with a booster shot every five years or less. If the wound is very dirty and if your tetanus boosters are not up to date or nearing the time for renewal, immunoglobulin may be given as a temporary measure.

Typhoid and paratyphoid Caused by related bacteria, typhoid and paratyphoid are uncommon in most temperate countries, although they are a constant threat in warmer places, especially the overcrowded holiday resorts around the Mediterranean, and wherever there is poor sanitation and food hygiene. Typhoid is dangerous and often fatal; paratyphoid is somewhat less severe. Both diseases cause very severe fever, followed by violent diarrhoea, and are largely preventable with vaccination. Two doses are given, several weeks apart, so your doctor needs adequate warning if you are going abroad on holiday. The immunity lasts for about three years before a booster is needed.

HYGIENE AND HEALTH

Infections may be transmitted by physical contact, by inhaling infected water droplets or by the indirect transfer of infections from faeces to the mouth.

It is often difficult to avoid the microscopic water droplets coughed or sneezed out by a person with a respiratory disease such as a cold or influenza. When you cough or sneeze, these droplets are shot out of your mouth and wafted for considerable distances. Common sense and courtesy dictate that you use a handkerchief or tissue to cover your mouth when you sneeze. If you have to travel or commute in crowded public transport, or if you work in conditions where you are exposed to many people in a restricted area, you are particularly at risk from this form of infection. Unfortunately, there's not much you can do about it.

However, you can reduce the chances of infection entering your body by mouth. Many bacteria and viruses enter the body in this way - polio, dysentery, cholera, food poisoning, typhoid, and so forth. They are shed in the faeces of an infected person, and are passed on to another person usually in contaminated food or drink if hygiene standards are poor. In some countries, sewage can contaminate drinking water, and flies with access to faeces may walk on food, spreading the infection in this way.

Measurements taken during a sneeze show that the air travels out of your nostrils at nearly 100 mph. This spreads droplets of moisture many feet around you, possibly carrying airborne viruses such as colds, influenza and other upper respiratory tract infections.

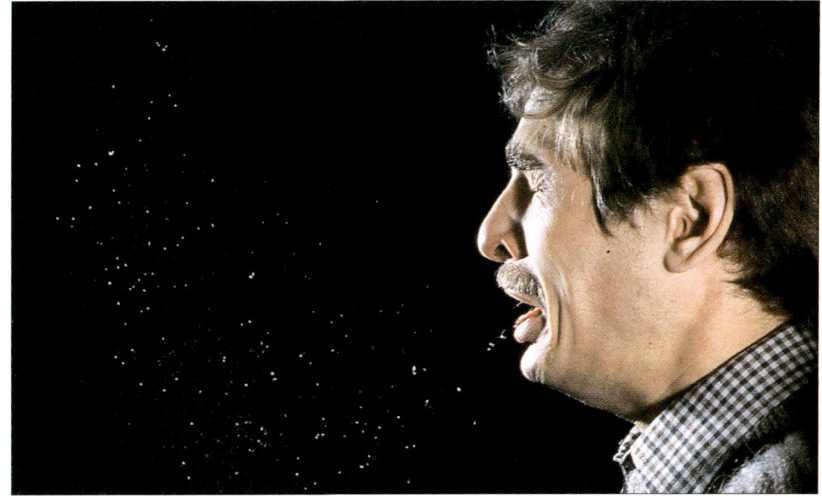

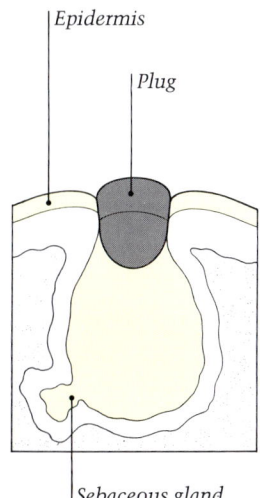

Epidermis

Plug

Sebaceous gland

Acne forms when excess sebum (the oily secretion from the sebaceous glands within each hair follicle) oxidizes and forms a plug in the follicle. The follicle becomes inflamed and the hair dies. Squeezing such a spot can force the infection back down the follicle and into the blood stream causing a boil to develop.

Food hygiene is important, even in the cleanest of kitchens. Bacteria proliferate in huge numbers on working surfaces, and in part-used canned foods kept for re-use. The wall can-opener is one of the most heavily infected spots in the home; the encrustation that can develop around the cutters will be composed of billions of bacteria.

Bacteria grow rapidly in meat, causing food poisoning. A common form of food poisoning is salmonellosis (named after salmonella, the organism responsible), which results in diarrhoea, vomiting and abdominal pain. The bacteria may be present as a natural contaminant of meat and poultry, and they reproduce at enormous rates in poorly cooked poultry or poultry that has been insufficiently thawed before cooking and does not cook thoroughly. Refreezing and reheating meat can also provide perfect conditions for the growth of these bacteria. Another form of food poisoning is that caused by staphylococci, usually from an infected cut or boil on a food-handler's skin. Staphylococci multiply in warm conditions and produce toxins which, unlike those of salmonella, are not destroyed by thorough cooking. The symptoms of staphylococci food poisoning are similar to those of salmonellosis.

Personal cleanliness is as much a matter of self-esteem as it is of health and hygiene. We produce more than a pint of sweat every day; much more in very hot weather or if we are carrying out some violent exertion. Most of this sweat is water, produced by the tiny eccrine or sweat glands which cover the body. In the armpits and groin are found a different type of sweat gland called apocrine glands. These produce a more oily sweat, which has an odour thought to play a part in sexual attraction. It is the secretions from the apocrine glands which are responsible for body odour, and this is why attention to personal hygiene in these areas is important for social reasons.

Acne Your skin is covered by millions of tiny sebaceous glands. The oily secretions may become trapped, solidifying into a blackhead or comedo and forming a plug. Inflammation may then set in, causing a reddish pimple and trapping pus beneath the head of the spot. This condition is called 'acne' and mainly affects the sebaceous glands of the face and upper trunk. It is not known exactly why the condition occurs, although it is certainly most common in people who have oily skins. Acne is an all too

Continued on page 110

BALDNESS

For many men, baldness seems to be a part of the natural ageing process and, despite the vast sums that have been spent on research, no one knows why. It seems to be partly the result of age and partly the result of activity of the male sex hormones. It is very much an inherited condition.

Hair loss probably starts at quite an early age, but it does not become apparent until sufficient hair has gone. It usually proceeds in a standard pattern: the hair on the crown thins gradually, while that at the temple hairline on each side recedes slowly until, inexorably, the bald areas meet. The hair at the sides and back of the head is usually retained. The condition has nothing to do with greying of the hair, and, despite popular mythology, neither greying nor baldness has anything to do with receiving a severe shock. There is a diffuse form of baldness, however, that can follow certain severe illnesses, although the hair usually returns gradually after a few months. Some drugs, especially the cytotoxic drugs used to treat cancer, cause hair loss, although again, the hair usually re-grows after the treatment.

Alopecia is a particular form of hair loss that can affect *all* body hair, including pubic hair and the hair in the armpits. It may also affect only small patches of the scalp. The cause is unknown.

So, unfortunately, nothing can usually be done about hair loss, unless a specific disease or treatment is involved. Some men accept baldness without too much distress: after all, in some cultures, it is regarded as a sign of virility. Wigs and hair pieces are sometimes worn, while some men seek transplant treatment, an expensive and lengthy process, which seldom produces very convincing results. It involves transferring small patches of the skin, complete with healthy hair, from the back or sides of the head to the bare portions of scalp. The loss of hair usually continues, however, and these areas too eventually become bald.

Bitemporal recession is the mildest form of balding and occurs in 90 per cent of men, usually during puberty.
Frontotemporal loss and thinning occurs in 60 per cent of men before they reach the age of 50.
Frontal recession at the temples is followed by thinning and loss at the crown of head. Rates of hair loss vary consideraby but an accurate estimation of the extent of loss can usually be made by studying male relatives in the previous generation.
Final stages During the final stages of balding the hair loss extends completely over the crown of the head. Baldness and excessive body hair occur together because both are under the control of the male hormone testosterone. However, neither is a sign of sexual potency.
Alopecia The cause is still not fully understood. Patches of complete hair loss occur on the scalp. When the hair re-grows it is often white for a few months.

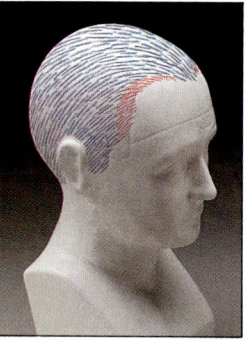

Bitemporal recession

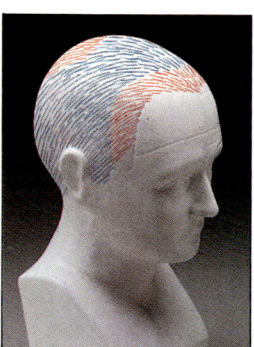

Frontal recession

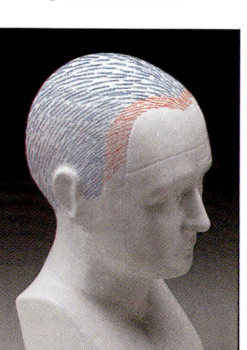

Frontotemporal loss

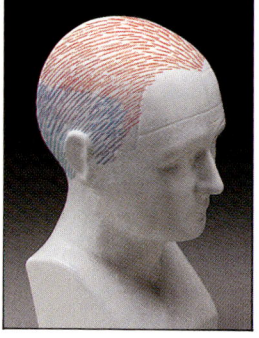

Final stages

Scarring (for example, following a burn) destroys hair follicles. The effect is irreversible.

During a hair transplant a plug of skin is punched out of an area of scalp where the follicles are still producing terminal hair. The plug contains all the underlying skin structures and a number of active follicles. It is then placed in a similarly punched hole at the front of the scalp. It is in fact a full-thickness skin graft. Complications such as scarring or infection may occur, and the active follicles may also die back; this treatment can have limited success.

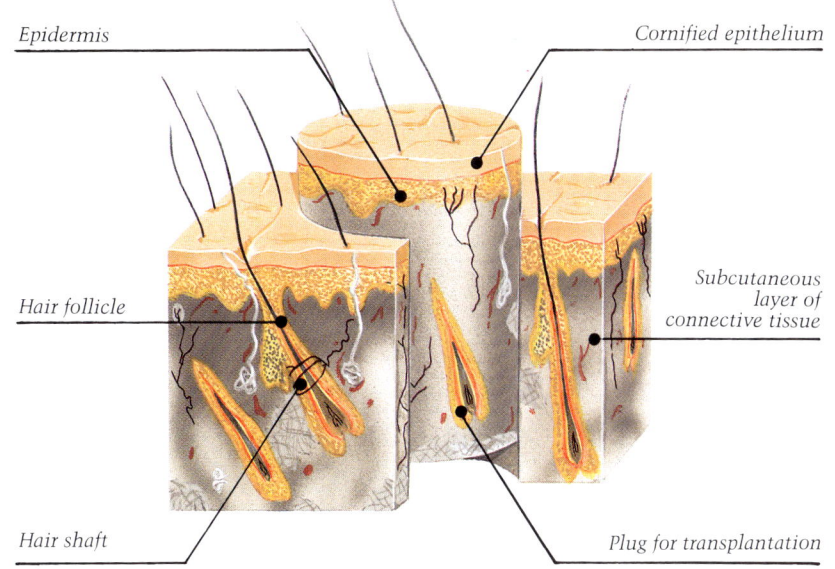

Epidermis

Cornified epithelium

Hair follicle

Subcutaneous layer of connective tissue

Hair shaft

Plug for transplantation

CAUSES OF HAIR THINNING AND LOSS

CAUSE	HAIR LOSS	TREATMENT
Seborrhoeic eczema *Excessive and scaly dandruff*	*Partial/temporary*	*Proprietary preparations*
Ringworm *A fungal infection of the scalp*	*Partial/temporary*	*Proprietary creams*
Strong shampoos *Containing selenium, a naturally occurring anti-dandruff mineral*	*Partial/temporary*	*Discontinue use*
Iron deficiency	*Thinning*	*Diet supplement*
Thyroid hormone deficiency	*Thinning*	*Replacement therapy*
Alopecia areata *Hair follicle disorder of unknown origin*	*Temporary/patchy*	*None*
Alopecia totalis *A more generalized alopecia*	*Total/usually permanent*	*None*
Chemotherapy *Anti-cancer drugs eg Cyclophosphamide*	*Temporary*	*Acceptance of side-effect*

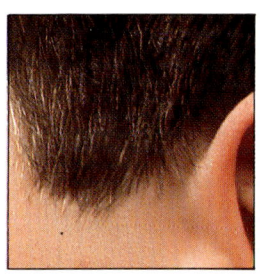

The follicles on the scalp produce *terminal hairs* which have a three-year life cycle. Between 100 to 300 hairs are shed from the scalp each day and at any one time one per cent of the follicles are in a resting state prior to producing new hair.

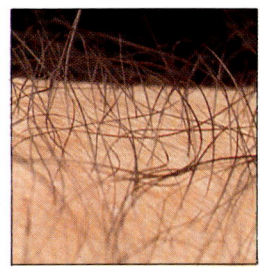

Vellus hair is the short, fine hair that grows on other parts of the body. Baldness begins when the follicles of the scalp produce vellus hair instead of terminal hair.

DENTAL CARE

Before cleaning your teeth, chew up a disclosing tablet, run your tongue over your teeth, then rinse your mouth out gently. The disclosing agent shows plaque up a brilliant red, particularly noticeable around the tooth margins. Clean all the red away.

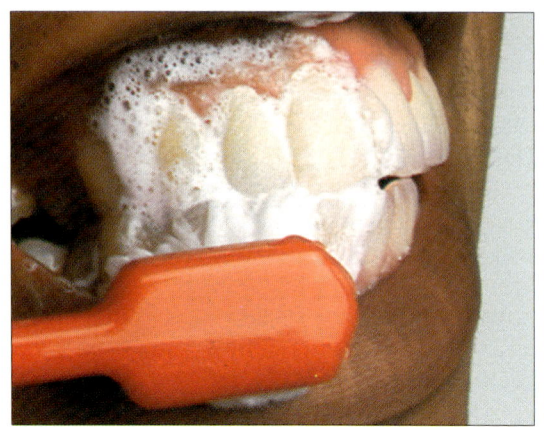

Use a flat-headed brush to clean your teeth and change it every two to three months. Brush from gum to tooth tip and pay particular attention to the backs of the teeth. Clean the tooth surfaces with a scrubbing action. You should brush for three minutes at least once, preferably twice, a day.

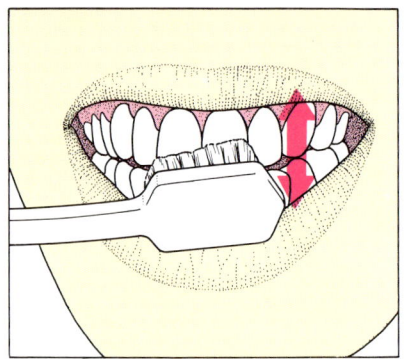
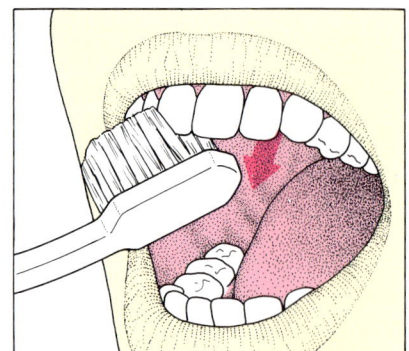

Floss is strong thread which can be used to clean plaque from between the teeth and beneath the gum margins. Hold it wrapped firmly around the fingers and stretch it between the thumbs. Work it gently into the gaps of the teeth, taking care not to jar it into the gum and damage it. Then work it gently up and down the sides of the teeth, easing it beneath the gum margin. Avoid any sawing action.

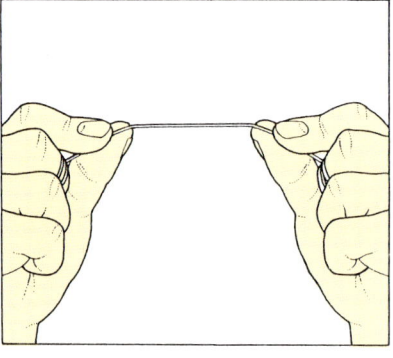
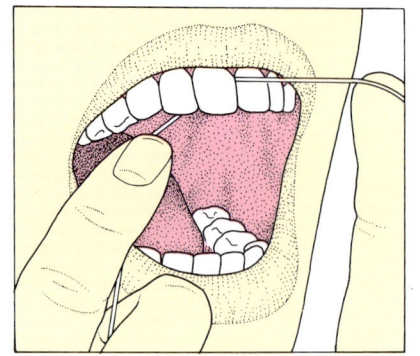

A small pointed stick of soft wood can be used to remove plaque from between the teeth.

A single tuft brush is useful for cleaning small, difficult areas such as a tooth that is overlapped by another. You can also reach the inside of the molars.

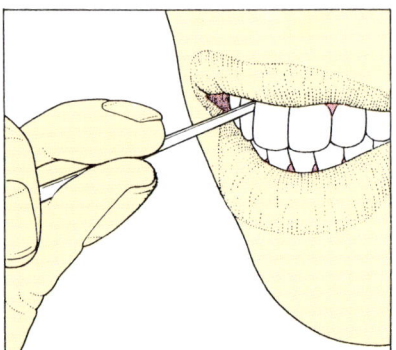
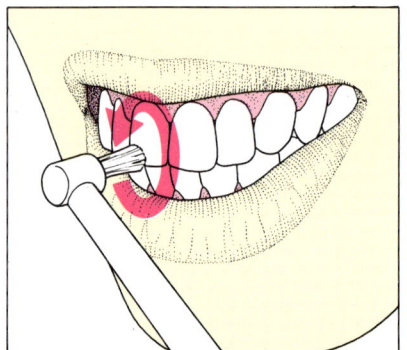

Continued from page 107

common feature of adolescence when drastic hormonal changes are taking place and the sebaceous glands are especially active. Contrary to popular belief, however, acne has nothing to do with over-indulging in sweets. Frequent washing with mild soap will help, and you should *not* squeeze spots, as this only damages the pores and can cause permanent scarring. Medication may be necessary in troublesome cases.

Dental hygiene Like many other parts of the body, the mouth is a rich breeding-ground for bacteria, which spread over the teeth in a transparent, sticky layer called plaque. The bacteria are nourished by the food we eat, and especially by frequent sugar consumption, like sweets and sweet drinks. Most of us eat too much sugar. The plaque bacteria break this sugar down into acid within minutes of our eating or drinking anything sweet, and the acid attacks the tough mineral forming the tooth enamel, which becomes softened and pitted, allowing bacteria to enter the layers beneath, creating a cavity and tooth decay.

Plaque bacteria also cause the deposit of minerals in the saliva around the base of the teeth, where your toothbrush may not reach. These build up into a rough stony layer called calculus, which gradually spreads down the tooth and beneath the gum surface. Bacteria can now enter the gap between gum and tooth, causing painful inflammation of the gum (gingivitis) and erosion of the bony socket, loosening the tooth and leading to its eventual loss. Gum disease is more prevalent among adult men than is tooth decay, which is more a problem in children.

Dental decay and gum disease are conditions that you can avoid. Cut down on sugar and you cut down on the food source for plaque bacteria, thus reducing the acid they can produce. Removing plaque by cleaning your teeth properly reduces both tooth decay and gum disease. Brush your teeth correctly with a medium-grade brush with round-tipped, nylon bristles; do not use a 'hard' brush. Discard and replace your toothbrush as soon as it becomes splayed.

You should also remember to use a toothpaste that contains fluoride. Fluoride, either in toothpaste or in drinking water, becomes chemically attached to the tooth enamel, changing its nature so that it is much more resistant to acid. The effects are most marked in children whose teeth are not fully mineralized or hardened, but, even in adults, fluoride can give worthwhile protection from decay. It can also be taken in the form of mouthwashes, drops or tablets, which can be bought from the chemist.

It is important to visit your dentist regularly so that any potential problems may be treated before they develop into permanent dental damage. Your dentist or dental hygienist can do an excellent job of removing unsightly and damaging calculus from inaccessible parts of the teeth, so helping to prevent gum disease. If you do develop a dental problem, don't delay in getting it treated. Tooth ache is obvious, but watch out for reddened or bleeding gums and soreness of the gum margin, which indicate gingivitis. If the trouble persists after a few days of careful flossing, it may require the attention of your dentist.

Poor dental hygiene is often painfully apparent to the owner of the mouth - and frequently to others who do not appreciate halitosis. Mouth odour is usually caused by the action of bacteria on food debris. It is also often an indication of gum infection. Smoking may make it worse - or at least, worse for other people.

EYE CARE

The human eye is a beautifully designed and intricate colour television camera, packed into a jelly-filled ball barely an inch in diameter. It has an iris to adjust the amount of light entering it, a lens to focus the rays, and a retina or screen consisting of about 135 million light-sensitive cells, each connected via the optic nerve to the visual cortex of the brain. Light rays from objects pass through the transparent cornea at the front of the eye, then through the pupil which is simply an adjustable aperture in the centre of the coloured iris. The light then passes through the transparent elastic lens which can be flattened by a ring of tiny muscles attached around its edge. These changes in the shape of the lens focus the rays into a sharp image onto the retina at the back of the eye which in turn sends coded impulses up the optic nerve to the brain.

It is not possible to 'strain' the eyes. The muscles that move the eyeball around within the socket are in constant motion day and night and never tire. The same is true of the muscles that adjust the shape of the lens.

It is a myth that reading in a dim light or watching too much television ruins your eyesight. As for sunglasses, many experts regard them as unnecessary. The pupil has the ability to shut down to the size of a pinhead in very bright sunlight and, combined with a mechanism by which the sensitivity of the retina can be adjusted, the eye can cope with an intensity of light 75,000 times as bright as the dimmest glimmer discernible. In dim light the pupil enlarges to allow in as much light as possible.

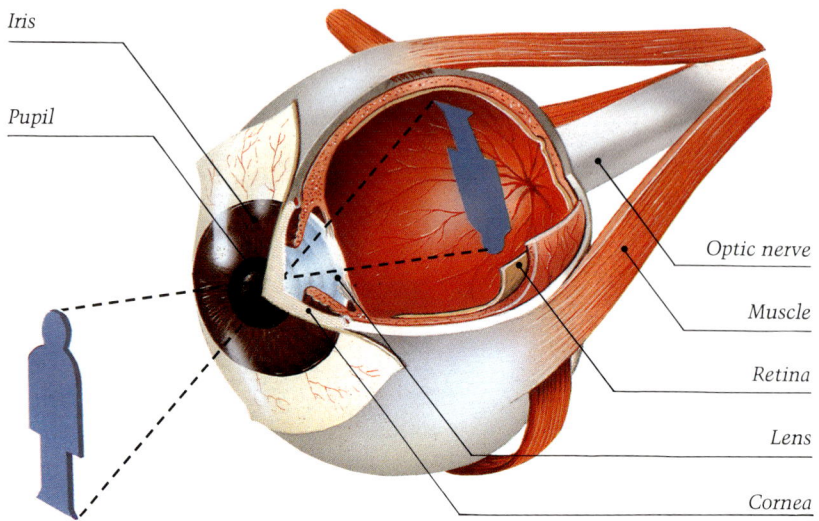

Iris

Pupil

Optic nerve

Muscle

Retina

Lens

Cornea

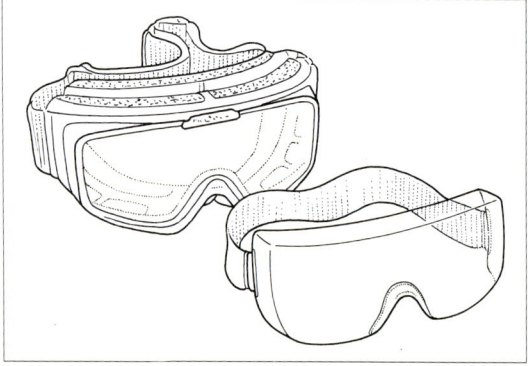

Eye protectors are designed for specific jobs, and it is important to choose the correct variety. To protect against flying particles such as masonry or metal splinters, plastic lenses are used because they will not shatter, but welders have tinted glass in the goggles because the hot sparks melt the plastic. Squash players can wear special protectors to prevent 'blow out' injuries to the eye.

LOOKING AFTER YOUR EYES

The eyes are constantly bathed with tear fluid produced by glands under the upper lids and wiped over the delicate surface of the eye with every blink. Crying, laughing, coughing, sneezing, vomiting, yawning, cold wind and a smoky atmosphere all make your eyes water. Tear fluid soothes sore eyes, flushes out any foreign material, and contains a mild antiseptic called lysozyme which helps to prevent conjunctivitis

(inflammation of the membrane which covers the eye). None of the proprietary eyewash preparations can do a better job. Some eyewashes claim to cure red eyes, but their effect is only temporary and wears off after about 20 minutes. Used regularly, the drug could permanently damage the delicate conjunctival lining. Cold water and cotton wool is probably the most effective treatment, but always use a clean swab for each eye. If

there is a minor infection present it can easily be spread to the other eye on the swab. A persistent or severe inflammation of the eye needs medical treatment.

Eyesight should be checked every two years even if you don't wear spectacles, and more frequently after the age of 40. An opthalmic optician not only tests your vision, but also assesses the internal and external health of your eyes.

EAR CARE

The ear is divided into three parts, the outer, middle and inner. The outer ear is the gristly flap which funnels sound into the ear canal at the base of which lies the eardrum. On the other side of this is the middle ear which is connected to the back of the throat by a tube which opens when you yawn or swallow, thus equalizing pressure on each side of the eardrum. The middle ear contains three miniature bones which transmit vibrations from the eardrum to a 'window' leading into the inner ear. The inner ear consists of a fluid-filled coiled tube containing 20,000 microscopic hair cells sensitive to minute fluctuations in pressure. Thus sound waves in the air are converted to pressure waves in the inner ear which send nerve impulses along the auditory nerve to the brain where we perceive them as sound. Ears need little maintenance other than keeping the outer ear clean. Never stick anything down the ear canal. This can compact the wax, and may even damage the delicate eardrum.

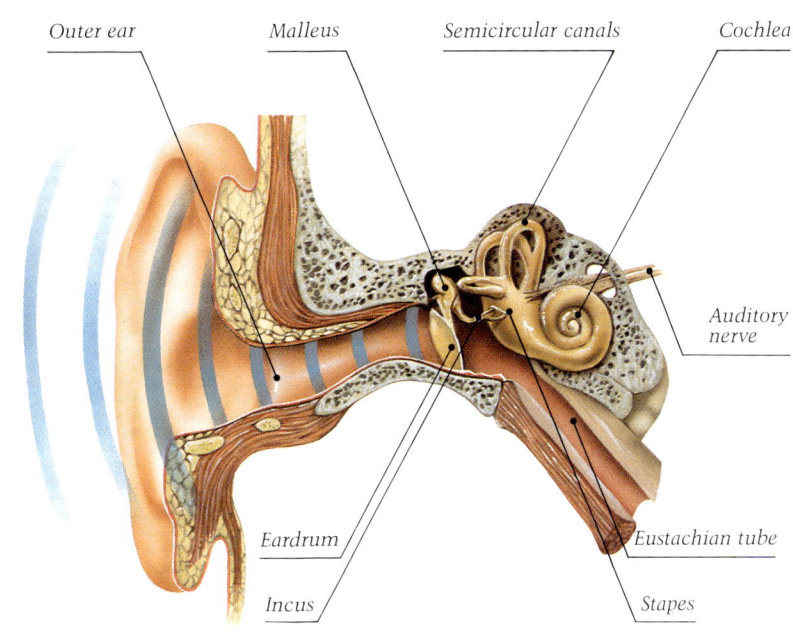

Outer ear · Malleus · Semicircular canals · Cochlea · Auditory nerve · Eardrum · Eustachian tube · Incus · Stapes

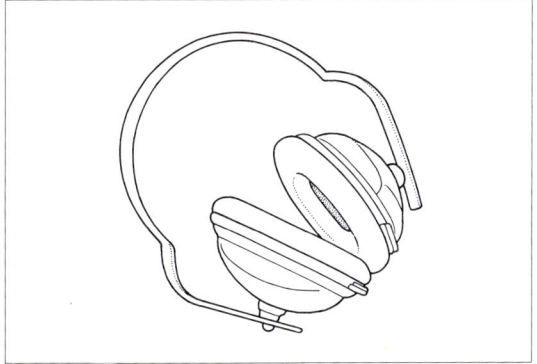

Ear protectors should be worn for any job that is carried out in sustained, loud noise. About 40% of workers exposed to 90 decibels of noise a day will suffer from 'conversational deafness' within 10 years.

● Protection from industrial health hazards, see pages 133-4

Loud, unexpected noise raises the blood pressure and quickens the pulse and breathing rate. Continuous noise can affect concentration, and hearing sensitivity can be reduced temporarily following exposure to loud noises for a short period of time. Continued exposure causes permanent and irreversible damage. However, the effects of exposure to different noise levels are cumulative, so that working in a noisy environment may not in itself produce deafness, but if you spend your evenings listenings to loud rock music as well, the total dose can cause deafness.

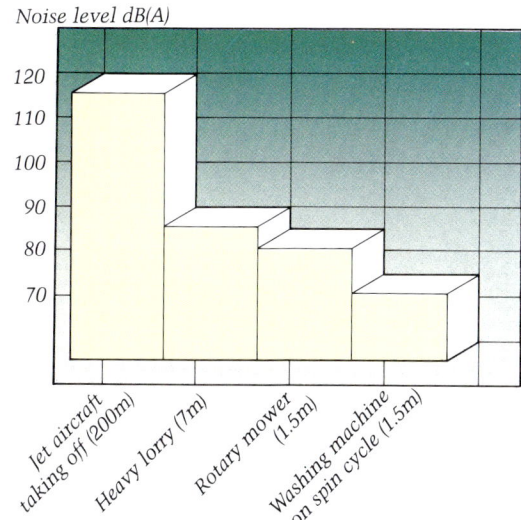

Noise level dB(A)

120 · 110 · 100 · 90 · 80 · 70

Jet aircraft taking off (200m) · Heavy lorry (7m) · Rotary mower (1.5m) · Washing machine on spin cycle (1.5m)

dB(A)	EFFECT
150	Instant damage or deafness
140	Pain and eventual deafness
90	Permanent hearing loss with time
80	Conversation only audible at a shout
55	Telephone conversation difficult
45	Relaxed conversation possible
0	Barely audible

LOOKING AFTER EVERYDAY ILLNESSES

By far the majority of infections and illnesses clear up on their own as your body adapts to the condition and learns how to fight it. For most of these minor illnesses, neither you nor your doctor can, or need to, provide curative treatment. What you can treat, or ask your doctor to treat, are the annoying symptoms of the disease.

A cough, for example, is one of the most common 'illnesses' doctors are asked to treat. It is caused by the body's attempts to remove something irritating the air passages. This may be sticky mucus, produced towards the end of a cold; or it could be caused by inhaling dust or a piece of food; or it could be simply a reaction to an inflammation of the air passages, causing the irritation that triggers off the cough reflex. Coughing is the body's way of removing or clearing an obstruction; it is a natural process and one that it may not be advisable to prevent. If you have a phlegmy cough, however, it may be worth inhaling steam, with a medicated vapour rub or added menthol, to loosen the thick mucus and speed its removal. A dry, irritating cough can often be soothed with an antitussive cough linctus.

Prolonged or chronic coughing may be a warning of something more serious. If your cough lasts for more than a week or so after a cold has cleared up, or if the mucus is very thick, copious, yellowish, greenish or blood-stained, consult your doctor. You should also see your doctor if you find it difficult or painful to breathe or if you develop a temperature.

Sore throats may also be self-treated. Most are caused by viruses, which are completely resistant to antibiotics and to medicated lozenges and gargles. They will soon be destroyed by your body's own immune system and usually clear up within a few days. If your throat has white patches on it, you may have tonsillitis or pharyngitis. These *are* caused by bacteria and should be treated by your doctor. Do not take old antibiotic tablets that are left in your medicine cupboard after a previous illness. These would probably be worse than useless.

For most sore throats, self-treatment is symptomatic. That is, you can relieve the pain and discomfort, while waiting for the inflammation to subside. Gargling with soluble aspirin, which is then swallowed, kills the pain in the throat and reduces fever (if there is a fever). Paracetamol may also be used but is less effective in reducing temperature. If your temperature continues to rise or if your throat gets worse, consult your doctor.

Diarrhoea is both uncomfortable and inconvenient, but for adults it is seldom a serious problem. It occurs when food passes through the digestive system too rapidly for excess water to be absorbed from the waste, so the faeces remain fluid.

Most attacks of diarrhoea are caused by viruses or bacteria, which attack the walls of the gut and cause inflammation, interfering with its normal function. This type of diarrhoea is common in summer when flies may spread infection to uncovered food. It is also the 'tummy bug' many people pick up when holidaying abroad. Every country has its own indigenous strain of 'bug', to which the locals are immune - as you will be too, after a few days of suffering.

Many remedies for diarrhoea are available, usually working by slowing down the normal movement of food along the gut, allowing more water to

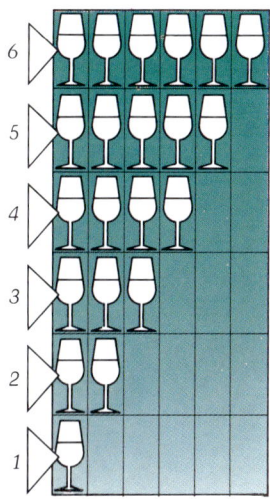

Number of standard drinks

1 2 3 4 5 6

No. of hours required for blood alcohol level to return to normal

A standard drink is a glass of wine, a pub measure of spirit or half a pint of beer. For each standard drink you have, it takes your body an hour to expel the alcohol, but longer to expel the other toxins which cause hangovers.

be absorbed so that the waste can become more solid. However, such remedies, including kaolin and morphine mixture, have the disadvantage that they also slow down the elimination of the causative organism, thus prolonging the problem. The best treatment for diarrhoea is the simplest: eat nothing for at least a day and drink plenty of water to replace lost body fluids. The disease organisms will have nothing to feed on, and the gut can quickly recover from the infection without having to work at digesting food.

However, you *will* need medical attention if the diarrhoea continues for more than three or four days, if there is continuous abdominal pain, or if your stools are black or blood-stained. It is particularly important to get medical advice if diarrhoea persists after a foreign holiday.

Vomiting is the stomach ridding itself of the part-digested food it contains. Apart from anxiety, or over-indulgence in alcohol, or travel sickness, the usual cause is a virus infection, and the condition seldom lasts for long. As with diarrhoea, eat nothing for 24 hours, drink plenty of water and, when you do start to eat, be cautious and at first take only modest amounts of bland food like cereal or toast while your stomach gets used to working properly again. Go to your doctor if the symptoms persist for more than three to four days, if there is continuous stomach pain or if the vomit looks like coffee grounds (due to bleeding).

Headaches These are probably the most common of the everyday problems to be treated at home. Generally they are only a minor annoyance, although occasionally they may be a symptom of another disorder. Most headaches are the result of tension and are caused by strain in the neck and shoulder muscles. The pain is usually experienced in the scalp, not the brain, for although the brain is made of nerve cells, it is completely insensitive to pain, while the meninges, which cover the brain, are very sensitive to pain.

Another form of headache is caused by the swelling of blood vessels. These are vascular headaches, but the causes are very similar to tension headaches. Constant stress, noise, worry, overwork or a hangover are all common causes of a headache.

If your headache is caused by a hangover, part of your problem is dehydration, and drinking plenty of water will help, preferably along with, or soon after, the alcohol. For other types of headache, first try to relax. If possible, get away from whatever has caused the stress. A hot bath may help you to relax. Then take a mild analgesic or painkiller, like soluble aspirin or paracetamol (there is no need to buy expensive branded painkillers: unbranded drugs are just as effective and only a fraction of the price). Always follow the dosage instructions carefully. If a headache lasts for longer than a few days or if you suffer severe headaches frequently, consult your doctor.

Migraine A recurring condition which can cause agonizing headaches, as well as other problems such as visual disturbances and nausea. It affects about one person in ten, and is most common among younger people. The causes are not properly understood, but it is believed that the arteries leading to the brain become first narrowed then dilated, and interfere with the normal blood flow to the brain. This in some ways resembles the cause of a vascular headache. It is known that certain foods can trigger off a migraine attack in susceptible individuals; chocolate, cheese, red wine and sherry are all implicated in this. In other people, stress or worry can precipitate an attack.

There is usually a warning period before a migraine attack when the sufferer can anticipate what is to follow. He may feel tired and low, with a vague feeling of malaise. Or, in some people, there may be quite severe visual disturbances such as flashing lights or jagged coloured lines. These preliminary warnings may immediately precede an attack, or may persist for many hours or even days before the migraine proper. The migraine itself is an intense gripping pain which can last for several hours, and is followed by a period of weakness.

Self-help can be useful to the migraine sufferer, who should avoid foods known to cause the problem or take steps to relieve stress when the warning symptoms are experienced. During an attack, most migraine sufferers find it beneficial to rest in a darkened room. There are several medical treatments for migraine, some of which control the abnormal dilation of the blood vessels supplying the brain. It is important to seek medical advice if you experience migraines, both to control the symptoms and to exclude related medical problems.

Migraine attacks are often heralded by vision disturbances. These may last from five to twenty minutes. They are caused by blood vessels in the brain and retina clamping down and some people experience numbness and weakness auras. The vascular headache then ensues. This is caused by dilation of the blood vessels within the skull which stretches the pain-sensitive fibres in the vessels' walls.

SCINTILLA

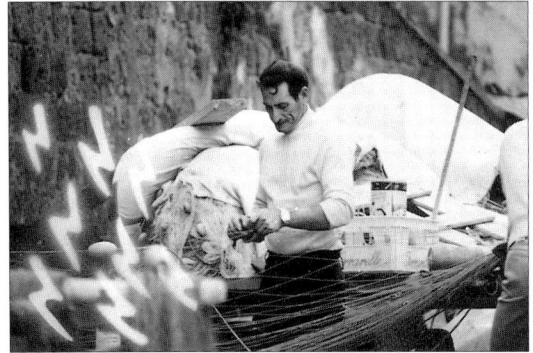

Bright arc of jagged zig-zags on one side obliterates object

HALF VISION

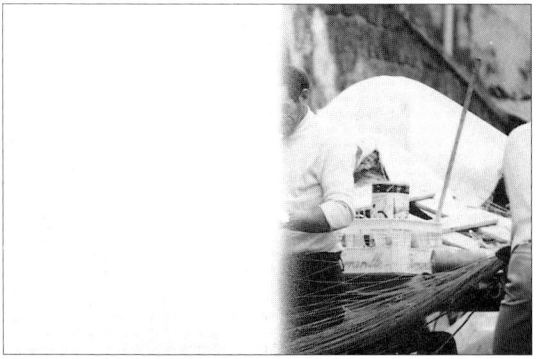

One side of object disappears completely

TUNNEL VISION

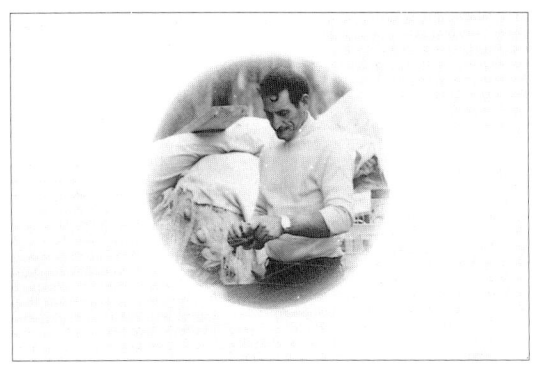

Outside edge of object missing

AURA

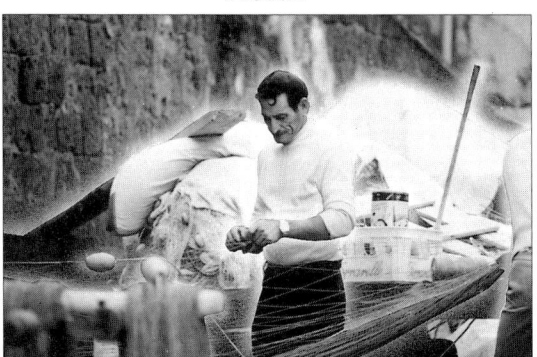

Edges of object look haloed

COLDS AND INFLUENZA

Both colds and influenza are caused by viruses (and cannot, therefore, be treated with antibiotics), but influenza is a much more severe illness, which certainly doesn't clear up in a couple of days. If you do contract influenza, you are likely to need a week or two to recuperate.

There are three influenza viruses, A, B and C, but it is A and B which cause interpandemic and pandemic infection waves. In 1977 a whole population had grown up without exposure to the H_1N_1 strain and the effects were again devastating. Experts predict which strain is current and vaccinate people who may be particularly at risk.

•**A₁ flu**
1947-57
Antigenic description: H_1N_1

•**Asian flu**
1957-68
Antigenic description: H_2N_2

•**Hong Kong flu**
1968
Antigenic description: H_3N_2

•**USSR/Russian flu**
1977
Antigenic description: H_1N_1

Colds can be caused by anyone of nearly 200 different viruses. After the infection you become immune to one virus, but there are still plenty of different viruses to which you haven't yet developed immunity. The result is often that you get one cold after another; each time, the infection has a different cause.

Cold viruses usually attack the nasal passages and upper throat. They may also infect the voice-box or larynx, causing laryngitis or, if they attack the lungs, bronchitis. Because there are so many different viruses, the symptoms vary widely. The running nose and streaming eyes, together with sneezing, are classic early symptoms. Later, catarrh, coughing and hoarseness are common, and perhaps even a slight fever. If you develop a high temperature the problem is likely to be influenza.

A cold lasts for varying lengths of time, depending on the virus involved. Unfortunately there is no cure, despite the pet remedies which may be recommended. All you can do is treat the symptoms. Keep yourself warm (but not too warm), drink plenty of liquids and take aspirin at the recommended dose to keep down your temperature. Don't bother to 'feed a cold'; this is another of those myths that don't work.

If you have a cold there's no point in bothering the doctor unless you already have some other serious health problem which you think may be affected by it; diabetes, for example. But if the symptoms last for more than a week or two, it is best to consult your doctor.

Influenza A much more unpleasant condition. The flu virus spreads into the bloodstream and the symptoms are chills and fever, often alternating, pains in the muscles and joints, headache, sore throat and, in the later stages, a hacking cough. Your temperature may soar to 39°C (102°F) or more, but will usually subside after about three days, leaving you feeling weak and wobbly for a week or ten days. Some doctors believe that the after-effects can last much longer than this.

Once you have contracted flu, there's no point trying to fight if off. Retire to bed, drink plenty of water or fruit juice and take aspirin or paracetamol at the proper dosage. If the symptoms continue or worsen after a few days, call your doctor. When the infection has run its course, you may feel low and depressed for a while. There is some evidence that taking multi-vitamin tablets *after* a flu infection may help speed recovery. High-dose vitamin C tablets have been recommended to prevent and treat both flu and the common cold, but very careful medical research has failed to confirm that they work.

Influenza usually occurs in epidemics, and it is highly infectious, being spread, like colds, in water droplets sneezed out by infected people, usually before they even realize that they are ill. Vaccinations are available, and these are often recommended for people known to be at particular risk (with lung disease, for example). However, most doctors can give influenza vaccinations on request, although the vaccination gives only partial protection, as there are several different flu viruses, and unless the vaccine contains the right ones, no proper immunity will develop. Flu viruses mutate every few years, so they will probably never be completely controlled by vaccines as the viruses are no longer recognized ·by the body's defences and are able to overcome any immunity that has been acquired. This mutation is called a shifting antigen, and it protects the virus from antibodies.

ALLERGY AND ASTHMA

Allergies such as hay fever and allergic rashes or itching are caused by the body's natural defences over-reacting to a substance that is not actually a threat to health. It is an exaggerated version of the normal immune response, called hypersensitivity, and it can develop after repeated exposure to a harmless substance like pollen or certain foods. The substance causing the problem is called an allergen.

The body's reaction can take many different forms and will depend on where exactly in the body the immune system clashes with the allergen. In hay fever, pollen is inhaled and the allergic reaction takes place largely in the nasal passages, causing fierce itching, swelling of the nasal membranes, copious mucus discharge and sometimes a slight fever. A food allergy may cause vomiting and, if the allergen is absorbed into the blood and carried round the body, there may be rashes and itching skin or headaches. Allergy to external contact can also cause rashes, which may lead to eczema, or eventually, to dermatitis.

The house-dust mite lives on the shed skin-scales of humans which fill the dust and dirt in every house. People can become sensitized to proteins on the mites, so that even dead mites can produce allergic symptoms of sneezing and runny eyes similar to hay fever; others get asthma on exposure.

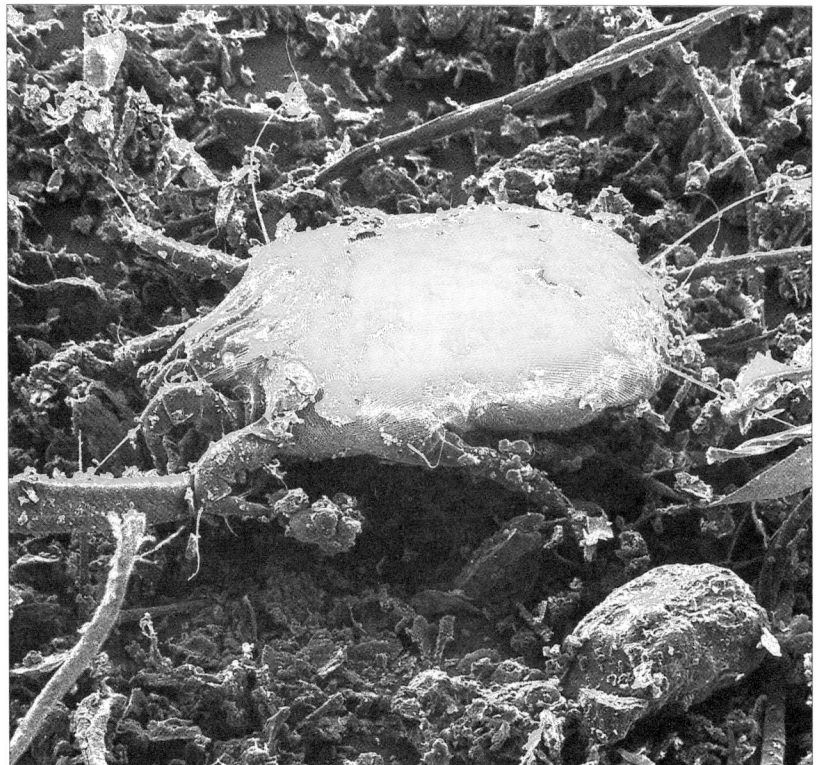

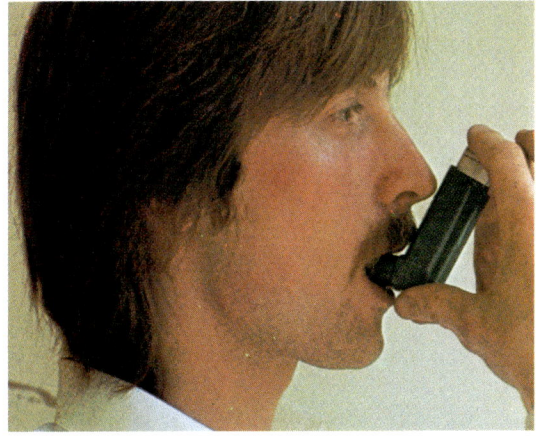

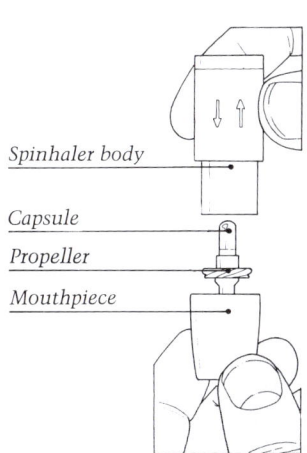

Spinhaler body

Capsule
Propeller
Mouthpiece

The aerosol spray (*above*) for controlling asthma is used by breathing out then spraying and inhaling to draw the drug deep into the lungs. A spinhaler (*above right*) propels the drug into the lungs and can be reloaded with a new capsule, inserted into the propeller. The capsule is then pierced as the body of the spinhaler is replaced.

Asthma An allergic condition, often caused by sensitivity to household dust or, more particularly, the millions of microscopic mites that infest dust and bedding. The reaction causes spasms or contractions of the muscles wrapped around the bronchi and smaller bronchioles carrying air in and out of the lungs. These airways become partly obstructed, causing wheezing and breathlessness.

Asthma usually appears in childhood, but it may sometimes appear for the first time later in life. Attacks are sometimes triggered by stress or exercise, or by exposure to obvious allergens such as animal fur or feathers. More often, however, an attack has no obvious cause.

When an attack begins, there is usually a feeling of tightness across the chest, followed by wheezing. It is usually harder to breathe out than to inhale. Occasionally the breathlessness can become so severe that the sufferer becomes blue unless immediate treatment is given.

Between two and three per cent of adults have asthma, but fortunately, modern treatments control the condition very well for most of them. A special inhaler containing a powdered drug called sodium cromoglycate has to be used regularly to prevent attacks, while drugs called bronchodilators should be taken if an attack has started.

Most asthmatics are perfectly able to control their condition by using the treatment prescribed by their doctor. Several famous athletes are sufferers. However, asthma is not a disease for self-treatment. There are no safe or effective herbal, folk or traditional remedies and, as asthma can be dangerous if untreated, proper medical supervision is absolutely essential. Usually an asthmatic will undergo a range of tests designed to identify any allergies that could precipitate an attack so that they may be avoided.

Other forms of allergy Some, such as hay fever, can be controlled by drugs called antihistamines, which are generally effective although they can cause sleepiness. Most of these drugs can be bought at the chemists, although you should check with your doctor before starting them. Some people can be 'desensitized' by a series of vaccinations containing the allergen, which gradually accustom the immune system to the allergen so that the hypersensitivity reaction no longer occurs. These vaccinations are not always effective, and they generally need to be taken for a considerable time before worthwhile results are obtained.

ARTHRITIS AND HOW TO COPE WITH IT

The constant use we make of our joints means that any problems with joints are apparent as soon as they begin to develop. Diseases affecting the joints are forms of arthritis, of which there are two distinct types: osteoarthritis and rheumatoid arthritis.

Joints allow bones to move against each other without causing damage. The smooth ends of the bone are covered with a layer of cartilage, a slippery, resilient material, which looks like milky plastic. Cartilage allows the bones to slide across one another without causing any damage, and with a minimum of friction.

This is called a synovial joint. Between the pads of cartilage in this joint is a fluid-filled bag called the synovial membrane, containing an oily, lubricating fluid, which allows the joint to move with very little friction.

Osteoarthritis Joints are capable of repairing normal wear and tear, at least for as long as the rest of the body repairs itself properly. But in osteoarthritis, the normal repair process breaks down. This may be due to wear and tear or to over-use; or it may be the failure of the repair process in old age. The condition is common among men who have jobs requiring repetitive exertion and among dancers and athletes. It is also very common in people who are grossly overweight and who are placing enormous strain on their hips and knee joints.

In osteoarthritis the smooth cartilage overlying the ends of the bones begins to wear out. It becomes hard and brittle, develops cracks and eventually starts to flake away. This causes pain in the joint and eventually restricts mobility. As the erosion continues, the ends of the bones are exposed, and the two bones in the joint grind together. This wears away the bone, and, as it attempts to repair itself, jagged spurs develop, which reduce movement still further. The lack of movement causes the muscles around the joint to waste, so the arthritic limb eventually becomes thin and weak.

Osteoarthritis is the commonest form of arthritic disease, and X-rays can detect its signs in at least nine out of ten people over the age of 40. Osteoarthritis can probably be regarded as part of the normal ageing process, and although it can be painful, the worst feature for most sufferers is the lack of mobility it causes. Fewer men than women suffer from this form of arthritis.

Rheumatoid arthritis Although this too affects the joints, it is a quite different disease. It is a systemic condition, affecting the whole system rather than just one or two joints. People with rheumatoid arthritis feel thoroughly ill, rather than just having local joint pain as in osteoarthritis.

Although its causes are not understood, rheumatoid arthritis is thought to be a disorder of the immune system, in which the body begins to attack itself. The synovial membrane, which produces the lubricating joint fluid, becomes inflamed and thickened, and the fluid in the joint capsule loses its lubricating properties. The whole joint becomes red and painful, and movement is difficult, particularly after a rest, as the whole joint stiffens up. The continuous inflammation can lead to bone damage and destruction of the joint. The systemic effects may be unpleasant, and often the onset of the disease is preceded by a general listlessness or weakness. This form of arthritis appears in acute flare-ups, which may diminish for a

Cervical spondylosis develops as a result of many years of wear and tear to the cervical vertebrae at the base of the neck. The discs of cartilage between the vertebrae become narrow and thin. This leads to pressure on the spinal nerves going to and from the spine.

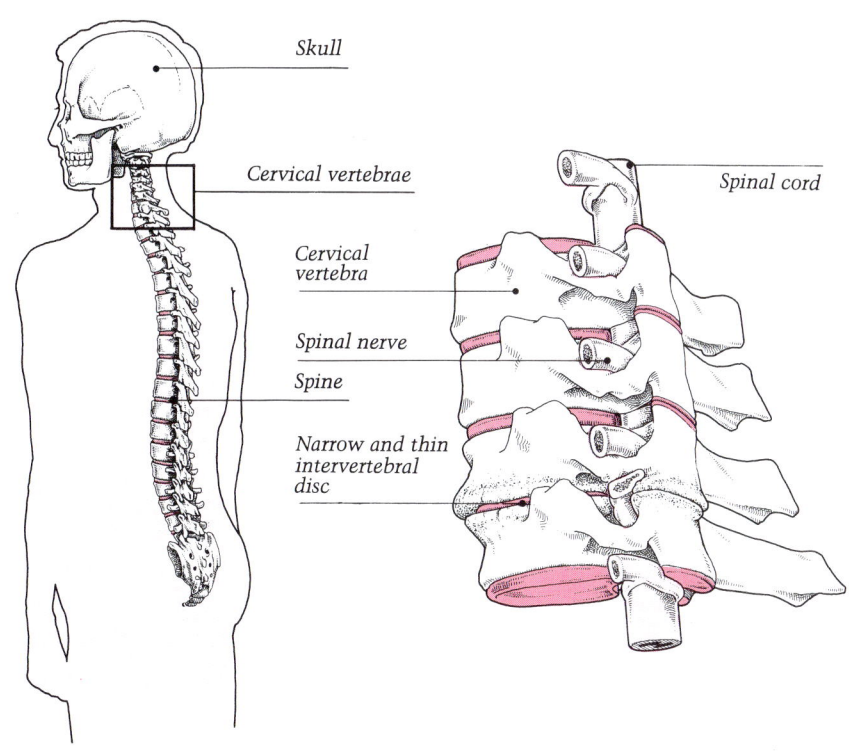

Skull

Cervical vertebrae

Spinal cord

Cervical vertebra

Spinal nerve

Spine

Narrow and thin intervertebral disc

while before the next episode. Unlike osteoarthritis, which generally affects the most active or heavily used joints, rheumatoid arthritis can attack any joint - even those in the spine.

Ankylosing spondylitis A disorder which is related to rheumatoid arthritis and specifically affects the spine. It affects ten times more men than women, usually attacking those in the 20 to 40 age group and, frequently, men who have led a very active life. Ankylosing spondylitis causes damage to the joints between the vertebrae, eventually making them fuse together and so preventing normal flexing of the spine. The problem usually starts in the lower back where the spine is attached to the pelvis, and gradually works up the spine. Like rheumatoid arthritis, ankylosing spondylitis is a systemic condition and affects various parts of the body. The sufferer may feel listless and have chest pains as well as the spinal stiffness and pain. Oddly enough it also causes iritis, a condition in which the eyes become painful and inflamed. Like other forms of arthritis, ankylosing spondylitis varies from a chronic course to acute flare-ups which need intensive treatment. If not controlled properly, it causes very severe spinal damage and can result in permanent deformity of the spine.

All types of arthritis are usually treated with aspirin or related analgesics called non-steroidal anti-inflammatory drugs (NSAIDs). These are related to aspirin and reduce the inflammation, which causes further joint damage, and help to control arthritic pain. Some much stronger drugs, which are used only in severe rheumatoid arthritis, may be prescribed by specialist arthritis clinics.

You can do a great deal for yourself if you are unlucky enough to suffer from arthritis. Your doctor will probably give you special advice on exercise and other helpful measures, and there are several patient organizations that can provide help and advice.

In general, if you suffer from osteoarthritis, you will be advised to rest and to lose weight to avoid putting any more strain on damaged joints. A walking stick can be used to take a lot of weight off the knee and hip joints, and regular gentle exercise of the type recommended by your doctor will prevent your muscles becoming weak through under-use.

If you have rheumatoid arthritis, the problem is largely to avoid stiffness, and gentle exercise such as swimming is very useful. Once more, your doctor or clinic will recommend the type of exercise most suitable for your condition. Obviously, in mild arthritis, more vigorous exercise is possible (and desirable) than in more severe disease, when the joint may already be badly damaged and could become even worse if you over-exercise.

The long-term prospects for arthritis sufferers are now very good. Drugs can control the pain of osteoarthritis and help relieve the stiffness, although the damaged joints cannot repair themselves. In rheumatoid arthritis, which affects about one person in every 200, at any age (even children), modern treatment can prevent the joint deformity that was

Hydrotherapy pools are of great advantage to the arthritis sufferer because the water supports the weight of the body allowing a much fuller range of joint movement than is normally possible.

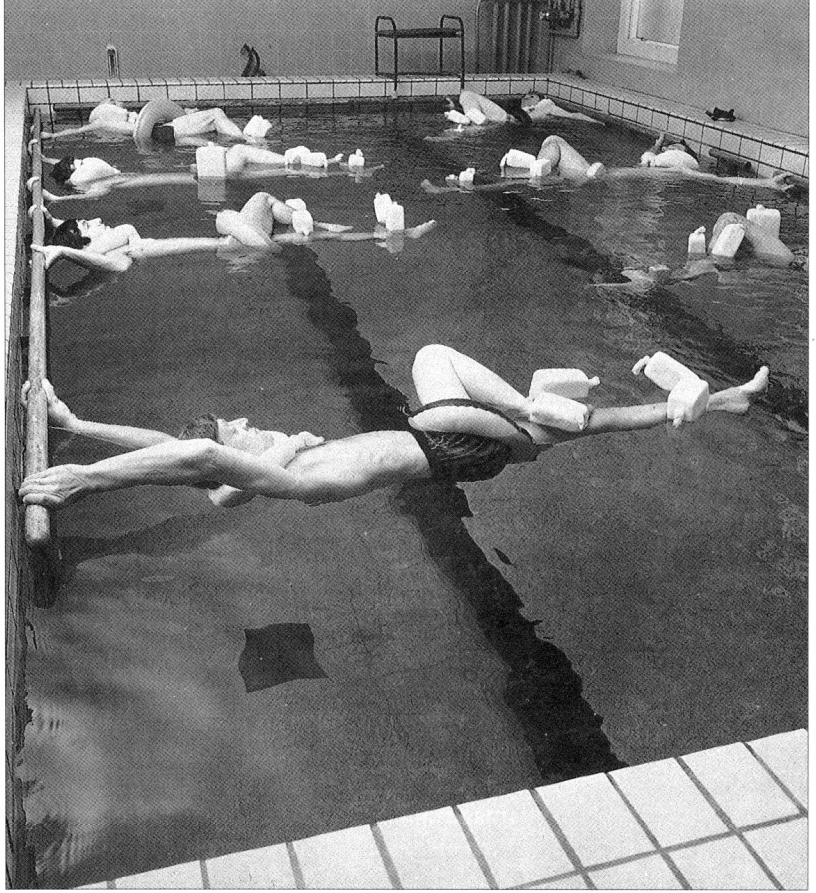

formerly common. About 45 per cent of sufferers recover completely from the first flare-up and never have another bout, and for most of the remainder, the disease can be kept well under control.

GOUT

Gout is another, less common, form of arthritis. More common after the age of 45, 95 per cent of all sufferers are men.

Gout is a metabolic disease: it is caused by a malfunction of the body chemistry, which results in tiny crystals of waste uric acid being deposited around and in the joints, especially those of the toes and hands. Uric acid is a common waste product, usually eliminated by the kidneys, and the reason for the malfunction is not known.

Although gout has traditionally been the subject of jokes, its symptoms are far from funny. The affected joint becomes painful, red and swollen, and the urine becomes discoloured. An acute attack can last for a week or more; it will then subside for a while before reappearing. There is also a chronic form in which there is continuous pain and inflammation. As the uric acid crystals continue to accumulate, the joint becomes permanently swollen and distorted, and there may also be kidney damage.

Diet is implicated in gout, and your doctor may ask you to cut down on certain foods, such as liver and kidneys, strawberries, rhubarb and alcohol, all of which are thought to raise blood levels of uric acid. Your doctor may prescribe pain-killing drugs, which reverse the balance of uric acid in your body; these drugs may need to be continued for life.

BACK PAIN — 'SLIPPED DISC'

Slipped disc is a term usually and inaccurately used to describe acute back pain. The true prolapsed disc is a quite severe condition, in which there is definite physical damage to part of the back. It affects twice as many men as women.

The bony vertebrae surrounding the spinal cord are hinged together to allow the back to bend. The vertebrae are separated by the intervertebral discs. These are made of rubbery material, with a jelly-like core, and they cushion the vertebrae while allowing some movement. The soft core of the discs becomes less resilient with age and, if put to severe strain, may burst out between the vertebrae causing a prolapse. More rarely, the disc actually breaks up. The damaged portions of disc, and the vertebrae themselves, press upon the nerves leaving the spine and can cause intense pain or tingling anywhere from the neck downwards, depending on the position of the prolapsed disc.

Treatment for acute back ache varies. Rest flat in bed for several days taking analgesics, until the pain eases off, and then very gently mobilize yourself. Some disc damage can be treated by wearing a corset to immobilize the back while the disc heals. More serious damage may need surgical treatment, removing part of the vertebrae or fusing two adjacent vertebrae together to prevent further damage (spinal fusion).

BACK PAIN

Numerous diseases are associated with being overweight or actually obese, including hypertension, heart problems, atherosclerosis and diabetes (see Chapter 2). These conditions seem to be caused by changes in our body chemistry, but others are caused more directly, by the effects of extra weight on the joints. One of the most common disorders of this type is low back pain, which is also widespread among men of normal weight and which probably affects about eight out of ten men at some time in their lives.

Pain and stiffness can develop suddenly or gradually and may be continuous or appear for only a short time. The cause of most cases of low back pain is thought to be an overstretched ligament or muscle in the spine, which causes nearby muscles to go into painful spasm. Sometimes muscles in the back or elsewhere can go into spasm for no apparent reason. This pain in the lower back is sometimes called lumbago, and it is often caused by heavy, unaccustomed exertion such as digging the garden or moving furniture or constant bending. The pain tends to be nagging and non-specific.

If you suffer from back pain, you should be careful about the loads you put on your spine. While the pain is actually there, you will need no reminder to avoid twisting awkwardly or lifting heavy items. More dangerous is the time when you don't have the pain and forget to be careful.

Aspirin is as good a treatment as any for any non-specific back pain, but you can do a lot to avoid further problems by taking deliberate precautions to protect your back. First and most obvious is to get rid of any excess weight that is increasing the work your spine has to cope with. Being overweight also causes people to move less freely, so they are more liable to cause themselves damage.

It has long been known that a relatively hard bed minimizes back problems. The so-called 'orthopaedic' bed is, in fact, a misnomer and is usually nothing more than an excuse for the manufacturers to over-charge. All that is required is a fairly firm mattress, or a board beneath the mattress to stop it sagging; or you could put your mattress on the floor. This stops your spine bending unnaturally whether you sleep on your side or on your back.

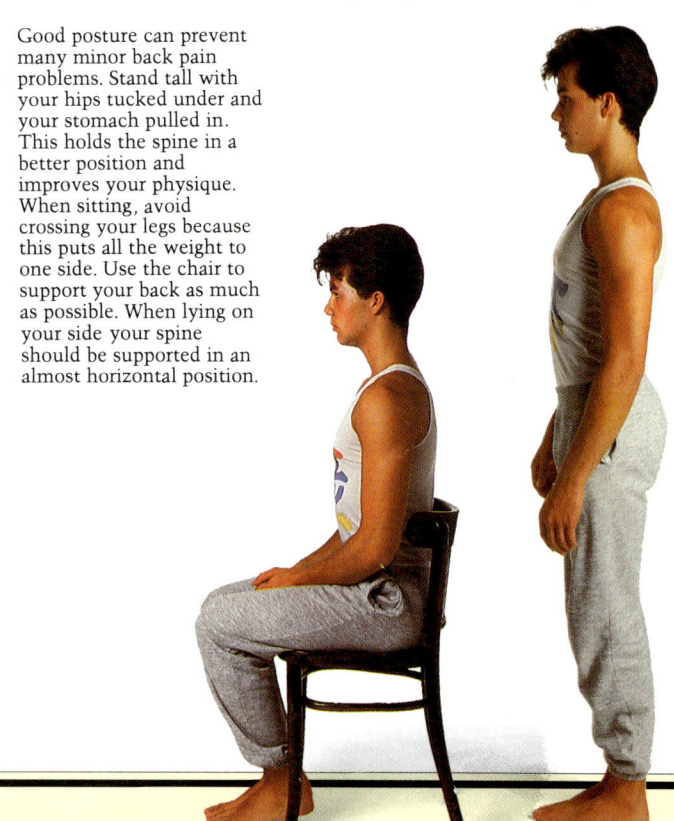

Good posture can prevent many minor back pain problems. Stand tall with your hips tucked under and your stomach pulled in. This holds the spine in a better position and improves your physique. When sitting, avoid crossing your legs because this puts all the weight to one side. Use the chair to support your back as much as possible. When lying on your side your spine should be supported in an almost horizontal position.

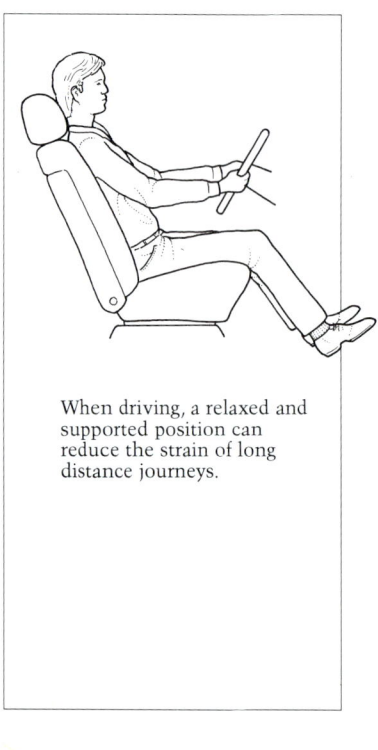

When driving, a relaxed and supported position can reduce the strain of long distance journeys.

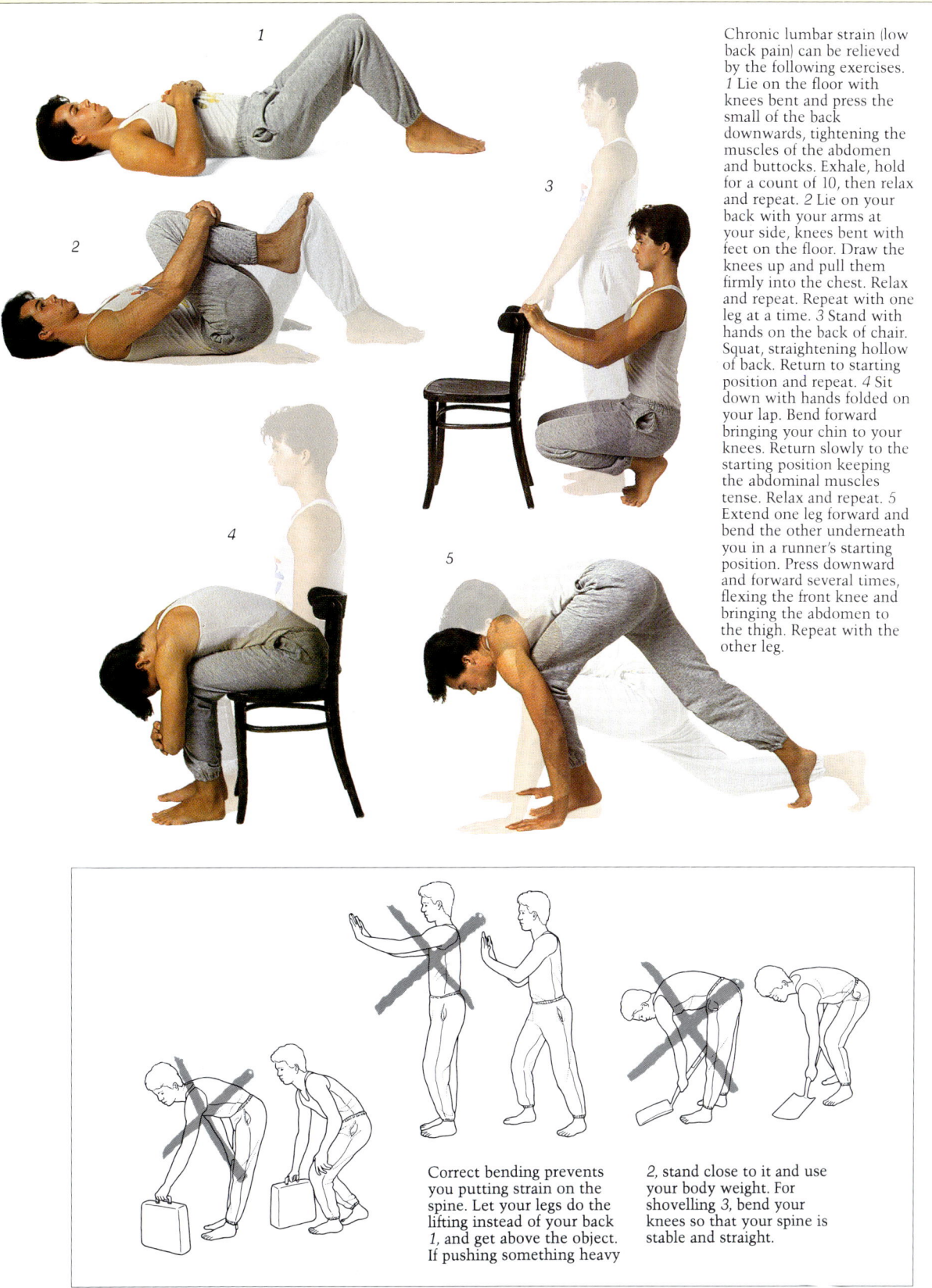

Chronic lumbar strain (low back pain) can be relieved by the following exercises. *1* Lie on the floor with knees bent and press the small of the back downwards, tightening the muscles of the abdomen and buttocks. Exhale, hold for a count of 10, then relax and repeat. *2* Lie on your back with your arms at your side, knees bent with feet on the floor. Draw the knees up and pull them firmly into the chest. Relax and repeat. Repeat with one leg at a time. *3* Stand with hands on the back of chair. Squat, straightening hollow of back. Return to starting position and repeat. *4* Sit down with hands folded on your lap. Bend forward bringing your chin to your knees. Return slowly to the starting position keeping the abdominal muscles tense. Relax and repeat. *5* Extend one leg forward and bend the other underneath you in a runner's starting position. Press downward and forward several times, flexing the front knee and bringing the abdomen to the thigh. Repeat with the other leg.

Correct bending prevents you putting strain on the spine. Let your legs do the lifting instead of your back *1*, and get above the object. If pushing something heavy *2*, stand close to it and use your body weight. For shovelling *3*, bend your knees so that your spine is stable and straight.

CANCER – THE RISKS AND THE TREATMENT

Cancer is the most feared of all diseases. It is common, often fatal, striking its victims without apparent cause. Yet much of this fear is misplaced, as a diagnosis of 'cancer' is by no means a death sentence.

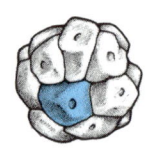

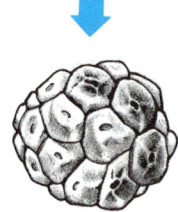

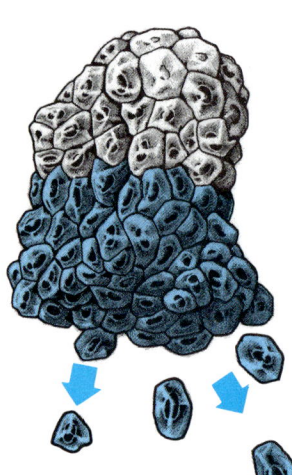

Cancer occurs when something disrupts the genetic coding of a cell. The genes within each cell carry a code which governs how and when that type of cell should divide. The messages sent by the genes can be altered by carcinogens (for example, tobacco or asbestos), by radiation or by certain viruses. The cells begin to divide quickly and at random. Eventually a malignant tumour sheds cancer cells into the bloodstream.

The word 'cancer' is often used incorrectly. A cancer is a malignant tumour, a lump of body tissue that grows and spreads uncontrollably. A benign tumour also grows but will fail to spread and so can usually be removed. The word cancer covers a whole group of diseases, as malignancy can develop in almost any type of tissue or part of the body. Its effects vary widely, depending on where it develops.

Most body cells are capable of reproducing themselves; in fact, they do so regularly to repair damaged or worn-out tissues. When a cell becomes cancerous, however, it divides and then continues to divide again and again without stopping, so that a colony of rapidly dividing cells is produced. These cells fail to 'switch-off' their multiplication, as would normal cells. As the tumour develops, some cancerous cells become detached and are carried away in the bloodstream or the lymph system, which drains fluid from the body's cavities. These cells lodge elsewhere in the body and start further colonies. The whole cycle occurs again and again. This spread of cancerous cells is called metastasis, and some cancers undergo this process more readily than others.

As a malignant tumour develops, it interferes with the function of nearby organs and may block or rupture blood vessels. But the causes of most of the effects of the disease are not well understood. Advanced cancer causes rapid weight loss and may also cause severe pain. Occasionally, these symptoms may appear and the sufferer may even die, before the tumour is big enough to cause any serious deterioration in the function of vital organs.

What causes cancer? The unfortunate truth seems to be, almost anything. It is thought that about 80 per cent of all cancers have environmental causes, chemicals in our environment called carcinogens that are capable of transforming a normal cell into the malignant form that divides so rapidly. Some well-known examples of carcinogen are tar from cigarette smoke, asbestos and some chemical dyes and solvents. A few rare cancers are caused by virus infections, and some researchers suspect that many more common cancers may eventually be traced to this source. There may also be a hereditary factor, and there are examples of families in which the condition is exceptionally common.

Nuclear radiation is another known cause. It is known to damage the genes within the cells, preventing normal reproduction of the cells. Other forms of radiation have similar effects, and ultraviolet light, experienced in strong sunlight, is known to cause the skin cancers that are very common in many tropical areas. They are also more common than usual among regular sunbathers, so skin cancer can be classed as an avoidable risk.

Food may be regarded as an environmental factor, and a diet rich in fat and low in fibre can predispose to bowel cancer, while high-fibre, low-fat diets reduce the risks.

Cancer kills one in eight of all people who die before the age of 35, and one in four of those who die above the age of 45. But the rate is falling rapidly for many forms of cancer: the cure rate for diseases such as bowel cancer and certain forms of leukaemia is now very good. The most common cancers in men are lung, stomach, prostate, colon, urinary system and leukaemia.

Because of the way cancer spreads, effective control or cure depends on diagnosing it as early as possible, before metastasis has spread tumours throughout the body. Because there are so many forms of cancer, the warning signs and symptoms are very diverse, but there are several warning signs that you should never neglect.

Lung cancer   Almost all cases of lung cancer start in the bronchi, the tubes carrying air into the lungs, and nearly *all* cases of lung cancer are believed to be caused by smoking; the three in a thousand victims who are not smokers will almost certainly have been exposed to cigarette smoke. The tar in cigarette smoke contains powerful carcinogens (cancer-causing agents), and it is thought that it starts the first cancerous changes in the walls of the bronchi, gradually spreading to the lung. As metastasis takes place, lung cancer can spread to the brain, bones, liver or elsewhere.

There is now no doubt that the more cigarettes are smoked and the earlier the habit starts, the greater is the risk of developing lung cancer. When you stop, the risk gradually diminishes until, after several years, you are no more likely to develop cancer than a life-long non-smoker.

Lung cancer usually becomes apparent when the following symptoms appear in conjunction: a smoker's cough, chronic bronchitis together with blood stains in the phlegm, perhaps breathlessness and occasionally chest pains. These symptoms are often masked by chronic bronchitis, and the condition is then recognized only when it has already metastasized to another organ. This happens in about one in eight cases of lung cancer and makes the condition difficult to treat in its later stages.

When lung cancer is diagnosed by chest X-ray, the diseased part of the lung can often be removed surgically, but this depends on early diagnosis, when the disease is confined to a small area. Chemotherapy may also be used, with powerful cytotoxic drugs, which can sometimes kill the cancer cells but have unpleasant side effects. Early diagnosis is essential if this serious condition is to be treated successfully.

Prostate cancer   Increasingly common among older men, this is an unusual cancer in that it can lie dormant for many years without causing any symptoms. Often, men dying from other causes are found to have a cancer of the prostate that has been quite unsuspected. Probably 15 per cent of men over 40 will have prostate cancer, although it will probably never develop and cause any problems. By the age of 80, nearly all men have it, but it kills only one man in every thousand, so cannot be regarded as a serious threat to life.

If it does metastasize, prostate cancer usually spreads to the bones, which is where it is usually detected. Prostate cancer is generally discovered when an enlarged prostate is being investigated, and an X-ray scan may be carried out to find if it has begun to spread to the bones. Radiotherapy may then be given but, if the cancer has not spread, your doctor will probably only make a regular check to ascertain that it remains dormant.

Cancer of the colon   One of the most common forms of cancer, in Britain it accounts for 14 per cent of all deaths from cancer. The cure rate is, nevertheless, very good and if it is diagnosed early there is an 80 per cent

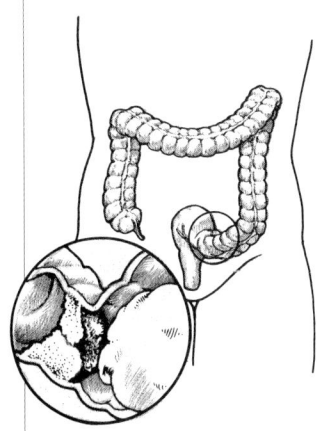

Cancer of the large intestine develops slowly until it obstructs the passage of faeces and causes bleeding and ulceration. However, it can be completely cured if the affected bowel is removed surgically at an early enough stage.

Men contract more of certain types of cancers than do women. Lung cancer is by far the most common cancer among men, but this is because until recently men smoked more than women. This table shows the number of mortalities in Britain in 1981 for the various types of cancer.

- Lung cancer
  29,810 mortalities
- Stomach cancer
  7,050
- Prostate cancer
  5,750
- Colon
  5,060
- Rectum
  3,640
- Pancreas
  3,340
- Bladder
  3,300
- Oesophagus
  2,580
- Leukaemia
  2,010
- Brain
  1,420
- Others
  13,980

More substances found to cause cancer in man have been discovered during the search for occupational hazards than by any other research programme and each represents high risks.

- **Farmers**
Skin cancer
Cancer agent: sunlight
- **Radiologists**
Bone marrow cancer
Cancer agent: radiation
- **Asbestos miners/workers**
Lung cancer
(also stomach, large bowel)
Cancer agent: asbestos
- **Sailors**
Skin cancer
Cancer agent: ultraviolet light
- **Chemical/dye/rubber workers**
Bladder cancer
Cancer agent: aromatic amines
- **Pesticide workers**
Lung and skin cancer
Cancer agent: arsenic
- **Coal gas workers/roofers/asphalters**
Skin, scrotum, lung cancer
Cancer agent: some oils, tar and soot

chance of complete cure.

The cancer develops in the wall of the bowel, forming a large tumour that interferes with bowel function, causing diarrhoea or constipation, with blood-stained faeces. If these symptoms are neglected, the tumour can metastasize to various other parts of the body. It is diagnosed by X-ray, after a barium enema, which outlines the bowel on the X-ray, so that the tumour can be located. A biopsy may be taken during a sigmoidoscopic examination. This procedure differentiates bowel cancer from polyps, which are harmless or benign swellings on the colon wall. However, these too may need to be removed to eliminate any chance of them later becoming malignant.

Treatment is usually by surgery. The affected section of the colon is cut out, and the healthy portions of the gut are rejoined. To give the damaged colon time to recover from the surgery, a temporary colostomy is often performed, in which part of the colon is brought out on the surface of the abdomen, and faeces are discharged through this 'stoma' into a disposable pouch. Sometimes the damage to the colon or rectum is so bad that a permanent colostomy has to be made. Although this sounds unpleasant, once the patient has learned to cope with this new way to evacuate the bowels, he can resume a normal life. Colostomies and similar operations may also be carried out in diseases other than cancer. A high-fibre, low-fat diet is prevention against cancer of the colon.

Cancers of the urinary system   Tumours of the kidney and bladder are relatively uncommon. Both cause colicky pains and are usually first noticed when blood is passed in the urine. In bladder cancer, there is usually low back pain, and a burning sensation when urinating. These cancers are treated by a combination of surgery to remove the tumour, and radiotherapy and chemotherapy to mop up remaining cancerous cells. Provided the condition is diagnosed and treated before it metastasizes, the cure rate is quite good.

Leukaemia   Like cancer in general, the word leukaemia covers a collection of diseases, of which three types affect adults: chronic lymphatic leukaemia, and chronic and acute myeloid leukaemia. (Acute lymphatic leukaemia is the form that primarily affects children.)

Myeloid leukaemia affects the white blood cells produced in the bone marrow, weakening and, in the acute form of the disease, destroying the body's defences against other infections. In chronic lymphatic leukaemia, it is the white blood cells in the lymph system which are affected, and the cancerous lymphocyte cells eventually invade other organs such as the liver and the spleen. These forms of leukaemia are rare conditions, chiefly found amongst the elderly. Treatment by chemotherapy and, in some cases, radiotherapy, can control their progress and keep them in remission for several years.

Skin cancers   There are several types of skin cancer which, unlike some cancers found in other parts of the body, are often possible to identify before they become established and difficult to treat.

Rodent ulcers, or basal cell carcinomas, occur most commonly in fair-skinned people who have had a lot of exposure to bright sunlight. They begin as a small lump, often with a raised border, and grow very slowly. Fortunately they do not metastasize to other parts of the body, and so are fairly easily removed by surgery. Squamous cell carcinomas are similar but

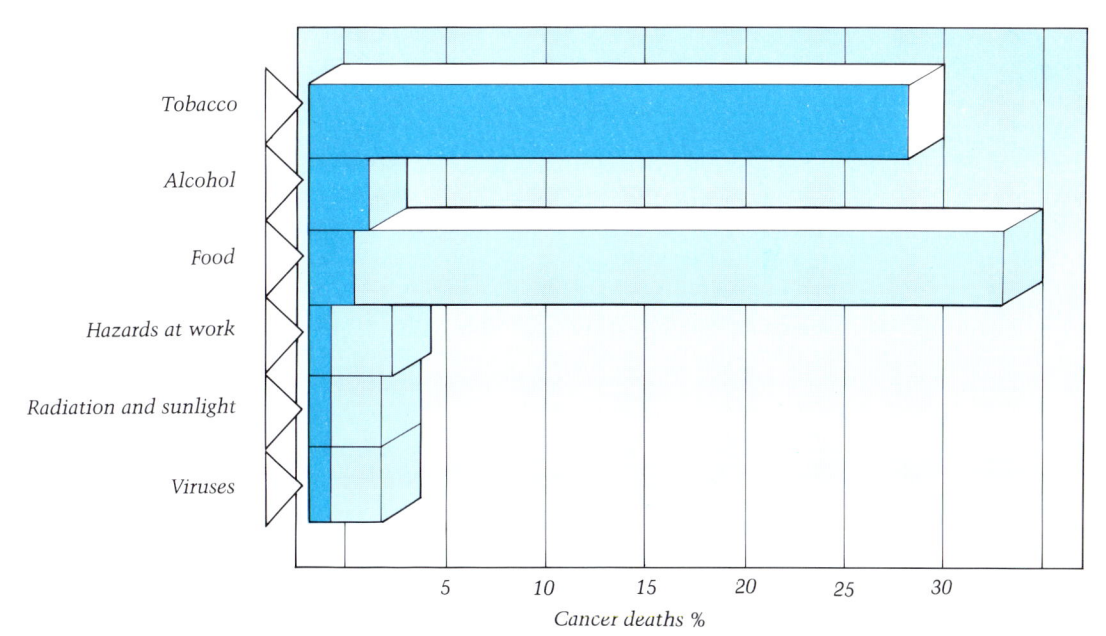

Tobacco

Alcohol

Food

Hazards at work

Radiation and sunlight

Viruses

5　10　15　20　25　30

Cancer deaths %

■ *Definitely preventable cancer deaths*　□ *Possibly preventable cancer deaths*

Cancer causing agents are being discovered all the time. Cancer from tobacco is now regarded as a definitely preventable disease and experts predict that in a few years time diet-related cancers may be preventable in the same way.

are more dangerous because they can spread if not treated promptly. They too are most commonly found in people who have been exposed to strong sunlight over long periods. Both rodent ulcers and squamous cell carcinomas affect about one person in every 1,500 every year. The cure rate for squamous cell carcinomas is about 90 per cent, which emphasizes the need for prompt treatment of any suspicious skin spot or swelling.

Malignant melanoma is a skin cancer which is prone to spread quickly. It usually develops from a pigmented mole which may have been present on the skin since childhood, or may appear in the liver spots found on the skin of old people. The danger signs are any new change in a mole which has been present for a long while. It may become lighter, develop a black edge or bleed occasionally. Any alteration to an existing mole should be promptly reported to the doctor. Once again, like other skin cancers, malignant melanoma is particularly common among middle-aged or elderly people who have spent a long time in sunny climates.

All of these forms of skin cancer are quickly diagnosed by taking a small sample of skin, usually under local anaesthetic. All are treatable if caught early enough.

Other cancers　Because there are so many different types of cancer, most of them quite rare, it is impossible to describe them all here. But it is important to emphasize that you should consult your doctor about any unusual symptoms you think may be a cause for suspicion. This does not mean that you should develop a cancer phobia, which is quite unnecessary now that so many forms of the disease can be controlled. If you stop smoking, reduce your alcohol consumption and improve your diet by reducing fat intake and increasing dietary fibre, you will be doing a lot to reduce the threat of cancer. If you are still concerned, it might be wise to limit your intake of foods which contain food colourings, preservatives and other additives too, although there are no *proven* anti-cancer benefits yet.

DIGESTIVE PROBLEMS

A multitude of complaints, some of which are avoidable, can affect the digestive system, and it is probably easiest to consider these problems in the sequence in which they are encountered as food travels through the digestive system.

Swallowed food passes down a short tube called the oesophagus before entering the stomach. Here, a mixture of powerful acids and enzymes start the process of digestion. The point at which the oesophagus enters the stomach is the site at which a painful, though seldom serious, condition called **hiatus hernia** can develop. This is caused when the diaphragm, the sheet of muscle separating the chest from the abdomen, becomes weakened. Instead of sealing the lower end of the oesophagus after the food has passed through, the weakened muscle allows the upper end of the stomach to bulge up through the diaphragm so that stomach acid can bubble up, burning the oesophagus and causing painful 'heartburn'.

Hiatus hernia seldom needs medical attention. Its effects can be reduced by eating smaller meals so that the stomach is not overfilled and by taking antacids to reduce the effects of acid on the oesophagus. Heavy lifting and bending are best avoided. You should, however, seek professional diagnosis just in case some other problem is involved.

Gastroenteritis The term actually just means inflammation of the stomach and intestines, and this can be caused by factors ranging from alcohol to infection. It causes nausea, vomiting and diarrhoea, and in the more severe forms caused by bacterial infection, there is usually also a fever. Remember that nausea and vomiting are the stomach's way of getting rid of a problem, and if the stomach wall is inflamed, it is in no condition to produce the powerful chemicals needed for digestion. Starving yourself for a short while gives it a rest while it can recover.

In any form of gastroenteritis, excess fluid loss is the greatest health risk, and it is essential to drink large amounts of water or diluted fruit juice. If the condition lasts for more than a few days, you should take special electrolyte mixtures. These are usually sachets containing the chemicals likely to be lost from the body when there is persistent diarrhoea; they can be obtained from most chemist shops.

Indigestion Although a common condition, this is not actually a disease at all but a symptom of a number of conditions. It is a feeling of discomfort caused because something is not right with the stomach or the way it works. Indigestion may be caused by eating particular foods; cucumber and onions affect many people in this way, and you will soon learn what to avoid. It can also be an emotional condition, with attacks occurring when you are nervous or stressed. In many cases, indigestion is caused by trapped wind, caused by air swallowed with food that has been eaten too quickly. Most people quickly adjust to indigestion, altering their eating habits to avoid discomfort. It is seldom a serious problem, although it can be a symptom of something that needs medical attention.

Peptic ulcers, which affect the stomach or the duodenum (the first part of the intestine) are common, especially among men: 90 per cent of all sufferers are male and one in five men will be affected. Only about 10 per cent of these ulcers form in the stomach (gastric ulcers), most being in the duodenum, the short length of gut connecting the stomach to the small intestine. The cause of ulcers is not properly understood, but it seems to be

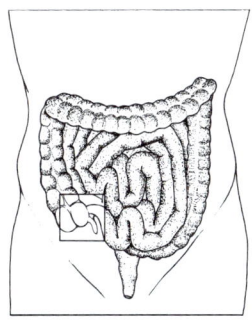

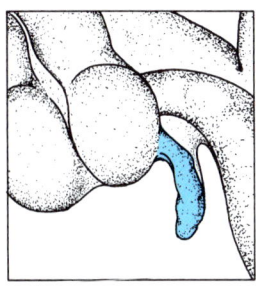

The worm-shaped appendix is the size of a little finger and lies at the point where the ileum of the small intestine leads into the caecum of the large intestine. It has no function in humans.

a failure of the mechanism protecting the stomach and duodenum from its corrosive contents. When the protection is breached, the acid and enzymes eat into the gut wall, causing severe burning pain. This pain is usually associated with eating, when the digestive juices are produced. Gastric ulcer pain is usually worse when food enters the stomach; duodenal ulcer pain when food leaves the stomach (about 2-4 hours after eating).

At first, peptic ulcers are uncomfortable and worrying, but if they are not treated they can be a serious threat to health. As they become deeper, ulcers bleed, and they can perforate right through the wall of the intestine, causing peritonitis or massive haemorrhage.

You should obtain medical advice. Effective drug treatments are now available, and your doctor will probably recommend that you take regular antacids to reduce the effects of stomach acid, that you change your eating habits, that you stop smoking, and learn to relax. This last point is very important, as it is known that continual stress is implicated in the development of ulcers. About half of all peptic ulcers clear up without medical treatment, but they often recur after a few years. Duodenal ulcers are especially common among heavy smokers, and a heavy alcohol intake makes both gastric and duodenal ulcers much worse.

Further down the digestive system is the appendix, which is positioned at the point where the narrow small intestine widens out into the colon, in the lower right side of the abdomen. It is a small, finger-like projection from the gut, with no digestive function, although in other mammals it is much bigger and plays an important part in digestion.

Appendicitis This affects approximately one person in every 500 each year, the appendix becomes inflamed and infected, usually after becoming blocked. The condition is often associated with a low-fibre diet, and is almost unknown in places such as rural Africa, where large amounts of fibre are eaten.

The symptoms of appendicitis are vague abdominal discomfort, which quickly becomes localized as a severe continuous pain in the lower right of the abdomen. Once appendicitis has developed, you will be in no doubt of the need for urgent medical attention, and the appendix can then be removed surgically. The so-called 'grumbling appendix' is probably nothing at all to do with the appendix; it is more likely to be caused by a general colonic sensitivity, known as irritable bowel syndrome, in which pain is caused by spasms of the intestinal wall. This condition is partly emotional in nature and may be aggravated by certain foods.

Diverticular disease, or diverticulitis, is an increasing problem. Diverticula, small pouches on the wall of the colon, occur in one in three adults aged over 65, although they do not always cause symptoms. Sometimes trapped faeces inflame and infect the pouch, which are then very painful. If left untreated, serious abscesses can result.

Like many other diseases of the developed nations, diverticular disease seems to be associated with our diet, especially with a low intake of fibre. It is thought that our low-fibre diet, which leads to chronic constipation in many people, forces the colon to work much harder to move hard pellets of faeces along. This causes unusually high pressure inside the colon, and its lining may burst through weak areas where the blood vessels enter, producing diverticula.

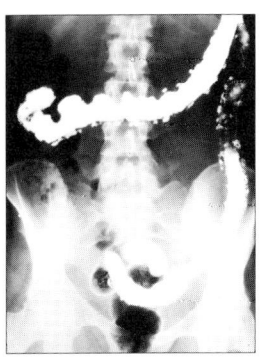

An X ray following a barium enema shows ulcers in the colon as white dots. The condition is ulcerative colitis.

If your doctor suspects that you have diverticulitis, he may carry out an X-ray after a barium meal or may conduct a sigmoidoscope examination, in which a flexible viewing tube is inserted into the colon to inspect its walls. **Inflammatory bowel disease (IBD)** A term covering both ulcerative colitis and Crohn's disease, two unpleasant and potentially serious conditions that are, fortunately, quite uncommon. Both cause long-term abdominal discomfort and, usually, blood-stained diarrhoea. They must be treated by the doctor, and treatment usually continues for life.

The last sections of the digestive system are the rectum and anus, through which faeces are discharged. This is the area affected by **haemorrhoids**, or piles, swellings of the veins in the walls of the rectum and anus, which are probably caused by straining as a result of constipation. This increases the blood pressure in these thin-walled veins, causing them to bulge and permanently stretch their walls. Most adults have haemorrhoids to some extent, but they do not usually cause any pain until they are enlarged. Eventually the damaged veins may bulge through the anus, and, being so thin-walled, may bleed and become very painful.

A switch to a high-fibre diet softens the faeces and means that less straining is needed when faeces are passed. Mild haemorrhoids sometimes clear up spontaneously with the switch to a better diet, but you may need medical or surgical treatment to shrink or remove them. Don't be put off from seeking medical help by the old horror stories of agonizing treatment. Modern treatment is quick and effective and usually gives a permanent cure, provided you take the proper dietary measures to prevent recurrence.

Many of these diseases of the digestive system are associated with an unhealthy diet, and diet is also thought to be implicated in causing **gallstones**, small pebble-like deposits within the gall-bladder, which is next to the liver. Men are only a quarter as likely to get gallstones as women but, with advancing age, they are still very common. Many people have gallstones without realizing it, but they occasionally block the bile duct leading to the duodenum and cause extremely painful biliary colic, sometimes followed by jaundice. Usually, however, the only symptoms are abdominal discomfort after eating fatty foods, which is when the gall-bladder normally passes bile along the bile ducts to help with the digestion of fat.

Gallstones can be composed of various substances, and among the more common forms are those based on cholesterol, a fat-like substance important in various cardiovascular diseases. Men with this type of stone usually have a high blood-cholesterol level.

If you do have gallstones, surgery may be required to remove them and your gall-bladder, thus preventing their recurrence. Some drug treatments help to dissolve certain types of gallstones, and a switch to a low-fat diet is usually recommended.

The liver is a large and very complex organ which has many different functions. It regulates the availability, storage and usage of chemicals throughout the body, and processes nutrients absorbed into the body from digestion. Any disorder which affects the proper function of the liver, the largest single organ in the body, is potentially serious.

Hepatitis A liver infection caused by viruses, and is actually two quite different infections. Hepatitis A is a flu-like infection caused when the virus is spread by contact with food or water which has been contaminated by infected sewage. As with other types of hepatitis, one of the symptoms is jaundice: a yellowing of the skin and the whites of the eyes caused by the failure of the liver to break down a pigment called bilirubin, which accumulates in the blood. Recovery is usually complete, though it may take several weeks, and the sufferer feels very weak for several months afterwards.

Hepatitis B is much more serious, and is usually spread by contact with infected blood. It is common among drug users who share contaminated hypodermic needles that have not been sterilized. The 'B' type can also be spread via infected saliva, semen, and vaginal secretions, and is therefore also a sexually transmitted disease. The symptoms are more severe than those for Hepatitis A, but recovery is usually complete. About one person in every 1,000 is a carrier of the disease, although they have no symptoms. Carriers and people who have previously suffered from Hepatitis B are not permitted to give blood, to avoid the risk of spreading the infection.

Cirrhosis Another form of liver deterioration, a scarring of the liver tissues which can follow Hepatitis B infection, or may be caused by alcoholism or some other medical condition. As more and more of the liver is affected, it loses progressively more of its function, at first causing weakness, nausea, and a tendency to bleed easily. In the later stages, when there is liver failure, the whole body becomes swollen, and there is deterioration of the mental faculties. There is little that can be done in the way of self-help. It is essential to remove the underlying factors which caused the problem, and this means medical supervision, usually to control a drinking problem.

OCCUPATIONAL HEALTH RISKS

In its broadest sense, the term occupational illness can encompass a huge range of diseases. Some of these are well known, and specific regulations are designed to protect workers from their effects.

Industrial health hazards Coal and stone dust have been known for centuries to produce a miners' lung disease called pneumoconiosis, which is the result of the lung's inability to rid itself of these materials. Similar types of lung damage have been caused by the constant inhalation of cotton dust or wood dust or, by farmers, of grain and hay dust. Most industrial premises where dust is generated are obliged by law to install air filters and provide appropriate protective clothing, including masks, to staff who are at risk from the materials they handle.

Some health risks have become apparent only after many years of use. Blue asbestos has recently been recognized as a cause of a rare but fatal form of cancer, and a common material used for years in garages to de-grease engines and car parts is now known to cause liver cancer. Large sums of money are spent on investigating the health effects of industrial materials, and many regulations cover their use. If you have any doubts about materials you may be handling, union officials or local health officers should be able to advise you.

Some occupations carry obvious risks - diving or steel erecting, for instance - but with proper training, the hazards are minimized. For example, only recently has it been realized that the constant use of vibrating tools like chain saws and road drills can cause a strange deterioration of the circulation of blood in the hands.

Noise is a definite occupational risk, and increasingly people in noisy jobs are offered, and sometimes obliged by law to wear, ear protectors or ear muffs. Prolonged exposure to loud noise causes eventual deafness and may also have psychological effects related to the high level of stress produced. Eye protectors are issued for use with certain types of machinery, where a single metal splinter could result in the loss of an eye.

Hernias (ruptures) often affect men who lift heavy loads. During violent exertion, the abdominal muscles may be tensed so much that the pressure from the organs in the abdomen forces them to bulge through the muscle sheet. There is usually a muscle weakness or tear at this point. Hernias can also occur elsewhere (see hiatus hernia, discussed earlier under digestive problems), but the lower abdominal type is most apparent, causing a large, often uncomfortable bulge. The bulge usually appears fairly slowly, and occasionally the doctor can push the contents back through the abdominal wall. More often a hernia will need surgical treatment to repair the torn abdominal muscles.

Hernias are at first only an inconvenience but, if a length of intestine is trapped in the extruded pouch, there can be serious after-effects, so it is always necessary to get medical treatment in the early stages.

Sprains Another type of injury commonly incurred at work. They are caused when a joint is flexed beyond its normal limits, and usually affect the ankle, after tripping, or the wrist, after a fall.

Joints are held together by flexible, strap-like ligaments; when bent too far, the bones simply lever these ligaments apart, tearing some of their fibres. The tissue around the joint is also damaged, and inflammatory fluid is produced, causing the joint to swell and become inflamed. This process can be minimized and the swelling reduced to some extent by putting the affected joint in ice-cold water or by placing ice packs around it. If you rest the joint as much as possible, the sprain should heal spontaneously in a few days, but it is important to avoid putting too much weight on a sprained joint while it heals and for a short time afterwards.

Dislocations These are caused in the same way as sprains, but are much more severe. A dislocated joint is levered apart and all or most of the retaining tissues are torn. Immediate hospital treatment is necessary, and the injured joint can take a long time to heal. Normally a dislocated joint must be completely immobilized while it heals.

It is not just industrial or manual work that carries health risks, however. Even a sedentary job can exacerbate back problems if your chair is not properly designed, but the most serious health risk of an office job is undoubtedly stress.

Stress causes the whole nervous system to operate at an unusual level of arousal and can lead to numerous emotional and physical problems. Peptic ulcers are a common health problem of the busy executive, together with anxiety and depression. In some jobs, alcoholism is an occupational risk too, and business lunches contribute to obesity and a generally unbalanced diet. Business executives suffer more than their fair share of heart attacks, and they are often subject to all the classic risk factors: over-working, over-eating, under-exercising, smoking and stress.

Death rates among men in different professions is a reflection of a number of factors. Accidents do account for some of the figures, but stress is now accepted as a serious contributor. This may be caused by noise, heat and chemical fumes, or psychological stressors. In general, manual workers die younger than white collar workers. Unskilled workers tend to suffer more from diseases such as cancer, heart failure and chest disorders. Shift workers tend to suffer from gastro-intestinal diseases, and although coronary heart disease is thought of as an executive disease, a survey in America showed that a group of skilled manual workers were two and a half times more likely to have heart attacks than were their managers.

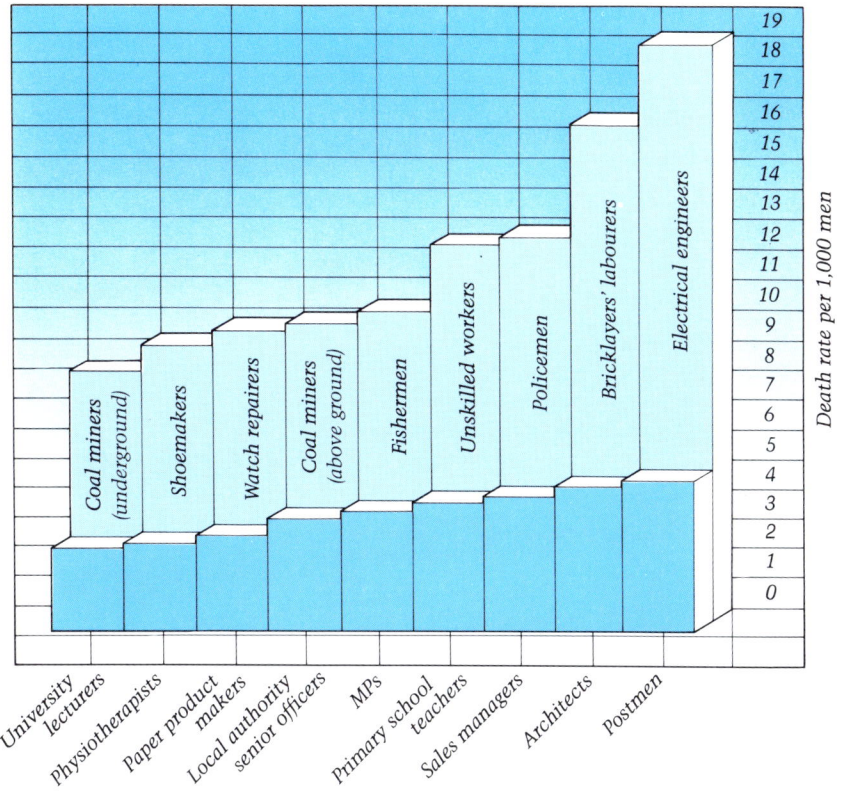

Death rate per 1,000 men

PROSTATE PROBLEMS

The prostate gland is found only in men in a fleshy mass encircling the urethra, along which pass urine and semen. It is actually composed of a mass of smaller glands, which pour their secretions into the urethra. The function of this liquid is uncertain, but it seems to contribute to the semen.

Most men over the age of 45 have some degree of enlargement of the prostate and, as the gland encircles the urethra, this can interfere with the flow of urine from the bladder. Eventually, the normally fleshy prostate becomes hard and inflexible, and the bladder can no longer force urine past it. This causes a weak, dribbly urination, even though there may be a frequent urge to pass urine. Urinary retention may occur, and the bladder becomes distended. A tubular catheter must be quickly passed up the penis to allow the bladder to drain, before back-pressure damages the bladder or kidneys. An additional problem may occur when the bladder no longer drains properly if stale urine accumulates and becomes infected.

Prostate enlargement affects one in ten elderly men but treatment is not always necessary. If the condition worsens, however, surgery may be required to remove part of the prostate, either by normal abdominal surgery or by operating from within the urethra itself. This usually cures the problem but sometimes affects sexual function as the nerves supplying the penis may be damaged. There may also be some dribbling of urine for a

When the prostate gland enlarges and restricts the flow of urine, surgical removal of the prostate gland usually solves the problems but this sometimes affects sexual function because nerves to the penis may be damaged. There may also be some dribbling of urine until the muscles have recovered their full function.

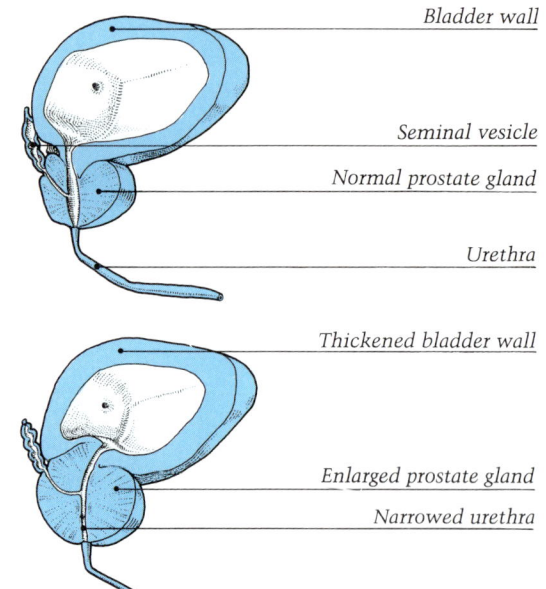

Bladder wall

Seminal vesicle

Normal prostate gland

Urethra

Thickened bladder wall

Enlarged prostate gland

Narrowed urethra

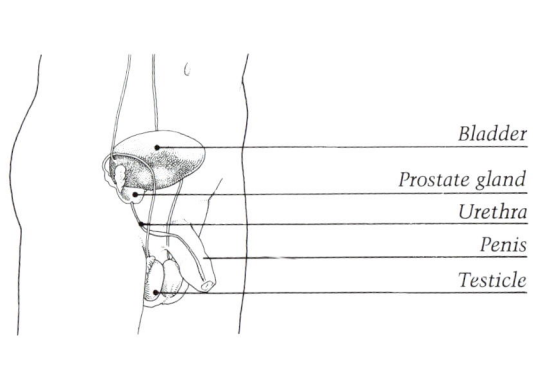

Bladder

Prostate gland

Urethra

Penis

Testicle

while until the muscles have recovered their full function. Another form of prostate problem is prostate cancer, which is discussed in the section on cancer, earlier in this chapter.

RESPIRATORY DISEASE

Our lungs are exposed to all sorts of hazards from the air we breathe, and sometimes from within our own bodies, as in asthma. Of all these conditions, the most common is bronchitis, the inflammation of the air passages carrying air into the lungs.

Bronchitis appears in several forms, and most people get acute bronchitis at some time in their life when a cold virus spreads down into the air passages. This sort of infection should clear up quickly, but it causes coughing and large amounts of sticky phlegm are produced. Acute bronchitis is a major problem for heavy smokers, who already have some degree of lung damage. It is usually self-treated, by aspirin, and cough medicines can suppress the cough reflex at night. Inhaling steam, with a towel over the head, can also help by loosening the phlegm.

Chronic bronchitis is quite different. Men are three times more likely than women to suffer from chronic bronchitis (although this gap is continually being eroded as more men than women are giving up smoking), and the disease is more common in Britain than anywhere else in the world, affecting over a million people there each year, 30,000 of whom are killed by the disease. The biggest single cause of chronic bronchitis is cigarette smoking, which eventually damages the linings of the air passages.

The disease starts so gradually that its effects are not at first noticed

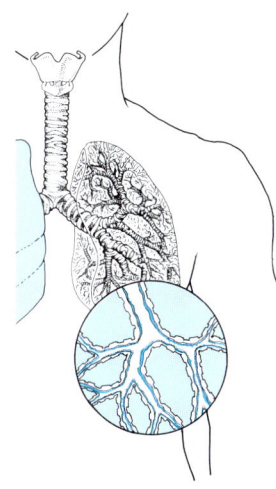

Bronchitis is inflammation of the bronchi and bronchioles of the lung. When the trachea and bronchi become inflamed production of sputum increases and this can become infected with bacteria. Inflammation may be caused by bacteria, as in acute bronchitis, or irritants, as in chronic bronchitis.

until inflammation of the bronchi starts to produce extra phlegm, causing a frequent 'frog in the throat' effect. Next comes a 'dry' cough (smoker's cough). The walls of the bronchi and smaller air passages are thickened, so that the air flow is restricted, causing shortness of breath on effort. Large amounts of mucus are secreted and obstruct the air passages. The infection that results from this obstruction brings on a racking cough and fever. In cold, damp weather, the symptoms are at their worst, often causing permanent breathlessness and making the sufferer susceptible to colds and other infections.

Chronic bronchitis is especially serious because the strain it puts on the respiratory system can lead to a form of hypertension, emphysema and heart failure. If you are diagnosed as having chronic bronchitis, you must take some sensible precautions: stop smoking and, if you are exposed to obviously polluted air, change your job. Your doctor may prescribe an inhaler, which will help to open up the obstructed airways, and drugs that help to remove the collected mucus in the lungs. You must be very careful if you contract any sort of lung infection, which may need medical attention.

Emphysema This goes hand in hand with bronchitis, affecting about one person in every one hundred. It is ten times more common in men than in women and, like bronchitis, it is associated with breathing polluted air - especially cigarette smoke. In emphysema the tiny air sacs, or alveoli, which absorb oxygen are attacked. Bit by bit they lose their springy texture and become stretched and distorted. Gradually the damage is such that they no longer absorb oxygen properly, and the sufferer may develop a barrel-like chest, as the body tries to compensate by increasing the lung size.

The symptoms of emphysema are increasing shortness of breath and a susceptibility to lung infections. Emphysema cannot be cured, as the lung damage is too severe. Life can be made more comfortable for the sufferer by the use of bronchodilator sprays, which improve the air flow into the lungs. It is essential to avoid sources of air pollution as much as possible, and smoking is, of course, strictly forbidden.

The other major respiratory disease, especially of smokers, is lung cancer, which is discussed in the section on cancer earlier in this chapter.

SEXUAL REALITIES

Sex is far more than just a means of producing children. For most couples, it is a vehicle expressing their love for each other, a special way of being close, a source of mutual comfort, an exciting pastime. It can also be used as an outlet for all kinds of frustration and an escape from worries. To get the most out of love-making, a couple need to be at ease with each other and with their bodies, considerate of their partner's needs, open in their communications, and prepared to be inventive. Unfortunately, for the majority of married couples, the sexual relationship falls short of their ideals. Problems range from total abstinence to intercourse which is boring, frustrating or even painful for one or both partners. Undoubtedly men's distorted attitudes and beliefs about sex are a majority contributory factor.

For men, sexuality is closely bound up with self-esteem. The 20-year-old who can boast of numerous conquests is generally admired and envied by his male friends. It is as if his manhood - and indeed his worth as a person - is measured by his success in seducing women. Although it may seem that his main preoccupation is with the opposite sex, his real gratification is in reporting back to his mates.

Most men grow out of this phase, but a number continue to look at sex as a way of proving their masculinity to themselves. Take, for example, the middle-aged business man whose effectiveness in the office is determined by his personal life at home. If his wife is cold and unresponsive to him, his confidence can slump. Or take the 50-year-old playboy who is continually taking younger women to bed in a futile attempt to overcome his inner sense of inadequacy. He may get a 'lift' from these experiences, but the effects are always short lived.

Why do men place such importance on their sex lives? Why do they often seem to see sex as an end in itself? The answers to both questions lie in men's upbringing. Throughout their schooldays, boys are encouraged to be competitive, particularly on the playing fields. Winners are revered; losers sink without trace. Not surprisingly, some come to see relationship with girls as yet another game, the aim of which is to 'score'. It is considered unmanly to admit to such feelings as warmth, tenderness and affection, and such an attitude is often reinforced by the cinema industry, which portrays 'heroes' as hard men who seduce and abandon women without a flicker of emotion.

The truth about men is very different. Beneath the machismo image lies a small boy who wants to be comforted and cared for; behind the cool façade there is a potentially loving person who is inhibited about showing how much he cares. Because they have been brought up to believe that emotions are unmanly, men are often reluctant to acknowledge these deeper needs - even to themselves. Sex may be the only vehicle they allow themselves for expressing tender emotions.

It follows from this that men are wary of intimate relationships. To feel strongly for someone poses a threat to their concept of being a man. Yet they have a need for sexual outlets on a regular basis. Their interest in pornography, stag nights, strip clubs, erotic videos and casual affairs can be explained as a wish for sexual excitement without personal risk.

The good news is that most men sort themselves out in time. They become bored with superficial erotica and realize that it does not meet their needs. When they find the right woman, whom they can trust with their emotions, they come to see sex in a different light. Nevertheless, it is a major task for a man to integrate his sexuality with his tender feelings while retaining his masculine identity. It is equally challenging for the woman in his life to make sense of his conflicts and contradictions, and for him to understand her needs, but this is the only route to a truly successful sexual relationship.

THE SEX DRIVE

Given that man's self-esteem is so bound up with his sexuality, frequency of intercourse is naturally a major concern. Am I getting my 'fair share'? Can I still perform as well as I used to? These are questions he can torture himself with, particularly when he hears others in the pub discussing their sexual exploits.

The precise role of hormones in determining the strength of an individual's sex drive is far from clear. It is known that the male hormone, testosterone, is responsible for producing such adult male characteristics as facial and pubic hair, fully developed sex organs, muscular build, deepening of voice and physical attraction to the opposite sex. However, there is by no means a one-to-one relationship between testosterone levels and sex drive.

Sexual release for men under the age of 40 is not restricted to sexual intercourse. Kinsey discovered that the younger the age group, the more varied the forms of sexual release.

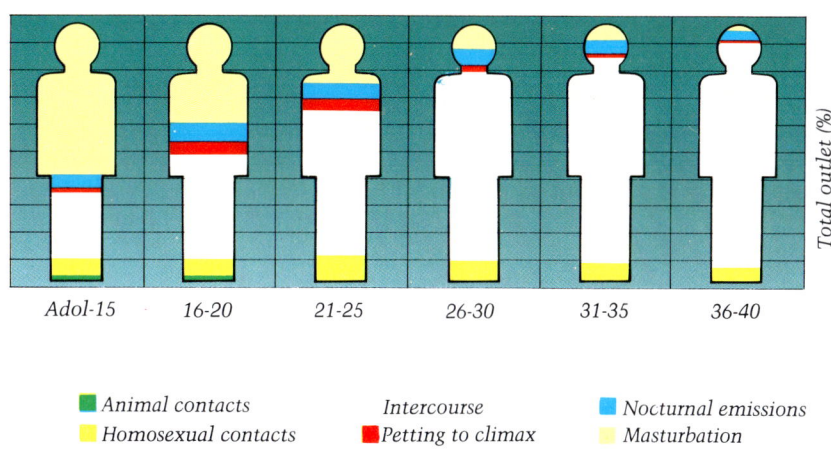

Total outlet (%)

Adol-15   16-20   21-25   26-30   31-35   36-40

■ Animal contacts   Intercourse   ■ Nocturnal emissions
■ Homosexual contacts   ■ Petting to climax   Masturbation

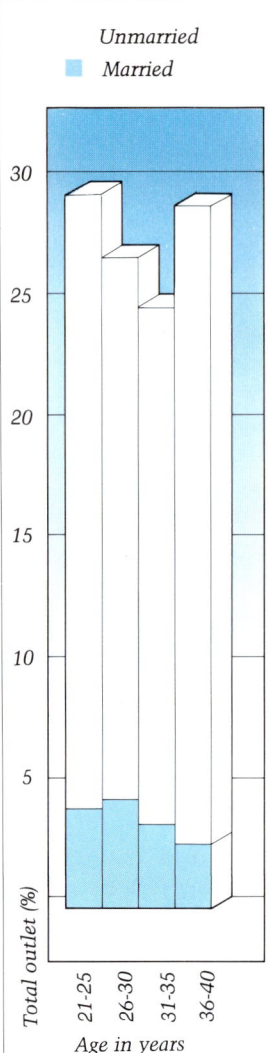

Unmarried
Married

Total outlet (%)

30
25
20
15
10
5

21-25 26-30 31-35 36-40

Age in years

Masturbation is common among adolescent men, but it is not limited to this age group. Single men of all ages find masturbation a satisfying form of sexual release. The chart shows that although married men get most of their sexual release through conventional intercourse, many still masturbate.

Leaving aside the small number of men who fail to develop properly because of a hormonal deficiency, the male body produces a more than adequate supply of testosterone to ensure adequate sexual functioning. This is true even in those cases where the sperm count is found to be low. We have to look elsewhere to account for variations in sexual appetites.

Fatigue, alcohol, nicotine and lack of exercise can all adversely affect man's ability to achieve and maintain an erection, even if his desire for sex is unaffected. As with other forms of physical activity, you need to be fit and healthy to get the most from your body. On the psychological side, a man's sex drive will suffer if he is constantly worried by problems at work or financial difficulties. Not suprisingly, many men report a dramatic increase in sexual activity while they are on holiday and away from their everyday pressures. Even more important is the state of his relationship with his partner. Resentment, bitterness and coldness towards each other are powerful antidotes to sexual interest on both sides. If he loses confidence in his sexual abilities for whatever reason, his interest in the opposite sex will lessen significantly.

By the age of 35 to 40, the sexual drive is less strong and most men are satisfied if they have sex two or three times a week. This level of desire remains relatively constant until they are well into their forties. In later life, the decline in sexual interest and potency becomes more noticeable. Most 60-year-olds are still sexually active but they rarely make love more than once a week. In their seventies, only about one in four still engages in regular sex.

Masturbation It has been estimated that about 95 per cent of adolescents masturbate on a regular basis. Masturbating provides the single man with a convenient means for releasing pent-up energies, and it is also a source of excitement, allowing him to fantasize about seducing 'unattainable' girls in the office or provocative models in the pornographic magazines. Stimulating a pleasurable part of the body can be a source of comfort for those who feel lonely, rejected or under stress. Others masturbate last thing at night to induce sleep.

Despite his preference for intercourse, the married man will usually continue to masturbate from time to time. When his wife catches him in the act she might feel rejected or disgusted. Does this mean he does not love her? Should he not have outgrown this 'filthy' habit? Usually there is a more simple answer. Given his need for regular sex, he may well choose to satisfy himself in this way rather than pressurize his partner into sex when she is clearly not in the mood. In the later stages of pregnancy and in the weeks after childbirth, masturbation is a harmless way of dealing with physical frustrations.

Myths about the dangers of 'self abuse' have existed for generations, the commonest ones being that 'it will make you blind' or 'it will drive you mad'. There is, however, no evidence whatsoever that masturbation damages a man physically or mentally in any way. Adolescents, who tend to stimulate themselves as soon as they are in bed each night, are particularly likely to worry about this strong urge, which they feel they cannot control. However, with the exception of the problem few who masturbate in public, masturbation should be seen as a perfectly safe and acceptable activity, which reduces physical and mental tension.

Turn-ons Most men become instantly aroused when their genitals are

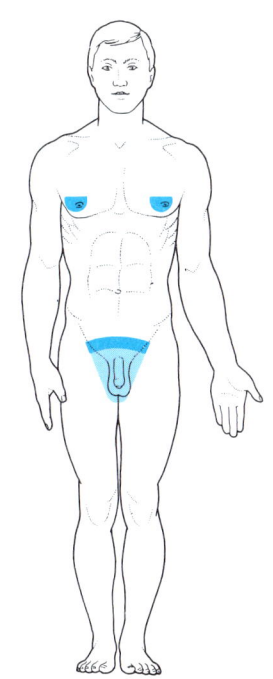

Moderately erogenous zone

■ *Erogenous zone*

■ *High erogenous zone*

Erogenous zones are areas of the body that can cause sexual arousal when touched and caressed. For a man, the genitals are highly erogenous, but other areas of the body such as the nipples can be moderately stimulating.

stimulated, regardless of whether or not they are feeling in the mood for sex. In this way they are different from the majority of women, who need to feel close or particularly attracted to their partner to respond to his touch. If a woman is feeling resentful towards her partner, she is unlikely to want sex with him or, at the very least, will become less easily aroused during intercourse. This is also a highly effective way in which she can show her disapproval. By contrast, if her husband is feeling moody, he can usually be stirred to action if she strokes his penis. It is as if his sexuality can function separately from his other emotions.

Affairs   Surveys have shown that about three out of every four married men have at least one affair at some time in their marriage. This is about double the rate found for married women. Presumably one reason why more men than women have affairs is that office life and business trips provide them with more opportunity for pursuing sexual relationships. Women who seek sexual fulfilment outside marriage rarely engage in more than two or three affairs, although these tend to be long lasting. In contrast, a husband who chooses to be unfaithful usually as sex with a considerably greater number of partners.

There are several reasons why so many men have affairs. One is sexual frustration. Women find it easier to go without sex than men, particularly if there are problems in the relationship. Given his persistent need for sexual outlets, a 'deprived' man can be easily tempted by the prospect of casual sex. Then the middle-aged man who engages in affairs is often seeking reassurance. He feels he has to prove to himself that, despite his receding hair-line and expanding midriff, he is still attractive to women.

Another reason could be male bravado, when a man feels under some pressure from his friends to join them in a spree or set himself up with a sexual adventure to prove that he is still 'one of the boys'.

The desire for novelty may cause some men to enter into an affair. Given his preoccupation with the female body, he may choose to have affairs simply in order to satisfy his sexual curiosity. Alternatively, a man may feel a need for excitement, and if his marriage has become jaded, both emotionally and sexually, he may look elsewhere for some sparkle in his life. Secret meetings with a willing partner in restaurants and hotel rooms can serve to break the monotony. Sex may be secondary to the need for an adventure. Similarly, if a man feels misunderstood at home, he may seek out a woman who is willing to comfort him - someone who will offer a port in a storm. Again, sex may be only incidental.

Perhaps the most important reason why men are likely to have affairs, however, is that they find it more difficult than women to 'give their all' in a relationship. If a man chooses to play the traditional role of strong, self-reliant breadwinner and head of the household, he may find it difficult to express his dependency needs within the marriage and so looks to someone else for tenderness, support and comfort. Alternatively, if he has been conditioned to think of sex as a recreational and impersonal activity, he may have problems combining his physical needs with his loving feelings. It can be argued that, because men seem to find it more difficult to integrate their various emotions than women, they are more likely to reveal different bits of themselves in different relationships. Only when they have resolved these various conflicts are they able to meet all their needs within a single intimate relationship.

Continued on page 144

SEXUAL ATTRACTION

Men are also extremely receptive to visual cues. They can quickly come to life when their partner changes out of baggy jeans and puts on a more glamorous outfit. A glimpse of a stockinged thigh or of a partially exposed breast can lead to an instantaneous erection. There seems to be a 'peeping Tom' in every man, which helps to explain his fascination for revealing dresses and exotic underwear. The huge profits made by 'soft porn' magazines and strip-tease clubs testify to his preoccupation with viewing the female body. For many men, however, the partially clad female is more attractive than the naked body.

Some men also tend to respond to women who tease them sexually or challenge their manhood in a provocative way, behaviour that seems to produce a 'cave man' urge to dominate the female. It is presumably bound up with the analogy of sex as a game. When his self-esteem is high and he is feeling confident in his sexuality, pre-sexual rituals of this kind can make him a passionate lover. However, given the fragility of his ego where sex is concerned, such a ploy can often backfire.

It would be wrong, however, to think that men are only turned on by their partner's appearance, her touch or feminine ploys. Strong feelings of romantic love can arouse them sexually in much the same way as women. A candle-lit dinner or holding hands in the park can lead to an intense desire for physical intimacy. Similarly, they can become aroused through comforting a loved one who is undergoing some distress. As they mature, men often become more receptive to atmosphere and intimacy and less easily titillated by more obvious sexual cues.

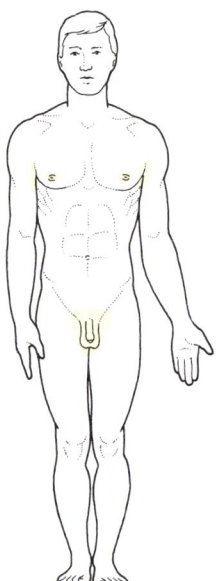

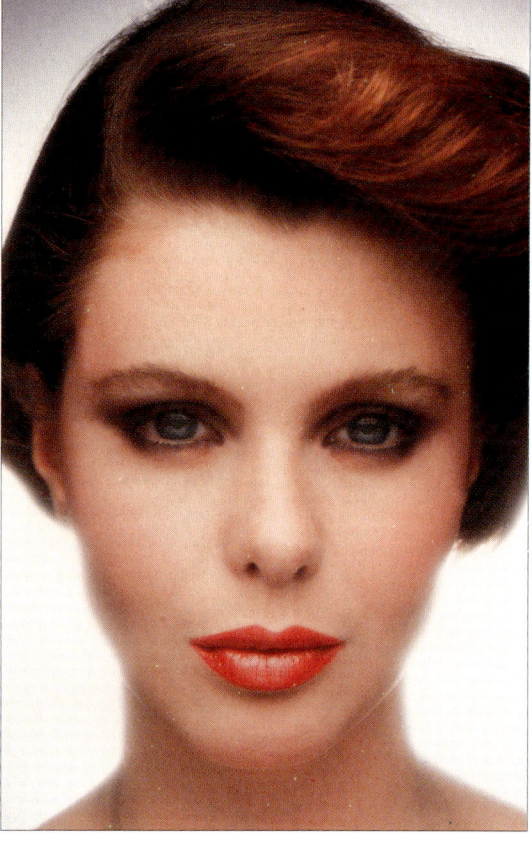

body hair in both males and females and these trap the scents to make them more powerful. Unfortunately, the wearing of clothes in most human cultures renders the scents stale and unattractive, making repeated washing and the use of deodorants a necessity. Experiments have shown that the male pheromone, androsterone, is attractive to women but arouses feelings of agression in men. Incidentally, blonde women produce stronger copulins (the female pheromone) than do brunettes.

Apocrine glands in the skin are concentrated around the groin, armpit and nipple areas. From puberty onwards they secrete, along with the sweat, chemicals called pheromones which are subconsciously recognized by members of the opposite sex as sexual messages. The areas where apocrine glands concentrate carry a higher density of

FEMALE	MALE
Shape *large buttocks, breasts and legs*	*ambitious • high alcohol consumption*
Shape *small buttocks, breasts and legs*	*perservering • higher social class*
Shape *big buttocks*	*ordered life • neat*
Shape *small buttocks*	*work orientated • uninterested in sport*
Shape *big breasts*	*extrovert • Playboy reader • masculine interests and hobbies • lower social class*
Shape *small breasts*	*introspective • low alcohol consumption • submissive • Christian moral code*
Shape *fat legs*	*low alcohol consumption • socially shy*
Shape *thin legs*	*low alcohol consumption • smoker • hobby magazine reader*

A group of men were shown silhouettes of different female shapes and asked which they preferred. Preference correlated closely with male personality type.

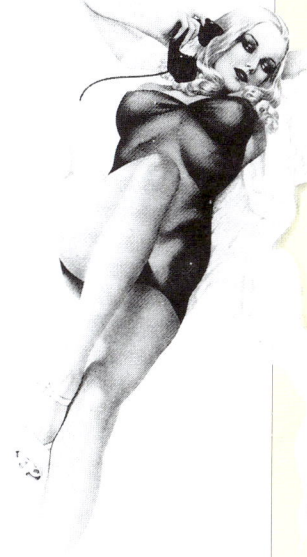

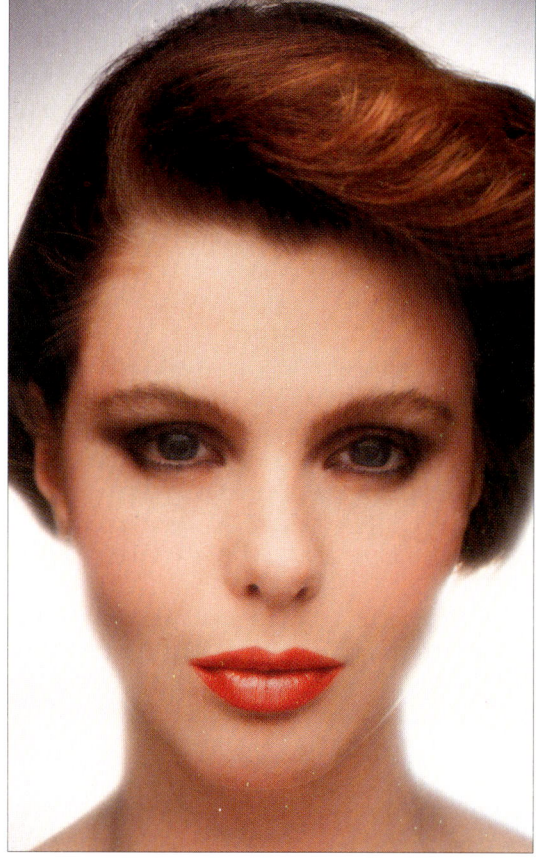

The pupil of the human eye narrows and widens in response to light stimulation. It also responds to emotional feelings. When a person looks at something he or she likes, the pupil dilates more than the light conditions require. A group of men were shown two pictures of the same girl, identical in every way except that one had normal pupils and the other had her pupils artificially enlarged. With very few exceptions the men in the study found the wide-pupilled girl more attractive but could not say why. The explanation is that a widening of the pupils implies that the subject likes what she sees, and is stimulated by her partner. Lovers spend much of their time watching one another's eyes during early courtship. From the earliest of times women used the juice of deadly nightshade berries to dilate their pupils and make them more attractive — 'belladonna' means 'beautiful lady'.

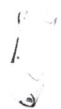

Leg length is often exaggerated to promote a woman as more sexy. This is probably because a girl's legs grow longer as she approaches sexual maturity and the artist exaggerates a natural biological feature.

Continued from page 141

The sexual response   Masters and Johnson, the celebrated authorities on human sexuality, have divided the male sexual response into four successive stages. Provided they are fit, healthy and have none of the anxieties about sex discussed later in this chapter, men go through each of these phases in turn when engaging in a complete sexual act.

The excitement stage   Once sexually stimulated by whatever means, a man quickly becomes erect. Such an obvious manifestation of desire can make his partner feel under pressure to respond. Unfortunately, many women wrongly believe that once the man is aroused, he will not be satisfied until he has reached a climax. However, in this early phase, the erection can subside without the man feeling unduly frustrated or upset.

The plateau stage   If the man continues to be stimulated, his penis will grow still further in size as more and more blood is pumped into it. If sex is interrupted at this point, he is much more likely to become irritated and moody, and these feelings can persist for some time afterwards. This is not just a question of the man acting like a spoiled boy because he cannot have what he wants. Without the release of tension accompanying the climax, his body is slow to recover from such intense physical excitement. He may also experience discomfort in the genital region. However, if sex proceeds normally, he will enter what Masters and Johnson call the phase of 'ejaculatory inevitability'. In other words, his body is committed to orgasm, and this event cannot be delayed through will-power or distraction.

The orgasm stage   The male climax normally lasts little more than a few seconds and ends abruptly. It is usually an extremely pleasurable sensation but not always so. Orgasm can vary from a virtual non-event to an experience so overwhelming that is almost frightening. A number of factors determine the strength of the orgasm. Generally speaking, a man experiences complete sexual release if he is relatively fresh and relaxed beforehand and is physically turned on by his partner. However, if he is distracted just prior to orgasm, or engages in a futile attempt to prevent ejaculation, it can be over in a flash. On the other hand, if he has gone without sex for a few weeks and is highly aroused, it can be so pleasurable as to be almost painful.

The resolution stage   The period immediately after orgasm is literally an anti-climax for a man. His energy and excitement evaporate very quickly, replaced by a wonderful sense of release and relaxation. Sometimes, though, the speed with which his bodily functions return to normal can leave him feeling flat and even morose. This is in direct contrast to his partner, who comes down from the heights much more slowly and wishes physical contact to continue for longer. Naturally she is upset if he stops abruptly, rolls over and falls asleep. His behaviour after intercourse depends on how close he feels to his partner, although it can also be affected by sexual hang-ups.

It is not uncommon for the adolescent or young adult male to remain erect after orgasm and to be capable of repeating the cycle almost without interruption. However, from the age of about 30 onwards, a man usually interruption. However, from the age of about 30 onwards, a man usually loses his erection altogether after orgasm. The length of this 'refractory period', during which he is physically incapable of intercourse, tends to increase with age. When he reaches his sixties, it may be several days before his batteries are fully recharged.

Aphrodisiacs   Since men have always been preoccupied with their sex drive, there is a long history of attempts to increase it through food and drugs. Oysters are just one in a long list of foodstuffs considered to have magical properties that will increase potency. However, chemical analysis has revealed that oysters consist of water, protein, carbohydrates and minerals - all of which are freely available in the ordinary diet. The Chinese favour powdered rhinoceros horn but, as this too lacks any special ingredient, it must also be relegated to the realm of folklore.

Although many men regard marijuana as a sexual stimulant, there is no evidence that it has arousing properties, although it may make the user more suggestible to sexual cues and give rise to the illusion of increased sexuality. Alcohol can increase desire but can, when taken in excess, interfere with performance.

There is more scientific support for the aphrodisiac effects of *yohimbine*, which is extracted from a tree native to Africa. Used primarily as a diuretic, this drug stimulates the lower-spine nerves, which control erections. However, given its various side-effects, doctors are understandably reluctant to prescribe it to increase libido. Cantharides (Spanish fly) should be avoided at all costs. Extracted from beetles, which have been dried out, this drug induces erections through causing irritation to membranes in the genital region. Apart from chronic physical discomfort, it can lead to severe illness and even death. It has recently been reported that the drug *L-dopa*, which is used to treat Parkinson's disease, has aphrodisiac properties. However, it too has side-effects that would discourage doctors from prescribing it to increase sexual appetites.

Since there is no magic potion for increasing libido, the most effective aphrodisiac remains a lifestyle involving plenty of rest, regular exercise, moderate alcohol intake and freedom from chronic stress.

SEXUAL HANG-UPS

The majority of healthy men seek regular outlets for their sexual urges, but many men have secret worries about intercourse which can lead them to suppress their sexuality. Most of these anxieties are psychological, often based on ignorance; and they can be overcome in time with reassurance and advice. Others, such as powerful ambivalent feelings of anger towards women or a desire to exert control over them, are deep-seated and require professional help.

Body image   The traditional image of a sex symbol is of a tanned, muscular 'hunk' with a forest of hair of his chest. Understandably, many men are ashamed of exposing their white, skinny ribcages or middle-aged paunches to the lady they are attempting to seduce, or even to their partner of long-standing. It is not unusual for a self-conscious man to undress quickly behind a chair and extinguish all lights before jumping into bed. This can be disconcerting to a partner who loves him 'warts and all', and in any case, women tend not to be so preoccupied with physical attributes as men and are inclined to respond emotionally and physically to the whole person.

Related to this is man's celebrated preoccupation with the size of his penis. Reference to these vital dimensions by comedians and in seaside

A number of men's hang-ups are based on myths about sex. Some of the most common are:

●**If a woman fails to reach an orgasm, she will feel dissatisfied.**
Although a climax adds significantly to the pleasure she gets from sex, her satisfaction is more closely bound up with her partner's overall approach to lovemaking.

●**The aim of sex is to achieve simultaneous orgasm.**
It can be equally pleasurable to come at different times so that you can enjoy each other's orgasm. Simultaneous orgasm is not common.

●**The bigger the man's penis, the more satisfied the woman will be.**
See sexual phobias, (right)

●**The 'missionary position' is the only normal way to have sex.**
Men should feel free to experiment with different ways of making love in the knowledge that what is right for both partners is perfectly acceptable.

●**Failure to achieve an erection is a sign of inadequacy.**
Most men can recall occasions when they failed to become hard, despite being in the mood for sex. This is usually because they are tired, stressed, intoxicated or too anxious to please. Provided they do not brood over this, it is unlikely to recur too often.

●**Sex during pregnancy will damage the baby.**
Sex is safe, assuming the woman does not have a tendency to miscarry, up until about the last month of pregnancy.

●**Men are past it once they reach sixty.**
As long as they are in good health, there are no physical reasons why men cannot have sex until well into their old age.

postcards is a sure way of raising a laugh in certain quarters. However, behind the humour lies considerable anxiety. 'Organ inferiority', as psychiatrists call it, discourages many men from entering into sexual relationships, and insecure husbands worry constantly about how they compare with their wife's former lovers. Yet the truth is that these fears are groundless except in the very few cases where hormonal deficiencies have interfered with the normal development of the sex organs. For most women, sexual satisfaction is more closely bound up with their partner's overall approach to love-making than with his physical endowments.

Phobias   Although physically attracted and emotionally attached to their partner, some men become turned off when confronted with the naked female body. Some of the more common aversions include the vagina, pubic hair, vaginal secretions and menstrual bleeding. To avoid experiencing acute anxiety or even panic attacks, the phobic sufferer tends to rush through foreplay, much to the dismay of his partner. Manual stimulation of the woman's genitals proves almost impossible for him, and active oral sex is regarded with total revulsion. Understandably, his partner can feel hurt and rejected, and even angry at his apparent selfishness as a lover. To prevent such misunderstandings from developing within a long-term relationship, it is always advisable to own up to one's hang-ups. An understanding partner can play an important part in helping gradually to reduce anxiety; mutual trust, and continued practice, combined with reassurance, are usually the key to solving to such simple problems.

A potentially more serious threat to sexual harmony is the fear of penetration. Some men are worried about entering their partner in case they contract venereal disease. Even if they are fully convinced of their partner's fidelity, they may nevertheless be preoccupied with thoughts that they can see to be irrational. Some are frightened in case she freezes and traps their penis inside her vagina. Although this is extremely rare, exaggerated accounts of such happenings tend to circulate freely in school playgrounds and readily feed into the adolescent's vivid imagination. Related to this is a primitive irrational fear that the vagina has 'teeth', which will bite off a man's sexual organ. Reassurance, combined with education in the physiology of women, is usually sufficient in such cases. However, occasionally, such a problem can be bound up with unresolved childhood conflicts regarding the man's relationship with his mother; if this seems to be the case, psychotherapy may be helpful.

A few men are unduly concerned about the process of ejaculation. This is usually the result of the guilt and embarrassment they experienced during adolescence concerning masturbating and wet dreams. As a result, they feel inhibited from producing semen in the presence of anyone else. To cope with this anxiety, some men learn to engage in intercourse without reaching a climax. Apart from the difficulties this creates for impregnation, such behaviour can be distressing for his partner, who feels that she is unable to satisfy him properly.

Performance neurosis   While women can have intercourse when only partially aroused, men have to achieve a full erection for coitus to occur. As a result, many men worry unduly about the strength and size of their penis during the sexual act. Such anxious thoughts are a sure way of losing an erection. When this 'failure' occurs, the man's anxiety then centres on the next time, making impotence almost a foregone conclusion.

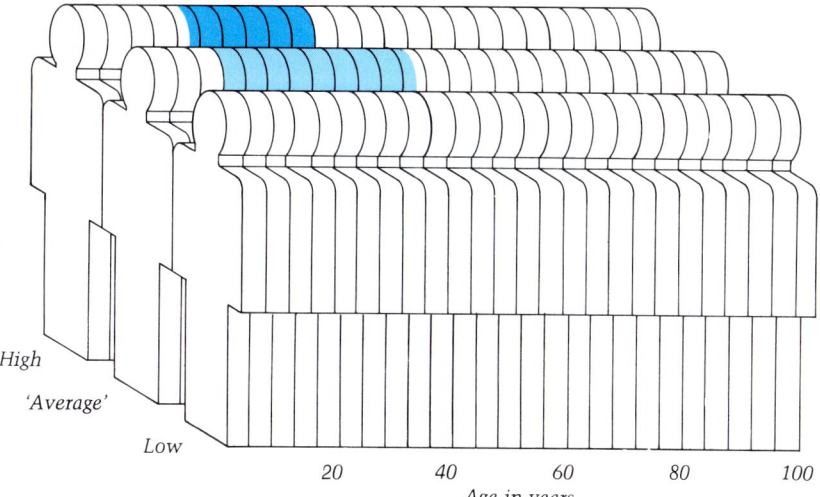

Male sex drive alters with age. If a man's level of inhibition is high, he starts to have sex late in his twenties and stops in his forties. A man with average sexual inhibitions has a reasonably long and plentiful sex life, whereas the man with low inhibitions starts having sex as a young teenager and if he stops at all, it will be when he is well into his seventies.

■ *Active sex begins late and stops early*

■ *A long and plentiful sex life*

Starts young and carries on throughout life

An equally common example of pressure to perform occurs when a man is so concerned to help his partner achieve orgasm that he fails to let himself go during intercourse. Since it is likely nowadays that his partner has had previous sexual experiences, the man feels the need to prove himself to be a better lover than her former boyfriends. He wants to avoid coming too quickly, leaving her frustrated. The problem here is that his partner would probably prefer him to be a passionate lover, whether she comes every time or not, to having him acting the part of a skilful technician. Moreover, most women are turned on by the obvious pleasure they are giving their partner and are more likely to reach orgasm under these circumstances. Even if a man does come early, there are other ways of satisfying his partner.

Fear of letting go   In most Western cultures, it is considered unmanly to get too excited. Expressions such as 'boys don't cry', 'stiff upper lip' and 'keep your cool' illustrate the commonly held view that 'a real man' keeps his emotions under control. Not surprisingly, therefore, many men find it difficult to let go during sex, particularly with their regular partner. They might act quite differently with a prostitute or with a woman they will never see again. However, they would be acutely embarrassed about letting their partner see them in a state of total abandonment and ecstasy. As a result, the pleasure they get from sex is limited.

Fear of intimacy   While men can feel inhibited about giving vent to their pleasurable feelings, they are even more guarded so far as the deeper emotions stirred up during sex are concerned. Exposing their dependency needs by begging to be comforted and held, or even sobbing at the moment of climax, would be seen as signs of weakness. If they do reveal such powerful emotions, they tend to withdraw into themselves afterwards, much to the dismay of their partner. It is as if they have revealed too much of themselves and are left feeling vulnerable and frightened. Sex is an area where the need for intimacy and the traditional masculine role come into conflict.

Fear of woman's sexuality   In their efforts to defend their fragile egos, many men feel compelled to dominate their partners during foreplay and intercourse. The fact that women have powerful sexual needs and feelings can be too threatening to contemplate. In extreme cases, the man always has to make the initial approach, keep foreplay to a minimum and use his body weight to suppress his partner's pelvic movements. He may even come quickly, because subconsciously he wants to prevent her from reaching orgasm. Since he refuses to discuss the matter, believing it is more manly to be thought of as an inconsiderate lover than be exposed as an emotional coward, she is unlikely to recognize that he sees her sexuality as a threat, and, understandably, she will feel resentful toward him.

Guilt   Despite their assumed bravado in relation to sexual matters, most men feel guilty about their desires and longings. This feeling usually arises in adolescence, when they are faced with the problem of finding secret outlets for their powerful fantasies within the sanctity of the home. They are worried about getting caught in the act and embarrassed by semen stains on the sheets. Any pornographic magazines are carefully concealed under the mattress.

Having learned to be secretive about their sexuality, they find it difficult to share this aspect of themselves with partners in their adult life. Few men find it easy to discuss openly their fantasies and desires with their partner, regardless of how loving and understanding she might be. By holding back this information, intercourse with her can quickly become boring and routine. For real sexual excitement, men often resort to their former secret habits and act out their fantasies with a mistress or prostitute.

SEXUAL PROBLEMS

We live in an age when sexual problems are discussed at length in the media and talked about with a frankness that would have appalled previous generations. Such openness is to be welcomed in that it helps to dispel much of the irrational anxiety and guilt surrounding the subject and encourages many unhappy couples to seek professional advice. Unfortunately, we have become so preoccupied with foreplay techniques, positions to adopt during intercourse and the frequency and duration of intercourse that we have created a new set of problems.

Many men, who were previously perfectly content with their sex lives, now have serious doubts about their abilities in this area. They worry that their desire is limited to once a week, that they come within five minutes and that they are old-fashioned in their approach to foreplay and intercourse. They may even be cajoled into seeking help by partners who have given them a low score on a sexual rating scale published in a women's magazine. Usually both they and their partners can be reassured by the knowledge that there are no yardsticks against which to judge sexual performance and satisfaction. 'If it's all right for you both, then it's OK,' is the usual advice.

However, if one or both partners are seriously dissatisfied with their sex life together, something has to be done, or the relationship may not be able to take the strain. It is advisable to discuss the problem with your doctor first, in case the problem is a medical one. This is particularly important in cases of impotence, since physical illness, psychiatric problems and

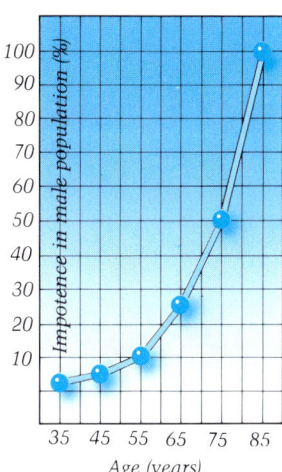

Total impotence affects a minority of men in their middle years but as age increases, so does impotence. Although physical deterioration plays some part in these figures, psychological factors are far more relevant. The men most likely to suffer from total impotence are those who were sexually inhibited when younger. Here old age is a good excuse to stop sexual activity. For others the opportunities for an active sex life no longer exist due to widowhood.

medication can all affect a man's ability to achieve an erection. Having excluded these possibilities, you might ask your doctor to refer you to a specialist for psychosexual counselling. Alternatively you could approach the local branch of the Marriage Guidance Council or the Family Planning Association and ask to be seen by someone with expertise in this area. This course of action is particularly recommended if you suspect that sex is only one of the difficulties in the relationship. However, many couples understandably prefer to sort out problems of such an intimate nature by themselves. Men are particularly reluctant to discuss personal matters with a third party. What follows, therefore, is a description of the most common male sexual problems, together with some brief advice on self-help.

Low libido If a healthy male, aged between 15 and 50, who is not unduly stressed, depressed or abusing alcohol, does not fantasize about sex, notice attractive girls or approach his partner for months on end, his desire for sex can be considered abnormally low. He may be moved to have sex occasionally, possibly after prolonged genital stimulation, but gets little pleasure from it. It's like sitting down to a meal when you are not feeling hungry.

It would be wrong to assume that a man is lacking in sexual desire simply because he appears uninterested in making love to his regular partner. He may be so anxious about letting her down that he avoids the situation altogether. Or he may find it difficult to have sex with someone with whom he is emotionally involved (see fear of intimacy, previous section). There is also the possibility that he no longer finds her attractive. Similarly, latent homosexuality (see page 000) can block all interest in women but need not constitute a lack of libido.

If a man is almost completely asexual, in terms of both his behaviour and his fantasies, in all probability he has deep-seated conflicts about his sexuality. Since these are likely to operate at an unconscious level, he may not even be aware that he has a problem. It could be that he is unable to reconcile his pleasure-seeking needs with his religious convictions. In such cases, discussions with a progressively minded vicar, priest or pastoral counsellor can prove helpful. Or the problem may lie in his childhood relationships with his parents. For example, unresolved incestuous fantasies and the guilt associated with them, can serve to suppress sexual feelings in adulthood.

Inability to communicate and show emotion is at the root of most sexual problems. Communication is the mainstay of treatment and this is best done with a referee. Couples are often too scared to say what they mean - sometimes it can make the situation worse - and it is usually better for a professionally trained party to be present. Talking your problem through with your partner can certainly help, provided, of course, that she is considerate and understanding and that you are honest with each other. If this does not produce results, consider asking your doctor to refer you to a psychoanalyst or psychotherapist who specializes in problems such as this. This may take a long time, could cost you a great deal, requires absolute commitment, and the eventual outcome is uncertain. However, if you manage to overcome your conflicts, you will end up being more effective in all areas of your life.

Impotence A more common problem is that the man is interested in sex

Impotence is usually caused by underlying psychological anxieties. However, some external factors do have an effect on a man's potency.

●**Work and emotional stress**
Effect: loss of libido
●**Alcoholism, diabetes**
Effect: erectile failure
●**Barbiturates**
Effect: libido loss and orgasmic failure
●**Psychological castration**
Effect: erectile failure
●**Anti-depressants**
Effect: ejaculatory and erectile failure

The steps of the sensate focus technique are as follows:

●Set aside a few hours each week when you will be free from all interruptions and distractions.
●Place a ban on intercourse, no matter how aroused you might become, for an indefinite period.
●Start with mutual bathing — a safe way to experiment with intimacy and great fun. Then take it in turns to stroke and caress each other, using massage oil if you so desire, but avoid the genitals.
●On later occasions, as you begin to feel more relaxed, include the genitals but do not place too much emphasis on them.
●When the man is regularly achieving a partial erection, the penis can be stimulated more vigorously.
●Agree to lift the ban but do not attempt intercourse until the occasion seems right.

Provided these guidelines are followed carefully, the probability of success is very high in most cases.

but is unable to achieve or maintain his erection when attempting intercourse. This can be caused indirectly by such physical illnesses as diabetes, multiple sclerosis and hepatitis, while disorders of blood vessels in the pelvic region can have a more direct effect on a man's ability to become fully erect. Commonly prescribed drugs, such as tranquillizers, anti-depressants and anti-hypertensives, can also interfere with his sexual functioning, as can alcohol and excessive cigarette smoking. However, if the man has erections at night or in the early morning, can masturbate successfully or have intercourse intermittently, then the cause is certain to be psychological - more than nine out of ten cases of impotence turn out to be psychological. Unexpressed anger and the need to control his partner by denying her her sexual satisfaction through impotence may be more difficult to uncover. In this situation, conjoint marital therapy is the key.

In the majority of cases, anxiety lies at the root of the problem. Moreover, even if physical factors are playing a part, there is usually an emotional component also. Unlike low libido, the cause of anxiety is usually self-evident. Sexual phobias, hang-ups and performance neuroses in particular, are frequently found in cases of impotence. The man is so preoccupied with his penis that he fails fully to involve himself in the sexual act. Asking himself, 'Is it hard yet?' is about the least erotic thought he could possible conjure up. The answer will almost inevitably be, 'No' and he has, in effect, reduced his sexual confidence still further.

Sensate focus is a technique devised by Masters and Johnson for overcoming problems related to orgasm, in both men and women. The aim is to help both individuals to get pleasure from touching and being touched while eliminating all pressures to perform. Impotent men are usually so preoccupied with getting an erection that they miss out on the sensual enjoyment of foreplay.

Premature ejaculation   Most men worry about ejaculating too quickly and so disappointing their partner. 'Did you come?' is the question they most want to ask her after they have reached a climax. If they suspect that she has not, they may feel deflated and tend to blame themselves for lacking 'staying power'. Many women occasionally - and sometimes regularly - choose to feign orgasm rather than go through the inevitable interrogation and post-mortem. In fact, the woman's ability to achieve orgasm depends on her mood, her feelings for her partner, her level of arousal during foreplay, how relaxed she feels during intercourse and the man's expertise as a lover. The actual duration of intercourse is not so important as most men believe. After all, if she feels unfulfilled when he comes, there are other ways in which she can be helped to achieve satisfaction.

Nevertheless, the man who regularly ejaculates within a few seconds of entry, or before doing so, clearly has a problem - at least with the particular partner in question.

Popular remedies include wearing a sheath, applying anaesthetic cream to the tip of the penis, consuming alcohol beforehand, masturbating a few hours in advance, thinking about one's bank balance or lying motionless during intercourse. Although all of these strategies can be effective in delaying ejaculation, they spoil the pleasure of love-making. The following two procedures have been shown to be successful and have none of the disadvantages of the home-made remedies. The aim, in both cases, is to

Common causes of premature ejaculation are:

- anxiety about coming too quickly
- excessive stimulation of the penis before entry
- infrequent sex, leading to over-excitement in the man when the occasion arises
- vigorous thrusting during intercourse
- an over demonstrative partner
- the man's ignorance of, or indifference to, the woman's needs

prove to the man that it is possible for him to delay ejaculation. In time he will feel more confident about his ability to control himself and will no longer have to rely on these procedures.

The first method is to modify the approach to sex to ensure that the man is as relaxed as possible both before and during intercourse. Foreplay should last for half an hour or more to enable him to overcome his initial excitement and control his urge to penerate quickly. During this time, the woman might stroke his penis and testicles gently but only on an intermittent basis. When attempting intercourse, she should move on top of him while he lies back in a comfortable position. Love-making should be rhythmic and gentle so that it is almost hypnotic. The more relaxed he feels, the less likely he is to come quickly.

The second is a modified version of the celebrated 'squeeze technique', which was popularized by Masters and Johnson in the 1970s. Here the woman stimulates the man's penis until just prior to the point of ejaculatory inevitability. When he indicates that he has reached that stage, she places her thumb on the frenulum with two fingers on top of the glans, and squeezes for about three seconds. This causes the man some discomfort, and he loses the urge to ejaculate. This procedure should be repeated immediately. It will be noted that the time interval will increase on the second occasion. If intercourse is then attempted, its duration should be significantly longer than usual. However it may require a number of training sessions before the effects become evident.

The effectiveness of both approaches depends on the extent to which the woman is willing and able to co-operate. Understandably, she may be feeling tense, resentful or uninterested in sex, and this will prevent her from becoming fully involved. She may well have problems of her own for which she too needs help. In either case, specialist help is required.

Retarded ejaculation   Although the ability to achieve an erection for an indefinite period might seem to be a positive attribute, it can cause problems. The woman might experience vaginal discomfort after a time and urge her partner to finish. She may feel hurt, rejected or inadequate because he finds it difficult to reach a climax. If she wants to become pregnant, his ejaculation difficulty will naturally cause her concern. This is particularly so in extreme cases where a climax is never reached, no matter how long sex lasts. Moreover, the man who is unable to produce semen may well worry about his virility.

Physical factors are unlikely to play a part except possibly where the man is never able to ejaculate by whatever means. Possible psychological causes are semen phobia and fear of impregnation. More usually, the problem is one of over-control. The man is reluctant to let go in the presence of his partner because he considers any form of emotional expression to be taboo. Or it could be that he previously ejaculated prematurely and has over-trained himself in the art of holding back.

The man should lie back, in a comfortable position, with strict instructions to engage in erotic fantasies throughout and ignore completely the actions of his partner. She meanwhile gently stimulates the penis, either orally or by hand. If choosing the latter, creams and lotions can be helpful. She gradually increases the speed and vigour of her movements until orgasm is reached. If this is unsuccessful, a vibrator might be used to help provide the pleasurable sensations he needs to reach a climax. It is important not to become discouraged if he fails to ejaculate on the first few occasions. He has to learn to let go and it may take some time before he feels sufficiently relaxed in this situation to concentrate fully on his sexual fantasies.

Once the breakthrough has been achieved, the problem may be solved and normal intercourse can resume. If not, the process should be repeated with the woman inserting the penis into her vagina at the point of ejaculatory inevitability. On succeeding occasions, the penis should be introduced at progressively earlier stages in the process.

METHODS OF CONTRACEPTION

On a 'first-night' occasion, do not just assume that she is on the pill - ask her. It may be a difficult question or seem inappropriate, in the heat of the moment, but a woman will appreciate your concern. If she is not using contraception and you do not have a sheath, then far better to wait rather than to risk making her pregnant.

In a long-term relationship be prepared to discuss contraception and to adopt the method that best suits you both. Advice is available from Family Planning clinics (see your telephone directory).

Remember that there is no perfect method of contraception. Each has drawbacks and a failure rate, and all require some motivation by the users. Most aim to prevent the sperm meeting the egg, or to stop the fertilized egg implanting in the womb.

Withdrawal *(coitus interruptus or 'pulling out')*   The man pulls out of the vagina before ejaculating. This method has a high failure rate - there is always some leakage of sperm before ejaculation. It may also cause frustration to both parties.

The rhythm method   This practice restricts sexual intercourse to the times in the menstrual cycle when the woman is less fertile. Conception is most likely to occur when intercourse occurs around the time of ovulation - 14 days before the next period is due - and is less likely further away from this time. So, just before, during, or just after a period are safer times, although this rule is not infallible.

This method only works if the woman has very regular, and therefore predictable, periods. It is made more reliable by combining calendar-watching with other methods of detecting the time of ovulation, such as temperature-taking and examining the consistency of mucus from the neck of the womb.

The failure rate obviously varies with the motivation and reliability of the user. It removes some of the spontaneity from love-making but it requires no special equipment or medical supervision. It is the only method approved by the Catholic Church.

Barrier methods   For the male, the condom, sheath or 'rubber' is very effective if used as instructed. It has the additional advantage of reducing the risk of acquiring (and passing on) a sexually transmitted disease. A new sheath should be used each time you make love and should be unrolled onto the hard penis before there is any genital contact. A separate spermicide is safer than relying on the one included by the manufacturer. The man should withdraw soon after ejaculation, holding the sheath in position on the penis to make sure it doesn't slip and allow sperm to escape.

In the female, the cap or diaphragm fits over the neck of the womb or across the upper vagina. It is very safe if used properly and with a spermicide. It should be inserted before sex and left in place for at least six hours afterwards. If sex occurs again during this time, more spermicide should be placed in the vagina and the cap left for a further six hours.

The vaginal sponge is a sponge impregnated with spermicide that fits in the upper vagina. It is a recently introduced method, but is not recommended as the failure rate seems to be high.

Intra-uterine contraceptive device (IUCD) or coil   This is a plastic device which may or may not contain copper. It fits inside the womb and prevents the fertilized egg from implanting. Threads project through the neck of the womb and allow the woman to check that the coil is in place. These strands occasionally cause the man discomfort during sex, but this is easily stopped by a doctor altering the length of the threads. Once fitted, no further effort is required except for an annual check. A few women experience side-effects of pain or bleeding and have to have the coil removed. It is not recommended for women who have not had children because of the risk of infection which can lead to infertility.

The pill   The most commonly used method of contraception, the pill contains small amounts of female hormones: either oestrogen and progestogen (the combined pill) or progestogen alone (the 'mini' pill). The combined pill is taken for three weeks out of four and works mainly by preventing release off the egg from the ovary ('ovulation'). A woman has her normal period a few days after stopping the three-week course and then restarts the pill. The progestogen-only pill is taken continuously. Its main effect is on the mucus at the neck of the womb, making it less penetrable to sperm.

Contraceptive devices vary in their effectiveness. The condom (sheath) *1* is 97% effective with careful use, as are the various intra-uterine devices for women *2*. The combined pill *3* is almost 100% effective and the mini-pill *4* is 98% effective. When used with spermicidal jelly *5*, the diaphragm *6* and smaller cervical cap *7* are 97% effective.

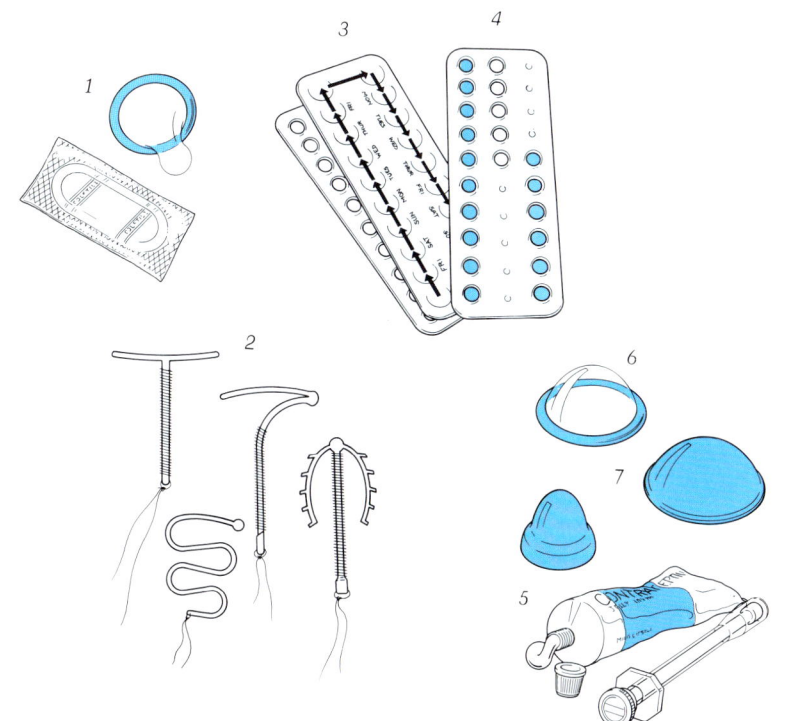

Most women have no problems on the pill; the few who do are the ones you hear about. The same hormones that are in the pill are secreted in much greater amounts during pregnancy, and so the side-effects of the pill are similar to those of pregnancy. However, it is safer to take the pill than to get pregnant. The pill is not given to women with certain medical conditions and can only be prescribed by a doctor. The combined pill is not suitable for women much over the age of 35, especially if they smoke, because of health risks.

Women on the pill must be able to remember to take the pill at about the same time each day. Tummy upsets, with vomiting or diarrhoea, or certain other drugs may interfere with pill absorption and make it ineffective.

The progesterone injection   An alternative to the pill, this is available to women who have problems remembering to take the pill each day. This 'depot' progesterone is given by intramuscular injection once every three months and is slowly released. It is an effective contraceptive but does produce side-effects, mainly irregular bleeding, in some women.

Female sterilization   This method prevents conception permanently. It requires a small abdominal operation, usually performed under general anaesthesia. The passage of the egg from the ovary to the womb is prevented by cutting and tying (or putting clips on) the Fallopian tubes. Any attempt at reversal has a low success rate and the method should only be considered if the woman is sure that her family is complete.

Male sterilization   Vasectomy has no effect on masculinity or sexual prowess as the testicles continue to work normally. Only the two tubes ('the vasa'), which carry sperm from the testicles to the penis, are divided. The operation is a minor one and is often performed under local anaesthesia.

The operation is not immediately effective as sperm are stored further down the exit route and these have first to be used up. This occurs most quickly by regular ejaculation, but alternative contraception must be used for sexual intercourse until three negative sperm counts have been obtained. Paternity occurs very rarely after this time and is then usually because the two ends of a tube have spontaneously reunited. However, attempts to reverse this operation, by re-joining the tubes, are not very successful.

Consider vasectomy only if you are certain that you would not want to father children regardless of how your personal circumstances may change, for example with divorce and remarriage, or the death of a child.

Morning-after contraception   Hormones taken in high dose and within 72 hours of unprotected intercourse are highly effective in preventing pregnancy but this method is only suitable for a one-off occasion and not for regular use. It is very much a 'last-ditch' method of contraception but men should be prepared to suggest it if, after intercourse, it turns out that no contraceptive had been used.

An IUCD fitted within a week of unprotected intercourse will prevent most pregnancies by stopping the fertilized egg from implanting in the womb and will also provide continuing contraception. Risks of bleeding and infection may be slightly increased by fitting a coil at this time.

Work continues on a pill for men and on new drugs for women, but there seems little prospect of a major contraceptive breakthrough in the near future.

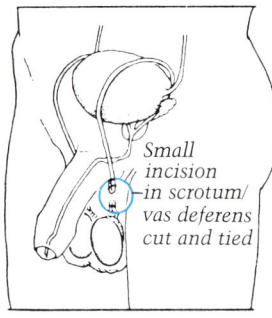

Small incision in scrotum/ vas deferens cut and tied

Vasectomy involves cutting the vas deferens on each side to prevent the sperm travelling from the testes to the penis for ejaculation. It is usually performed under a local anaesthetic but is not fully safe for 3 months after the operation.

SEXUALLY TRANSMITTED DISEASES

While it is true that almost any infection can be acquired at the time of intercourse, one wouldn't normally classify the common cold or influenza as 'venereal diseases' just because they had been passed on in that way. There are, however, many conditions which can be rightly labelled as sexually transmitted since sexual intercourse is the prime or only method of acquiring them.

The sexual act is one which lends itself particularly well to the transmission of disease since germs, be they bacteria, viruses, or other micro-organisms, are brought into direct contact with susceptible, or 'infectible' parts of the anatomy. While the traditional venereal diseases such as gonorrhoea and syphilis no longer pose a serious threat to general health, thanks to the advent of antibiotics, a whole host of new infections, including hepatitis and the HIV virus (which may lead to AIDS), has been recognized as being sexually transmitted. Many of these infections are predominantly found amongst practising male homosexuals.

It is unusual for there to be any indication that a prospective sexual partner is suffering from an infection. Indeed, it is the very lack of symptoms in both sexes that makes control of these diseases so difficult.

What, then, can be done to minimize the risk of acquiring or transmitting infection? Casual sexual encounters are traditionally, and in fact, the most chancy and this is reflected in the higher numbers of cases amongst men whose work takes them away from home and family or regular partner. Prostitutes, particularly abroad and in spite of 'licences' and 'regular medical examinations', are another likely source of infection and should be viewed accordingly. The use of a condom in all such encounters is a very effective way of reducing the risk.

There is no evidence that extra cleanliness, washing or urinating after intercourse, or the use of antiseptics or disinfectants in any way cuts down the risk of infection.

As important as the avoidance of infecting yourself is the avoidance of transmitting your infection to others. Because, in general, there is a significant time lapse, known as the incubation period, between catching an infection and showing any symptoms, the vast majority of infections are passed on unwittingly. Women are more likely have no noticeable symptoms than men and to be all the more surprised to learn that they have an infection.

If someone has been at risk, it is important therefore not to have intercourse with *anyone else* until a reasonable period has elapsed, to give time for symptoms or signs to develop, or for a clinic to be visited for a check-up.

Having said that, it remains true that, for the man at least, there will usually be signs and symptoms of infection and these will be dealt with under general headings of urethritis, spots and sores, itching and lumps.

Urethritis Urethritis literally means inflammation of the urethra, which is the pipe leading from the bladder, where urine is stored, to the tip of the penis. This pipe is used both for urination and the passage of the sperms and secretions which make up the ejaculate. Inflammation reflects the body's healing process and may either be a reaction to infection or to trauma. There are several infectious causes of urethritis in men, the most common of which are NSU (Non-Specific Urethritis) and gonorrhoea.

Gonorrhoea   This is one of the 'classical' venereal diseases and used to be responsible for much suffering and some nasty complications. Now that there are effective antibiotics, particularly penicillin, these problems are things of the past.

The two main symptoms are dysuria: discomfort or pain when passing urine; and urethral discharge: pus or fluid coming out of the penis. In days gone by, the dysuria was fairly severe but this is rarely seen today. Indeed, only about half of men with urethral gonorrhoea notice any discomfort at all and this tends to be mild. The discharge that is seen in most cases starts as a slight dampness but rapidly progresses to become profuse, thick and white or off-white. It used to be thought that the dysuria and discharge would be seen very soon after the infection had started - within a week in most cases - but it seems that nowadays the incubation period can be a lot longer than that. This means that lack of symptoms two weeks, say, after a risky sexual encounter does not exclude infection.

Gonorrhoea can also infect other parts of the body, the rectum in homosexuals and the throat also. Infection of these two sites often goes unnoticed although rectal infection may give a feeling of dampness at the anus and pus may be noticed on the faeces.

In a few cases (usually when the infection has been allowed to last for many weeks without treatment) gonorrhoea may spread to involve the testicle on one or other side giving great pain and swelling in the scrotum. In some people the infection gets into the bloodstream and may infect joints and cause slight painful spots. It must be stressed that these complications are extremely rare.

Although gonorrhoea has become less sensitive to antibiotics over the years, it is still readily treatable, usually with penicillin, and in most uncomplicated infections a single dose of antibiotic is adequate.

Non-Specific urethritis   NSU or NGU is much more common than gonorrhoea and is, in general, a milder infection. The incubation period may be quite long - several weeks - and some men who are infected do not develop any symptoms at all. The bacterium most often causing NSU is called *Chlamydia trachomatis*, less important in men than in the women in whom untreated infection may lead to involvement of the Fallopian tubes and subsequent infertility. The germ may also cause eye infections in adults and children.

Like gonorrhoea, NSU can produce dysuria and urethral discharge but these symptoms are much milder. The discharge may be very scanty, sometimes only present first thing in the morning. It is unusual for the pus seen in gonorrhoea to be found with NSU. Treatment of NSU is a course of antibiotics, usually tetracycline or erythromycin, for two weeks.

NSU has gained a reputation for being unresponsive to treatment and difficult to eradicate. One of the reasons for this has been over-treatment in the past by doctors, coupled with the minimal symptoms that are present. Once a person's mind has been concentrated on the possibility of infection, it may be hard to discount some minor irritation or slight dampness which may simply indicate continued healing of the urethritis. There is no doubt that *Chlamydia* is eradicated by the treatment outlined above; mild persistence of symptoms following the course of antibiotics does not mean that the treatment has failed. However, it is quite possible to catch any of the sexually transmitted diseases more than once and for this reason it is important that any sexual partners are examined and treated before intercourse is resumed.

NSU can be transmitted by homosexual intercourse and, in addition to urethritis, there may be a non-specific infection of the rectum.

During the treatment for NSU, and also gonorrhoea, it is important not to have any further sexual intercourse until the course of antibiotics is finished. Doctors used to ban the drinking of alcohol in all cases of urethritis but there is no evidence that this has any effect on the ultimate cure, although the symptoms may be aggravated by any alcohol that is excreted in the urine.

Other causes of urethritis   While NSU and gonorrhoea make up most of the cases of urethral infection, there are other causes, the most common of which is *Trichomonas vaginalis* (TV). This infection is responsible for fewer symptoms in men than in women, in whom an offensive vaginal discharge is found, often with much soreness. It is quite hard to diagnose in men and many cases are given the same treatment as for NSU. In practice this may not matter since it appears that many men will naturally eliminate the infection during the two-week period of treatment.

Often TV will be first diagnosed in the woman and it is common practice to give the same course of antibiotics to her sexual partner - a five- or seven-day course of metronidazole. This is one antibiotic that does not mix with alcohol.

There is a longer list of other causes of NSU, including viruses such as herpes and warts, but together they make up only a small percentage of cases.

SPOTS AND SORES

Syphilis   The first thought that crosses many people's minds on discovering a sore on the genitals is that it must be syphilis. This diagnosis, today, is in fact very unlikely. For reasons that are not clear, syphilis is almost entirely confined to practising male homosexuals - the few cases in women being passed on to them by a bisexual partner. There is some indication that even homosexual syphilis is on the decline, probably because patterns of casual sex have changed with increasing awareness and fears of AIDS.

Syphilis goes through several stages once it has been caught, the first, or primary, stage being the development of a hard, painless sore. This is usually found on the penis or point of first genital contact (lip, anus, cervix) and can appear up to three months after infection. If untreated there will be progression to the secondary stage in which there is often a non-itchy rash which covers the whole of the body. This rash is very obvious and consists of a mass of copper-coloured spots - even on the soles of the feet. It is accompanied by enlargement of lymph glands in the groin, armpits and elsewhere. These nodes are painless.

The disease then enters a 'latent' phase when there are no signs of infection at all. Even those people who have not been treated very rarely progress to the later stages of syphilis when the heart and blood vessels and nervous system are involved. Only a minute number of such late cases are seen today.

Syphilis at all stages can be readily diagnosed, and excluded, by a simple blood test which is routinely performed on all patients who attend a clinic specializing in sexually transmitted infections. Treatment is by a series of penicillin injections.

Herpes simplex   Herpes is a more common cause of sores and has acquired a largely unjustified reputation thanks to ill-informed scare-mongering by the media. The herpes virus is one of the most common in the world and a majority of adults will have been exposed to it, and infected by it. There are two sub-types of virus: Type I, which usually causes infection around the lips and mouth ('cold sores'), and Type II, which more often infects the genitals. Either type can, however, be found at either site.

While it is true that, like many other viruses, herpes cannot be 'cured', in most people it doesn't cause any symptoms or signs of infection and leads to no problems. In a minority of those infected there may be recurrences of sores after the initial infection but in very few are these anything other than a temporary nuisance.

If infection occurs for the first time in adulthood (and it can be shown that most people are infected by the virus at an earlier stage), it may produce multiple, painful ulcers which heal naturally within a few days. It is unwise to have any sexual contact when there are obvious signs of an outbreak because that is when the virus can be passed on, but otherwise life can, and should, go on as normal.

Herpes is the one sexually transmitted infection that can appear to arise 'out of the blue' in a faithful relationship. This may occur after oral sex when a man or woman has a mouth infection and transfers it to their partner's vulva or penis. For this reason fellatio or cunnilingus should be avoided when cold sores or mouth ulcers are present. Recurrent attacks of herpes tend to be less severe than the first attack and usually become less frequent as time goes by.

There are several obscure tropical infections that are very rarely seen in the UK which can cause spots and sores, and some other rather more mundane conditions which may give rise to anxiety. Vaginal thrush (see below) may lead to small red patches on the penis following intercourse; and scabies, which is caused by a small mite, can lead to itchy spots on the foreskin and glans penis. Most men who attend a clinic because of spots or sores have neither syphilis nor herpes and are in need of reassurance rather than medication.

ITCHING AND LUMPS

Candida albicans (thrush)   Candida is a yeast-like fungus which commonly infects the vagina in women. It is a very potent stimulator of itching in some people and may cause red spots on the penis and itching which is particularly noticed after sex. It is a minor infection and is readily treated - the most important factor being treatment of the woman (who may have no symptoms) to prevent further attacks in the man.

Tinea cruris   Dhobie's itch or 'crutch rot' is a fungal infection which spreads in the groin and upper thigh and leads to discolouration of the skin and intense itching. It is not a sexually transmitted disease but is often mistaken for one. Antifungal cream or ointment rapidly clears this infection.

Genital warts   Warts, genital or otherwise, are caused by a group of viruses, the human papilloma viruses, and have taken on an increased significance in recent years since they have been found to be associated with a risk of development of cancer of the cervix in women. They come in different shapes and sizes but seem to prefer a warm, moist environment and are therefore seen more frequently in uncircumcised men, under the foreskin. Treatment is unsatisfactory and may involve painting podophylline or acid onto the warts, or freezing or burning them off. They are sexually transmitted and other infections such as NSU may also be present. They are best dealt with at a special clinic.

Crabs The crab louse, or *Phthirus pubis* to give it its proper name, is a sexually transmitted infestation which gives rise to itching in the pubic area. The female louse lays eggs (nits) which are cemented to the pubic hairs and there may be a heavy infestation before the nits or adults are noticed. The adult louse measures about a millimetre across, is flat and slow-moving. It may look like a small mole on the skin.

Although fairly horrifying to discover, crabs are not in themselves of medical importance but, since they are sexually transmitted, they indicate the risk of other STDs and should therefore prompt attendance at a special clinic to make sure that there are no other infections. They do not survive for long away from the human body and are unlikely to have been caught from dirty linen.

Infections of homosexuals A combination of rectal (as opposed to vaginal) intercourse and sexual practices such as anilingus, exposes the male homosexual to a wider spectrum of disease. This is not to say that these infections are never seen in heterosexuals, simply that they are much less common.

Syphilis has already been mentioned as a predominantly homosexual disease these days and to this must be added Type B hepatitis, gut infections and Human Immuno Deficiency Virus (HIV, formerly known as HTLV III) which is responsible for the development of Acquired Immune Deficiency Syndrome (AIDS).

Hepatitis B used to be thought transmitted only by blood transfusions and other contact with infected blood; hence the high rate of infection amongst intravenous drug abusers who share needles. Since the 1970s, however, it has been recognized that homosexuals, perhaps because of trauma to the back passage in rectal intercourse, are also very likely to become infected. There are also several infections of the bowel, including dysentery, which are much more common in homosexuals.

HIV Infection Although most people refer to this infection as AIDS, it is more accurate and helpful to talk about HIV infection since most of those infected do not progress to AIDS. However, while the large majority suffer no ill-effects at all, the virus remains in the body and those who are infected remain infectious for the rest of their lives.

AIDS was first recognized in the United States in 1981 but it is now clear that infection with the virus has been around for some years. It appears that the virus first emerged in central, sub-Saharan Africa, possibly in Zaire. Because there were many French-speaking Haitians in that country, the infection may have been carried back to Haiti and thence, transmitted to American homosexual tourists, carried to New York. From there it spread rapidly to the homosexual community on the West Coast in San Francisco and Los Angeles. The infection reached Europe both from the USA and as a result of direct spread from Africa reflecting the many historical, colonial connections between the two continents.

There are certain groups of people who are categorized as 'high risk' and these include male homosexuals and bisexuals, intravenous drug abusers, haemophiliacs and the spouses or sexual partners of these.

Transmission of HIV occurs when infected blood is transferred from an infected person. It is thought that the trauma of rectal intercourse explains the greater risk to homosexuals than heterosexuals. The virus has been found in many body fluids that have been examined, including semen, tears and saliva. However, there seems to be little chance of transmission of infection from these, blood being the vehicle for transmission.

HIV infection can be likened to a pyramid of conditions with AIDS at the top, representing the small percentage of infected people who progress this far. The base of the pyramid represents the large majority who have been infected but suffer no illness or ill-effects.

HIV Disease   HIV acts by attacking certain cells in the body, primarily a type of white cell in the blood called a 'T-cell'. These cells are part of the body's immune defences and are important in the development of antibodies to infections. The virus also has a particular affinity for cells in the central nervous system. The result of infection in some people is that they are no longer able to fight off infections, called 'opportunistic' infections, which do not normally cause any problems in healthy folk.

Following infection with the virus, there may be a short flu-like illness with fever and aches and pains; and a few people develop signs of infection in the nervous system, and encephalitis which rapidly gets better. Most notice nothing amiss and, unless tested for the antibody to the virus, will remain unaware of their infection.

Up to 35 per cent of those infected will eventually progress to physical symptoms of disease and may be categorized as PGL or ARC. Persistent Generalized Lymphadenopathy (PGL) describes those in whom lymph glands all over the body become enlarged and remain so for a long time. The patient need not feel unwell, although there may be evidence from laboratory tests that their immunological defences are affected.

A number of patients progress from PGL to AIDS Related Complex (ARC) in which there is weight loss, fever, fatigue, diarrhoea, and minor infections, such as thrush, which infect the mouth and throat. Patients with ARC often feel unwell and run-down and need medical support and care.

Acquired Immune Deficiency Syndrome (AIDS) is the end-stage of HIV disease and carries with it a poor outcome. There have been no reports of anyone with AIDS being cured and about half of those diagnosed as having AIDS in the United Kingdom have so far died.

The most common 'opportunistic' infection is a pneumonia caused by a bacterium, *Pneumocystis carinii*. This is probably a widespread organism to which all of us are exposed but it is only in those whose defences are lowered that it leads to life-threatening infection. AIDS patients are also more likely to suffer from tuberculosis.

Several cancers are seen more often than usual in AIDS cases, the most common being Kaposi's sarcoma. This is a tumour which produces brown or purple slightly hard blotches on the skin and mucous membranes but which also multiplies inside the body to affect internal organs. Various other tumours are more common in AIDS, particularly those associated with lymph glands. In many cases there is a combination of opportunistic infection and tumour.

The first thing to recognize is that there is no blood test which tells whether or not someone has AIDS. What there is, however, is a test which tells whether there are antibodies to HIV, and current thinking suggests that the finding of such antibodies means that the virus is always present. However, a positive antibody test does not signify that AIDS is present. As stated above, *only ten per cent* of antibody-positive people go on to develop AIDS.

How catching is this virus? If one were to believe all that is written in the press, analogies with bubonic plague would seem to be understatements. Fortunately, nothing could be further from the truth. There is a wealth of evidence which demonstrates that it is almost impossible to become infected unless you belong to one of the high-risk groups. Heterosexual transmission of the virus certainly can occur but it is extremely uncommon.

Normal, non-sexual contact with an infected person is perfectly safe. It is not possible to catch the virus from sharing cooking utensils, knives and forks or lavatories with an infected person, and there have been no cases contracted from touching, kissing or being in close contact. The unfortunate sufferers from this disease have the added burden of being treated like pariahs by friends, relations and colleagues at work but this, perhaps understandable, reaction has absolutely no medical or scientific justification.

In the United Kingdom we are lucky to have a network of clinics which deal, amongst other things, with sexually transmitted diseases. These used to be known as 'special', 'VD' or 'clap' clinics and were often situated in basements or huts as far away from the main hospital as possible. They are now known as genito-urinary medicine clinics to reflect the fact that many patients who attend do not have infections, and the stigma which used to be attached to attendance has diminished.

These departments have open access, there being no need for referral from a GP, and are all happy to screen worried patients who have been at risk. Another service performed by these clinics is contact-tracing - of vital importance in preventing the spread of sexually transmitted diseases. The keynote of a clinic is total confidentiality and patients' notes are kept separate from the general hospital files. If in doubt, go and have a check-up.

INFERTILITY

When a healthy couple in their twenties or early thirties are attempting to produce a child, on average they will take about four months to conceive. 80 per cent of such couples succeed within a year, and eventually 90 per cent will conceive naturally, leaving 10 per cent who will remain childless unless help is provided.

The important thing is not to worry if, having decided to start a family, conception does not occur right away. Unnecessary anxiety can inhibit the process of conception and the delay may therefore be lengthened unduly. However, if after two years of trying, the woman has failed to become

The vigour with which a normal sperm swims varies. It is stimulated by the hormone androgen but a sluggish movement may mean that antibodies have developed in the semen which prevent full movement.

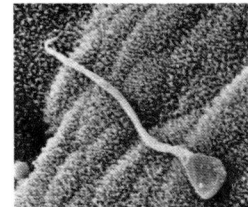

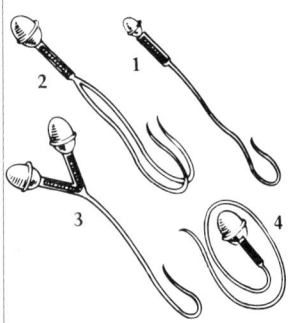

A variety of different sperm abnormalities including *1* small heads, *2* two tails, *3* two heads, *4* curly tails. As much as 20% of the sperm ejaculated may have one of these. Such sperm are unable to make satisfactory progress but the high proportion of fit sperm make up for this.

pregnant, medical advice should be sought.

Infertility is usually an extremely distressing experience for both partners. the onset of yet another menstrual cycle is a source of great disappointment to them and an atmosphere of gloom can pervade until just before the next period. Their sex life can suffer as the strain begins to tell. Naturally frustrated that they cannot get on with the business of starting a family, they become irritated with each other. They feel envious of their friends, who seem to talk about nothing but their babies, and make excuses not to see them. Above all, they can feel dejected at what they see as an inadequacy or a defect in their make-up.

Men are particularly reluctant to acknowledge that the problem may lie with themselves. As they see it, to be sterile is not to be a 'real' man. To maintain their self-esteem, they tend to blame the woman for once again failing to become pregnant. Having ejaculated in the vagina, many feel that they have done their bit and that the failure to conceive must therefore be their wife's responsibility. Yet it has been estimated that the man is entirely responsible in 3 out of 10 cases and plays a contributory role in a further 20 per cent.

Causes of male sub-fertility   Although it is true that the higher a man's sperm count, the more chance he has of conceiving it is nevertheless not uncommon for men whose sperm count is well below average to produce children. In cases where it is suspected that a low count is contributing to infertility, an effective technique is AIH (Artificial Insemination by the Husband). The first spurts of semen from a number of ejaculates are collected and frozen over a period of time. This sperm-rich concentrate is then thawed and introduced into the womb at the time of ovulation.

If a man is impotent, ejaculates before entry, or fails to reach a climax during intercourse, then obviously conception is unlikely to occur. Under these circumstances, the couple should undergo psychosexual counselling or use an appropriate self-help procedure described earlier in this chapter.

It follows that if a man rarely makes love to his wife, the chances of her becoming pregnant are slim. What is less commonly recognized is that if the man engages in some form of sexual activity each day, his ejaculate will contain less sperm. To ensure that his count remains at its highest, he should allow a delay of at least 72 hours between ejaculations.

In practical terms, to maximize the chances of conception, you and your partner should follow these guidelines:

● Do not worry if you are unsuccessful at first. If you have intercourse two or three times a week then it will be about six months, on average, before you conceive.

● When making love, your partner's hips should be supported by a pillow to ensure deep penetration.

● Afterwards, advise your partner to lie on her back for half an hour or so to keep the semen close to the neck of her womb.

● Leave at least three days between ejaculations to keep your sperm count high; it is highest on the third day.

● Make your sex life as enjoyable as possible. This will increase the quantity of sperm produced. If necessary, consult a psychosexual counsellor.

● Make time for sex between the 11th and 16th days of your partner's

MALE INFERTILITY

Men are reluctant to acknowledge that an infertility problem is due to them, but in three out of ten cases the man is reponsible. The following table shows the effect of these problems.

Anatomical causes

Pathological causes

Environmental causes

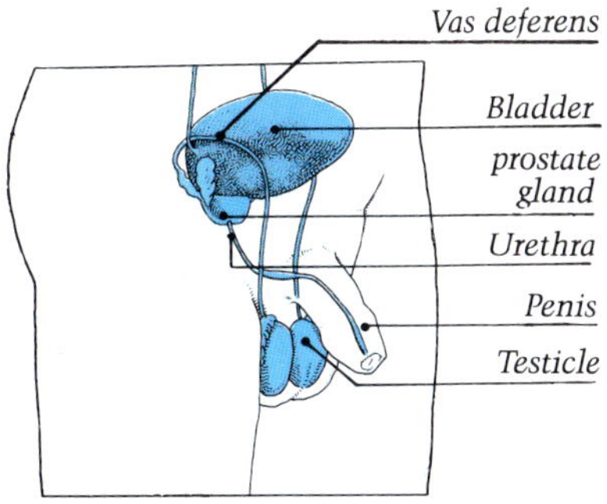

Vas deferens
Bladder
prostate gland
Urethra
Penis
Testicle

PROBLEM	SPERM COUNT	TREATMENT
Varicocele *Enlarged (varicose) veins around the testis*	Low	Semen quality increases after surgical removal of the vein
Vas blockage *Caused by venereal infection or, more rarely, tuberculosis infection*	Absent	Surgical intervention
Vasectomy *Surgical cut of the sperm-carrying duct as a contraceptive measure*	Absent	Reversals are successful in 40% of men
Retrograde ejaculation *Sperm goes into the bladder instead of down the penis*	Normal	Sperm must be removed from bladder and separated for future AIH (artificial insemination by husband)
Undescended testis *Testis remains in abdomen instead of descending into the scrotum*	Absent	None if left untreated until after puberty

PROBLEM	SPERM COUNT	TREATMENT
Mumps/other febrile illness/ injury through accident or surgery	Low	Semen quality usually improves within three months
Gonorrhea *Venereal infection*	Absent	Vas deferens blockage needs surgery
Age	Low	After 40 fertility decreases

PROBLEM	SPERM COUNT	TREATMENT
Lead, arsenic, zinc, radiation	Low or absent	Prevent further exposure
Excessive heat in working environments	Low	Foundry workers remain at risk
Alcohol, barbiturates, cannabis, other drugs	Low	Stop drug

cycle, when she is most fertile.

Genital disorders   Undescended testicles is a developmental condition which can only be treated successfully if diagnosed at an early age. There is no known treatment for Klinefelter's syndrome, a chromosomal abnormality impairing the growth of the testicles, which in turn fail to produce mature sperm.

A number of other conditions may affect fertility, for example, if the testicles are bruised or knocked severely, the sperm count may drop for a time before returning to normal. If they become twisted, it may remain permanently low unless medical help is sought right away.

It is widely known that an attack of mumps or another virus after puberty can make men sub-fertile but only relatively few are permanently affected. A varicose vein around the testicles may kill off sperm through overheating, although this can usually be rectified with surgery. If the vas deferens becomes blocked through TB or a venereal disease, surgery can prove effective. (A similar operation is used to reverse vasectomy and this is successful in about 50 per cent of cases.)

Although malnutrition is an extremely rare occurrence in our society, some cases of infertility are caused by a poor diet; this is usually associated with alcoholism. Exposure to certain pesticides, industrial fumes, and some types of drugs - including nicotine - can lower the sperm count. And glandular disorders, such as an underactive thyroid gland, may also cause sterility. If you have reason to suspect any of these conditions you should seek medical advice.

HOMOSEXUALITY

In most respects other than its orientation the sexuality of homosexual men resembles that of the heterosexual male. For most gay men, as for most heterosexuals, their sexuality is an enjoyable and fulfilling part of their lives. When homosexual men have problems with sex these problems, too, resemble those of heterosexuals. Like them, gay men have conflicts to resolve between a need for love and tenderness and a need to prove their sexual machismo.

Gay men vary in the strength of their sex drive, and may have similar anxieties about potency, the size of their penis, and their sexual performance and relationships. It has been found that the same principles of sex therapy can be used for gay couples as in heterosexual relationships. It appears that the differences in sexuality between men and women are much greater than those between heterosexual orientations.

It is generally estimated that between five and ten per cent of men are exclusively or predominantly, homosexual. The Kinsey investigation into male sexual behaviour found, however, that one in three men has a homosexual experience leading to orgasm at least once in his life. Although it thus appears that homosexuality is common and attitudes to it have shifted radically in the last 40 years, most people are still reluctant to discuss homosexuality openly and the only reference to it is often in the form of jokes or derogatory comments. Any male whose appearance or behaviour deviates markedly from the masculine stereotype is scorned by

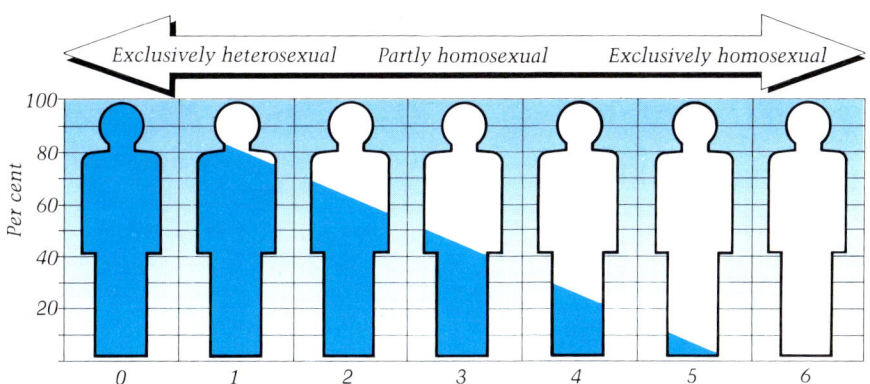

Homosexual experience is not confined to homosexual men. The Kinsey investigation found that a wide spectrum of sexual experience exists between the truly heterosexual man at one end of their scale (1-6) and the committed homosexual man at the other.

other men or, at best, is laughingly referred to as a 'queer' or 'poufter'. In spite of the fact that effeminacy is not a prerequisite for a homosexual, nor are such characteristics limited to gay men and that a gay man is as likely to be a lorry driver as a hairdresser, these stereotypes persist. This hostility and prejudice is not only due to ignorance, however, it also masks considerable anxiety on the subject. Most men, if pressed, will admit to being physically attracted to members of their own sex from time to time. However, since it is taboo in traditional male circles to raise the issue, a person can easily feel different from others in this respect and, therefore, become anxious and defensive. His anxieties about his own sexuality are projected on to other people.

In our society it is socially acceptable for a female to describe another as attractive. Womens magazines carry photographs of models advertising fashionable clothing and lingerie. With the exception of body-building publications, men's magazines rarely contain pictures of males. Thus those who experience homosexual attraction have conflicts and guilt feelings about their sexuality which they cannot share with others. Apart from denial and ridicule, they may attempt to cover up their anxieties by showing exaggerated sexual interest in the females. If their predominant sexual orientation is heterosexual, then in fact they are probably just being more honest with themselves than the majority of their friends.

'**Coming out**'   This hostility, born of fear and anxiety, can have very damaging effects on the man who is predominantly homosexual. Born and brought up in a world in which heterosexuality is seen as the norm and homosexuality as a disease, a sin, or at best a disability, he learns to see himself as irreversibly flawed. His sexuality, a central and vital part of his self-identity, is either derided or ignored. Unless he is very fortunate he sees no models of a successful amalgam of sexuality and a loving relationship on which he can base his own aspirations.

This process, whereby a person brought up in a society which sees him as a second class citizen internalizes the values of that society, learning self-denigration and self-hatred, could be compared with the experience of black people in a white-dominated culture. It differs, however, in that whereas a black person is always openly and irrevocably seen to be black, there is no external sign of homosexuality. The gay man, therefore, can grow up not only unable to accept his own sexuality, but also unaware that there are many millions of men who share his sexual orientation.

Many men repress their homosexuality so firmly that they themselves may not be conscious of it. They may merely experience a lack of heterosexual fantasies or attractions, and perhaps an embarrassment about being in close physical contact with other men. Homosexual fantasies otherwise suppressed may emerge in dreams.

The process whereby an individual overcomes the social and internalized pressures against homosexuality is sometimes referred to as 'coming out'. First, a man has to recognize and accept his own homosexual feelings - coming out to himself. If he wishes to express his sexuality in sexual relationships, as most gay men do, then he will need to share this discovery with others - to come out with them. For the integrated person this means not just sexual partners and others in the gay sub-culture, but to some extent at least family, friends and workmates. Even in a supportive environment this exposure of sexuality can be stressful to a man and is a burden which heterosexual men do not have to face.

Fortunately, in recent years the gay community has developed an infrastructure of social groups and telephone help lines which can help gay men deal with these obstacles and make a satisfactory adjustment to their sexuality.

Causes of homosexuality A wide variety of theories has been postulated to 'explain' homosexuality. One theory is that if a boy's first sexual experiment involves a member of the same sex, the excitement of this event will remain with him and he will always have a secret wish to repeat the experience. Psychoanalysts argue that the nature of the boy's relationships with his mother and father will determine his sexual preferences in adulthood. Physiologists offer complex theories about testosterone levels at different stages in the child's development. None of these, however, have proved satisfactory. Until we understand more about the causes and mechanism of sexual attraction in general, then it seems improbable that we will be able to explain any specific sexual preference.

These theories were developed in the belief that homosexuality was a mental illness and that it could be treated. These treatments were offered until comparatively recently, and homosexuals accepted them in an attempt to conform in the same way that black people still use skin lighteners to become more socially acceptable. They were not, however, successful, either in changing sexual orientation or in prompting sexual adjustment. Most psychologists and psychiatrists have abandoned treatment in favour of counselling designed to help the gay man take a positive view of his sexuality. This change parallels a shift from a disease concept to seeing homosexuality as part of the spectrum of human experience; neither better or worse than heterosexuality, merely different.

Gay sexual behaviour The gay scene has a reputation of promiscuity, though this is of course one of many possible gay lifestyles, and many gay men are celibate, monogamous, or in stable relationships. There is no doubt that after the traumas of coming out many gay men behave like children let loose in a sweet shop. The more immediate and impersonal nature of the male sexual response discussed above means that casual sex is perhaps more readily available in an all-male context. It is often suggested that the absence of the social structures of marriage, the family and children, makes it more likely for gay relationships to break down when the going gets tough. There is no doubt that without the steadying influence of children, homosexuals are more easily prey to alternative relationships. The hostility of a heterosexual world, or at least the lack of support and recognition given to gay relationships, is also said by some to make it harder for them to last. The absence of such structures can, however, also be a strength; gay couples are free of the rigid expectations of men and women in marriages and are free to define their own relationship in a way which suits them as individuals. In spite of the obstacles, a large number of gay men do seem to achieve loving and fulfilling sexual relationships which are an enriching part of their lives.

SEX IN THE LATER YEARS

It is indisputable that, in his old age, a man becomes less capable of having sex. Many stop trying, believing the popular myth that sex is strictly for young people. If a man does make an attempt, he may well have problems getting an erection and will probably lose it, from time to time, during foreplay. This can be embarrassing and frustrating for him and may well irritate his partner. It is all too easy for him to give up and conclude that he is past it. As a result, he can be left with a feeling that this is yet another of life's pleasures that has passed him by.

• Personal relationships, fitness and well-being in the later years, see *Mature Health*, pages 189-197.

Some useful hints to help you enjoy sex in the later years are:
● Keep your sex life going before the effects of old age set in. This helps you to stay young and tolerant.
● Take regular exercise and cut down on alcohol and tobacco to keep yourself fit. An improved self-image is vital to a good sex life.
● Even if you do not feel much like intercourse, cuddle your partner regularly. Closeness, and the warm expression of affection, are what matter most.
● If you have developed a physical disability, be imaginative and find ways of overcoming it. Ill or disabled people need love even more.
● Do not be embarrassed about using sexy videos or magazines in order to become aroused. Ask your partner to wear the clothes that used to excite you.
● Do not be discouraged when you lose your erection. There's always another time!

Most men are biologically capable of having sex until well into their nineties. In fact, many of those who have given up intercourse still masturbate from time to time. Given that an active sex life can act as a tonic, it is important for older men not to let themselves become discouraged by the occasional failure. Much of the advice contained in the 'sexual problems' section earlier, is particularly relevant to them and can produce quite remarkable results with people who thought their loving days were over. They may just have to work a little harder at the various exercises.

It is often said that older men make the best lovers. There is every reason to believe that this can be true. They are usually less concerned with their penis and their performance and get more pleasure from touching and being touched. By involving the whole of their body, they can get more out of sex than they did in their youth, and they are more considerate of their partner's needs, tending to put themselves out to increase her pleasure.

Moreover, they may well have got over the false idea that masculinity is determined by the frequency of sex and the strength of a man's erection. As a result, their self-esteem is not at risk every time they approach their partner. More important still, the effects of their early conditioning may well have worn off, and they can find themselves able to achieve a level of intimacy unknown to them in their earlier years. By, at last, being able to combine their loving feelings with their physical needs, many men get much more out of their sexual relationships in old age.

STIMULANTS, RELAXANTS AND YOU

In the strict sense, a drug is any substance that can intentionally affect the body or mind of the person who takes it. In practice, of course, drugs are of different types. Medicinal drugs are designed to treat a particular disease or symptom, such as aspirin for pain or digoxin for heart failure. Recreational drugs, such as cannabis and LSD, have no established medical use. In between the two extremes are numerous drugs that, although having medical uses, also have a potential for abuse, which makes their control very difficult. Heroin, tranquillizers, sleeping tablets and some stimulants fall into this category.

For the purposes of this book, we are considering only the mind-altering drugs taken for recreational purposes. The use and abuse of these drugs generally follows a pattern. First they are introduced and widely used because of their pleasant effects. Eventually it becomes apparent that their use causes ill-effects in some users, and legislation is introduced to restrict the use of the drug, which then becomes 'a drug of abuse'. This pattern has been seen with opium, morphine, cannabis, heroin, cocaine and several of the more recent introductions such as LSD. In recent years, however, there has been a tendency to make illegal the use of new drugs that seem to have a potential for abuse, often before real evidence of their harmful nature can be presented. This is largely an attempt to obviate the growing drug problem, and to prevent experimentation in search of new drug experiences.

WHY DO WE USE DRUGS?

Probably all cultures take drugs in some form or another, but the social and psychological pressures that cause us to depend on them are complex. It is clear, however, that in any society, some people are more likely than others to come to depend upon drugs.

Several terms used to describe the response to drugs need to be clearly understood, to avoid confusion about the effects of drug-taking. *Dependence* is the need to continue taking a drug and with some drugs may develop after only a few doses. *Physical dependence* means that it is necessary to continue to take the drug regularly to avoid unpleasant physical withdrawal effects, such as vomiting and severe tremor.

Emotional or *psychological dependence* is the need for mental support from a drug, to cushion the user from reality or to enable him to experience its pleasant effects. This emotional dependence is the prime motive for most drug-taking, extending drug-taking into our every-day life. *Withdrawal effects* are the unpleasant physical effects that appear when you stop taking a drug that causes physical dependence. The effects usually fade after a few days but are often temporarily very unpleasant. *Addiction* implies that dependence has developed. It is now not a frequently used term, but is popularly used to describe only physical drug dependence.

To distinguish them from 'medical' drugs, the drugs used for recreational purposes are often described as 'drugs of abuse'. Apart from its application to those drugs restricted by law, this phrase is misleading. Are tea and coffee 'drugs of abuse'? Are alcohol or tobacco? They are all drugs, capable of causing physical and emotional dependence. Aspirin, one of the most widely used pain-killers, has no known recreational use but is subject to more 'abuse' than any other drug. It is taken in vast amounts, often for the wrong reason, and causes demonstrable risks to health when misused. But it is not classified as a 'drug of abuse'.

So why *do* people take drugs, when there are widely recognized health hazards attached to their use?

The primary motivation and certainly the initial cause is peer group pressure - the desire to conform with the group you are in or, if you are young, with the group you aspire to join. In a social group, for example, the non-smoker or non-drinker can be made to feel an outsider, and subtle pressures are exerted to take part in the social activity of passing round the cigarettes or buying a round of drinks. There are many social occasions when the pressure to conform is almost irresistible. A glass of sherry is automatically placed in your hand at a wedding reception, and at many business meetings, gin and tonics are dispensed with a bland assumption that everyone present will be drinking.

Many young people are educated into the use of acceptable social drugs such as tea and coffee in early childhood; some are introduced by their parents to the smoking habit. A child brought up in a household where the parents smoke or drink will obviously be highly receptive to the habit himself.

In later years, the motivation for experimenting with drugs changes. For many young people, the very fact that the use of a particular drug is theoretically restricted to an older age group, as is the case with tobacco and alcohol, gives the drug a particular glamour. And the glamour is even greater when the use of a drug is actually illegal. Perhaps we all harbour secret resentment when something is banned, and the feeling that authority is keeping a pleasant experience away from us only makes us more curious.

A mixture of rebelliousness and curiosity encourages the young to experiment with drugs. Some try all the available drugs, and some people believe that there is an inexorable progression through cigarettes, alcohol, glue-sniffing and cannabis that leads eventually to 'hard' drugs like cocaine and heroin. This process is not automatic, however. Most young people who try glue-sniffing do not progress to harder drugs, and progressively fewer users are involved at each step towards 'harder' drugs.

Subtler pressures affect adult drug usage. Many men begin to take drugs to avoid physical stress, and some become emotionally, sometimes physically, dependent on their use. Tranquillizers and sleeping tablets are common examples of drugs that are taken initially for their medical effects but that may gradually become drugs of dependence. Taken in this way, they are *not* recreational drugs, unlike their occasional use by experimenting teenagers.

In some social circles, the use of cannabis is as acceptable as the smoking of cigarettes, and the motivation for its use is probably much the same: that is, peer group pressure and the desire to conform. A decade ago, LSD was used in the same way, but this drug is now much less fashionable among adults; its often severe psychiatric complications are now widely accepted.

In all these forms of drug-taking, initial effects are pleasurable. With some drugs, tolerance develops quickly, and progressively larger amounts are needed to recreate the initial effect. This can quickly lead to physical dependence, when high doses are taken at frequent intervals.

A drug may relax the mind, or make the user feel more alert, or induce a feeling of intense pleasure or lightheadedness. With the mildest drugs, such as tea or coffee, the physical effects are almost imperceptible, and it is often the rituals accompanying the habit that give most emotional comfort to the user. Hence the careful procedures for making tea, which are especially prevalent in Eastern countries (although British tea-making can be equally ritualized), or for preparing brewed coffee.

The mixing of alcoholic drinks, with the careful admixture of ice and other ingredients, is also important to the user, as are the rituals of finding a cigarette, carefully lighting up and tapping off the ash to a smoker. The offering of a cigarette to a woman and the panache with which a light is produced was a potent sexual gesture in the 1950s.

Some psychologists believe that these are all so-called displacement activities. That is, they are activities that distract our attention from some stressful event by giving us something else to concentrate on. This form of drug-taking can actually be useful, therefore, and help us to relax.

When drug-taking becomes potentially dangerous is when it becomes an emotional crutch, used to insulate us from reality. There is a definite association of drug-taking in various forms with social deprivation or with stressful occupations or situations. These forms of drug-taking are socially determined. Alcoholism is very common in areas of high unemployment. Tranquillizer abuse is common in stressful occupations. And in show-business, where long and irregular hours may be worked, cocaine is often used to increase alertness. Doctors and dentists, too, are particularly susceptible, working as they do in high-stress occupations with easy access to many drugs.

Using drugs for their emotional effects can lead to mental problems, but, as tolerance increases and larger doses are needed, most drugs also cause some physical deterioration. Smoking, alcohol and many of the 'harder' drugs cause demonstrable physical damage, and this is discussed in detail later in this chapter. Equally important are the disruption of family life and the effect on work performance resulting from the emotional and physical changes caused by drug dependence. Often, it is a deterioration in work or social interactions that first provides a clue to members of the family or friends that a man is using drugs to the detriment of his health or emotional well-being.

With the exception of the few socially acceptable drugs, the drug user is in potential conflict with the law. If he uses illegal drugs, he may be exposed to pressure from the supplier to try 'new' drugs or to buy larger amounts than he really needs. The cost of the drugs is such that it may be necessary to sell some in order to raise money for the next purchase. The user then becomes a pusher, and he will attract much heavier penalties if caught and prosecuted. A prosecution for using or supplying illegal drugs usually leads to dismissal by an employer, thereby increasing the stresses that probably led to the habit in the first place. With hard drugs it can lead to imprisonment.

It is not possible to explain why some people are able to cope with the effects of every-day drugs without needing to progress to stronger doses, while a few individuals move on to become alcoholics or hopeless addicts in the traditional sense, often with multi-drug use. However, drug use does appear to be commoner among psychopathic and highly aggressive individuals.

YOUR EVERYDAY DRUGS

Most men would be highly indignant if it were suggested that they were dependent on drugs. But could you face the day without a cup of tea or coffee? Could you finish off a meal in a restaurant without a cup of coffee?

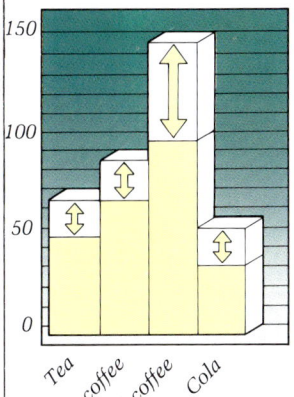

Caffeine per cup (milligrams)

150

100

50

0

Tea
Instant coffee
Brewed coffee
Cola

The amount of caffeine present in drinks varies.

Tea and coffee are not technically drugs in themselves, but they contain caffeine, which is. You will find caffeine in tea, much more in coffee, and it is present in cocoa and chocolate, as well as in cola drinks and various cold remedies. Caffeine is a powerful stimulant, and the amount present in two cups of coffee is sufficient to overcome drowsiness and often to prevent sleep for a while.

A medicinal dose of caffeine, which would be taken for its stimulant effect is, in comparison, 200mg. A moderate dose of caffeine (about two cups of brewed coffee) improves alertness, and at the same time, increases the amount of stomach enzymes and acid produced. Ideally, therefore, coffee should be drunk *before* a meal, and the Chinese may drink tea throughout a meal to allow the caffeine to increase the flow of gastric juices.

Taken in higher doses, caffeine can cause problems. If you drink more than eight cups of coffee each day, you are at increased risk of peptic ulcers and heart disease. In addition, cancer of the bladder and kidneys is more frequent among heavy tea and coffee drinkers.

Drinking this much coffee each day (or taking the equivalent amount of caffeine in other drinks) can also bring on the first signs of caffeine toxicity: anxiety, irritability and headaches are common warning signs of too much caffeine intake, as are muscle tremors, which cause the hands to tremble slightly.

Very large amounts of caffeine (15 cups of coffee or more a day) can cause quite severe physical effects, such as ringing in the ears and visual disturbances, but these are very rare.

In these every-day drinks caffeine is mild, predictable and generally perfectly harmless, unless taken in excessive amounts. Yet caffeine is undoubtedly a drug of dependence. If you are used to taking more than five cups of coffee daily (370mg caffeine), abstaining will make you irritable, sluggish and tired, and may cause headaches. These symptoms are a clear indication of physical dependence. Emotional dependence is very strong, and many men find it impossible to give up coffee, even when strongly advised to do so for medical reasons.

Because tea contains proportionately less caffeine than coffee, dependence is not usually so strong, and it is possible that tea is drunk more for its social aspects than for its caffeine content. Coffee, too, it has to be said, is primarily a social drink and usually not knowingly used as a source of caffeine.

Therefore, although caffeine is technically a drug, the social benefits of its use in every-day beverages clearly outweigh any health or emotional hazards. The exceptions are those few people who fail to recognize or accept their dependence and who, as they become tolerant of the effects, take ever-increasing amounts.

Death rates and smoking habits were studied in a group of male doctors revealing that the risk of premature death decreases in direct relation to the amount of cigarettes smoked.

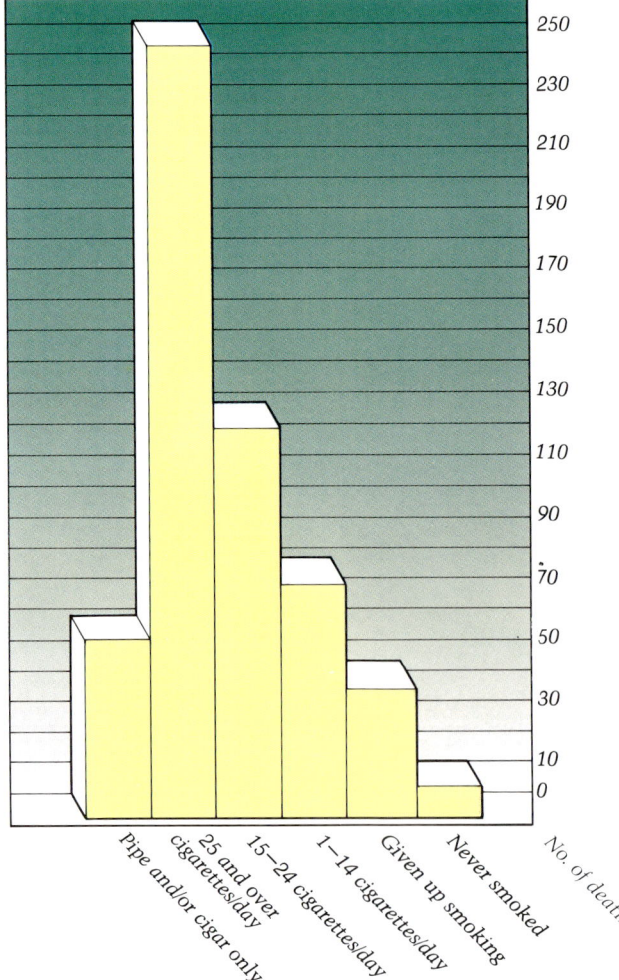

THE PROVEN DANGERS OF SMOKING

By now, there can be few who do not accept that smoking is hazardous to health. Many men will, however, attempt to defend their addiction to the habit and never admit in public that smoking is harmful. In recent years, attitudes to smoking have changed markedly. From being socially acceptable among a majority of adults, smoking is now in decline among men and is a minority habit.

For many smokers their habit is a classic example of drug dependence. It produces a very strong emotional dependence: some smokers need a cigarette to overcome stress or to provide a moment of relaxation after a meal. It is a powerful social tool: offering cigarettes in a group helps to 'break the ice' and establish fellowship among members of the group. And the small rituals associated with smoking, such as fumbling for the pack, tapping the end of the cigarette to consolidate the tobacco and frequently flicking off the ash, are all reinforcing aspects of the habit.

Yet smoking also produces a physical dependence. A smoker deprived of nicotine undergoes a true withdrawal syndrome. He is restless, irritable and depressed and has a strong craving for another cigarette. Tolerance develops too, as with other drugs of dependence, so consumption increases to achieve the same effect. One specialist in drug dependence has said that smoking is at least as strongly addictive as heroin. And in some aspects, the effects of smoking may be as bad as heroin, even though the habit is perfectly legal. Remember, heroin seldom kills its users by its toxic effects alone; other factors such as malnutrition and infection are the usual causes of mortality associated with this drug. But there is a direct relationship between the smoking of tobacco and deaths from cancer and other diseases.

SMOKING-RELATED DISEASES

Diseases caused by, or related to, smoking probably result from the combined effects of the mixture of chemicals present in tobacco smoke. Some are well known and recognized by most men as a common sequel to a lifetime of smoking. Others are less obvious, but no less damaging.

Lung cancer is the most common lethal form of cancer in Britain, causing 40 per cent of all male cancer deaths. It can be directly related to the number of cigarettes smoked and to the number of years that the habit has persisted. The disease usually starts insidiously. It is painless and will have been present for a considerable time before the smoker becomes aware of such symptoms as shortness of breath, sharp chest pain or coughing blood. Unfortunately, this often means that the disease is already well advanced and that it may have spread to other organs. Surgery to remove a cancerous lung is not always possible, and, as the disease does not respond so well to the chemotherapy used to treat other cancers, it has a high mortality rate. Fewer than one person in twenty with lung cancer survives long enough to be considered 'cured'. The number of people dying from lung cancer is closely related to the total number of smokers in the population, and one in six men who are heavy smokers can expect to die from lung cancer.

Continued on page 178

SMOKING THREATENS YOUR HEALTH

In Britain alone, one in six people dies prematurely because of smoking. Of those men smoking more than 20 cigarettes a day, 40 per cent will die before retirement, compared with only 15 per cent of non-smokers. Or, looked at another way, the 20-cigarettes-a-day man has chosen to shorten his life by five years, losing five minutes of life for every cigarette smoked.

The committed smoker may argue that he knows many healthy old people who have smoked all their lives, and the multinational tobacco companies can argue that the case against smoking is not 'proven'. But it is not possible to gainsay statistics collected from huge numbers of people in many country.

Smoking kills. And those it doesn't kill, it may well cripple.

Tobacco is a complex substance. When it burns, it produces a mixture of materials that can have varying effects on the body when they are inhaled into the lungs, and absorbed into the blood. Cigarettes are worse than cigars and pipes in this respect, as cigarette smoke is almost invariably inhaled. Smoke from cigars and pipes is less likely to be inhaled but, as their smoke usually contains more of the harmful substances, smoking these may simply mean that the user is substituting diseases of the mouth and throat for the lung disease more typically associated with cigarette smoking.

Tar has been shown to cause cancer in animals and scientists believe it has the same effect on humans. Irritants in the tar cause other damage to the lungs apart from cancer, and these include a narrowing of the tiny tubes within the lung tissue known as bronchioles. Smoking also paralyses the tiny cilia (hairs) which waft mucus and impurities up from the lung to the throat. Without these, the lungs have no way of ridding the tissue of the tar that collects in the lung. Tar accumulates in the unsmoked butt of a cigarette, so the shorter the cigarette is smoked, the greater will be the exposure to the effects of tar.

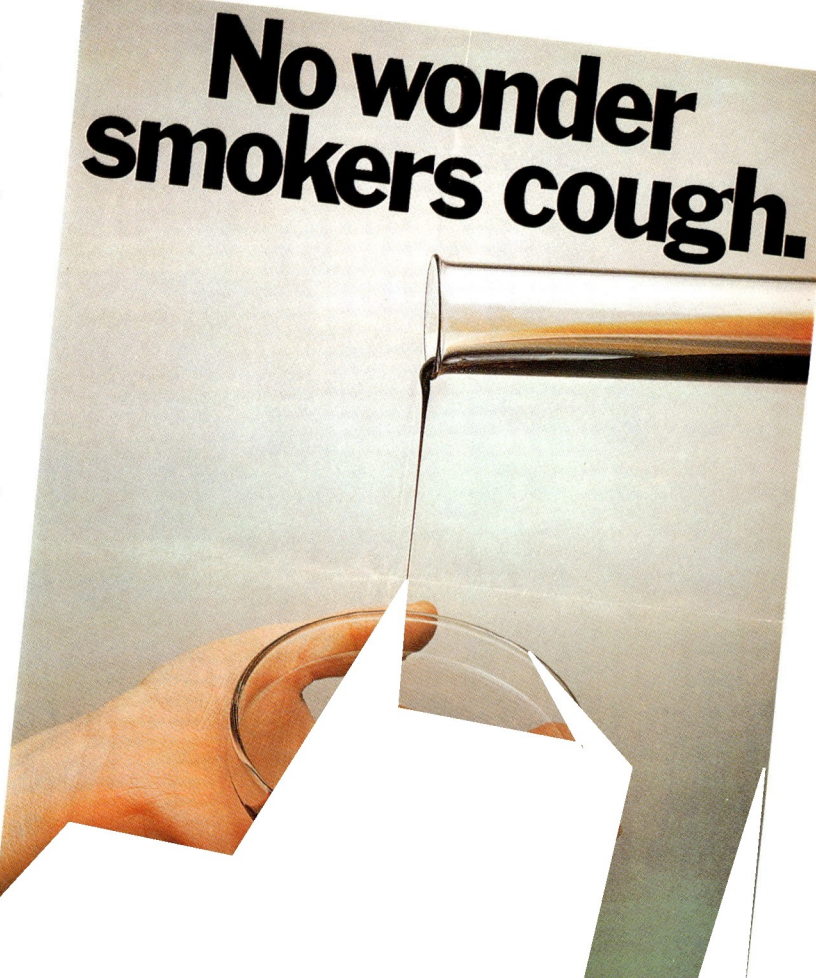

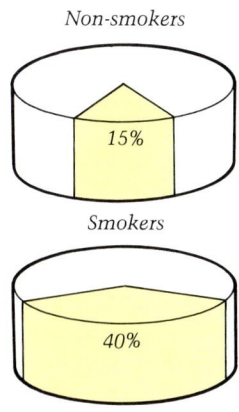

Non-smokers

15%

Smokers

40%

40% of heavy male smokers die before they reach retirement age, compared with only 15% of non-smokers.

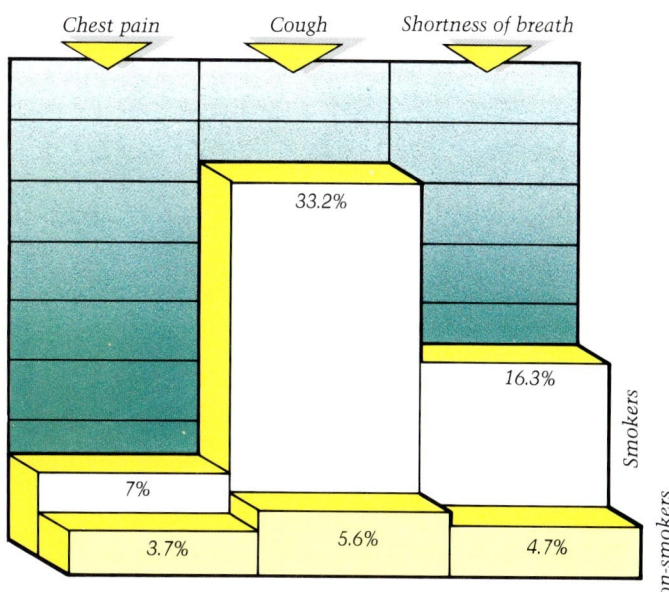

Chest pain   Cough   Shortness of breath

33.2%

16.3%

7%

3.7%   5.6%   4.7%

Smokers

Non-smokers

Smoking does not just kill, it also increases the frequency of many irritating and sometimes debilitating common complaints.

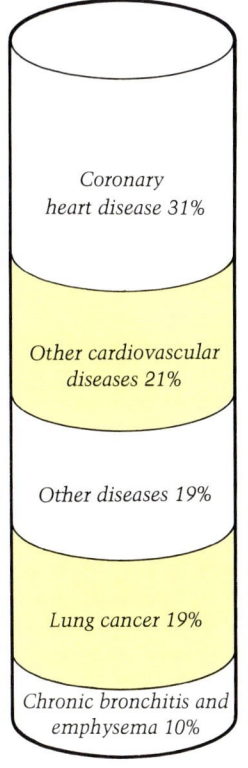

Coronary heart disease 31%

Other cardiovascular diseases 21%

Other diseases 19%

Lung cancer 19%

Chronic bronchitis and emphysema 10%

Causes of early deaths among smokers.

The connection between cancer and smoking has received so much publicity that few people realize smoking causes a variety of other life-threatening diseases. In fact, a heavy smoker is much more likely to suffer cardiovascular disease than lung cancer.

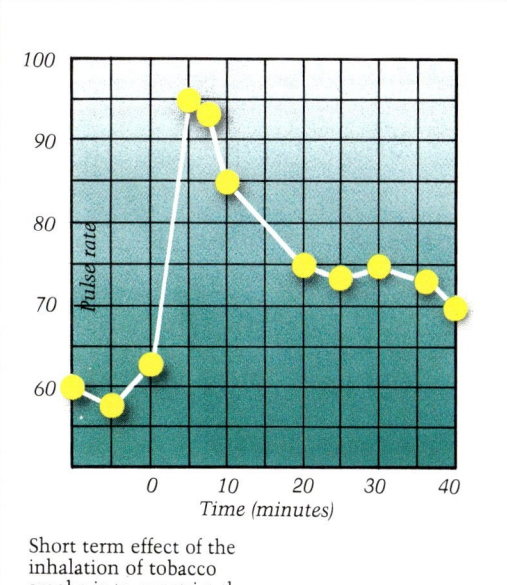

Pulse rate

100
90
80
70
60

0   10   20   30   40
Time (minutes)

Short term effect of the inhalation of tobacco smoke is to constrict the blood vessels and cause an immediate rise in blood pressure. This in turn increases the pulse rate and the carbon monoxide in the inhaled smoke decreases the oxygen-carrying capacity of the blood.

STRATEGIES FOR GIVING UP SMOKING

Now that the risks from smoking are so well known, most smokers want to give up. In fact, two out of every three smokers admit to wanting to give up the habit, although many will have tried and failed. Yet many smokers do succeed in breaking their dependence, which is why between 1960 and 1984, the number of male smokers fell from 61 per cent to 36 per cent, and in Britain at the time of writing there are ten million people who have managed to give up.

Giving up is seldom easy, but the rewards are substantial. Almost immediately, there is an improvement in general health. The smoker's cough briefly worsens, as the lungs begin to clean themselves properly, but, within a week or so, the condition of the lungs and circulation improves. This means that the risks of contracting a respiratory infection or cold will also be reduced.

Nearly every smoker has tried to stop at some time, but most have lapsed. For all but the lucky few, a definite strategy to stop smoking is important, and will-power plus plenty of encouragement from friends and family are crucial.

Because most people know that tar has been implicated as a cause of lung cancer, many smokers have consciously switched to low-tar cigarettes, helped by legislation requiring the tar content to be specified on the pack. Unfortunately, for a variety of reasons, this scheme has not proved entirely successful. It has been shown that the nicotine content of cigarettes parallels their tar yield. High-tar cigarettes deliver large amounts of nicotine; low-tar cigarettes provide low nicotine levels. Because the smoker varies his method of smoking to deliver the amount of nicotine demanded by his habit or dependence, he will simply smoke more low-tar cigarettes, so that the cumulative amount of tar inhaled is much the same. Or, worse, he will inhale more deeply, or hold the smoke in his lungs for longer, producing much the same result - a high tar intake.

Filters are not the answer either. They do not remove tar effectively, and they encourage the smoker to continue to smoke the cigarette right down to the butt - just where most of the tar has accumulated.

So what is the most effective way to give up smoking and to remain an ex-smoker? Several ways have proved successful, but for any of them to work properly, you will have to analyse *why* and *how* you smoke. For example, do you smoke to relieve tension or nervousness? Or is smoking an accompaniment to a cup of coffee in the morning, or the end of a meal in the evening? You are going to have to break both your addiction to nicotine and your emotional dependence on smoking. If you are conscious of your smoking rituals you may be able to break them by avoiding the situations that cause you to reach for the cigarettes.

ALTERNATIVE METHODS OF GIVING UP

Nicotine chewing gum may be prescribed by your doctor, especially if you are a heavy smoker. When chewed slowly, this releases enough nicotine to curb the craving, without carrying the hazards of tar. Like any other form of smoking cessation therapy, this works best when your doctor also gives detailed counselling. Some smokers find other successful routes such as hypnotherapy and acupuncture. The latter is best not tried except with medical advice and then given only by a properly qualified practitioner. For those who really find giving up a problem, some doctors run clinics where groups of smokers discuss their problems with each other and trained health professionals. The success rate achieved by these groups is quite high. Aversion methods include 'flooding' until smoking causes vomiting, and medication which makes cigarettes taste disgusting.

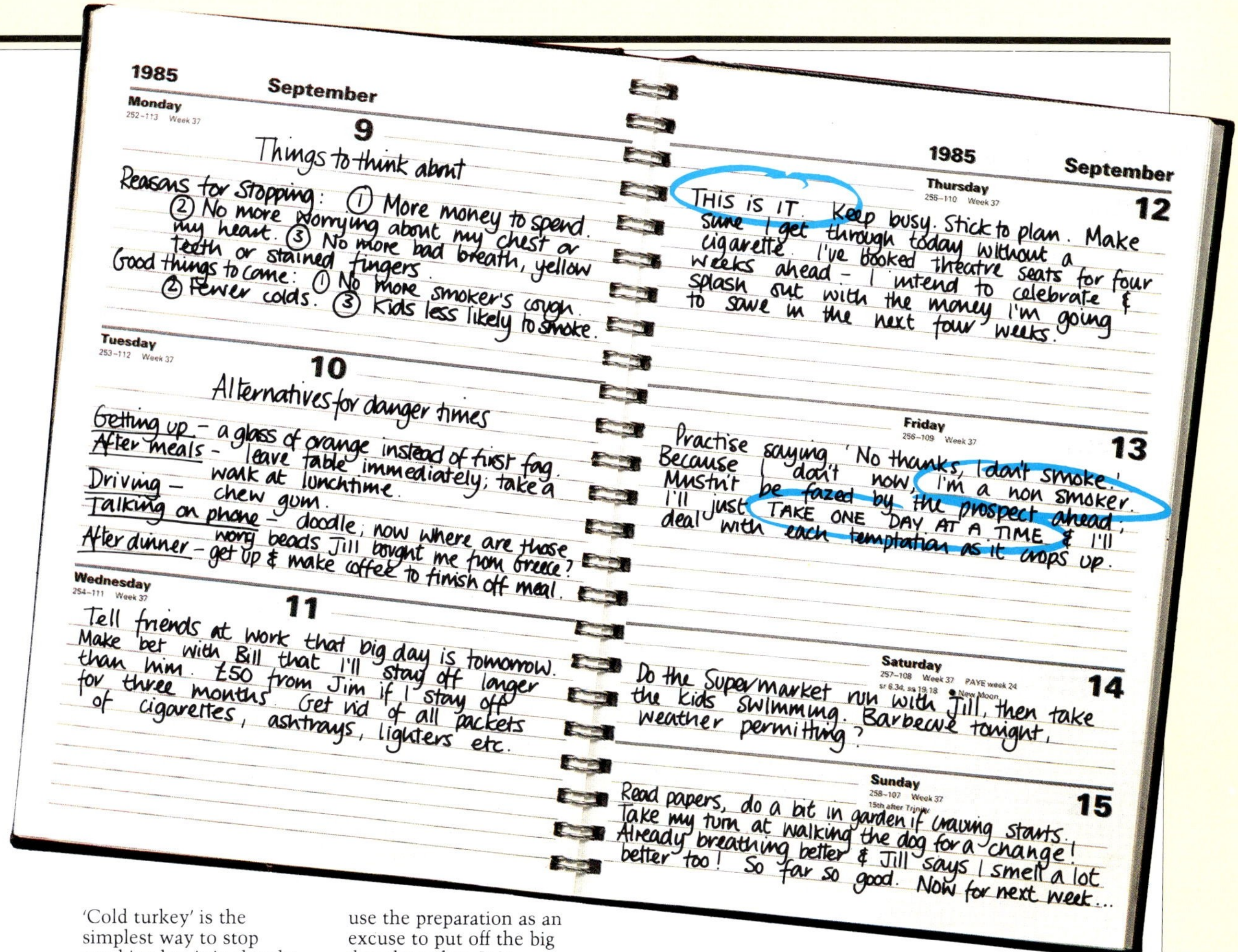

1985 September

Monday 252–113 Week 37

9

Things to think about

Reasons for stopping : ① More money to spend.
② No more worrying about my chest or
my heart. ③ No more bad breath, yellow
teeth or stained fingers.
Good things to come : ① No more smoker's cough.
② Fewer colds. ③ Kids less likely to smoke.

Tuesday 253–112 Week 37

10

Alternatives for danger times

Getting up – a glass of orange instead of first fag.
After meals – leave table immediately; take a
walk at lunchtime.
Driving – chew gum.
Talking on phone – doodle; now where are those
worry beads Jill bought me from Greece?
After dinner – get up & make coffee to finish off meal.

Wednesday 254–111 Week 37

11

Tell friends at work that big day is tomorrow.
Make bet with Bill that I'll stay off longer
than him. £50 from Jim if I stay off
for three months. Get rid of all packets
of cigarettes, ashtrays, lighters etc.

1985 September

Thursday 255–110 Week 37

12

THIS IS IT Keep busy. Stick to plan. Make
sure I get through today without a
cigarette. I've booked theatre seats for four
weeks ahead – I intend to celebrate &
splash out with the money I'm going
to save in the next four weeks.

Friday 256–109 Week 37

13

Practise saying 'No thanks, I don't smoke,
I'm a non smoker.' Because I don't now.
Mustn't be fazed by the prospect ahead.
I'll just TAKE ONE DAY AT A TIME & I'll
deal with each temptation as it crops up.

Saturday 257–108 Week 37 PAYE week 24
sr 6.34, ss 19.18 ● New Moon

14

Do the supermarket run with Jill, then take
the kids swimming. Barbecue tonight,
weather permitting?

Sunday 258–107 Week 37
15th after Trinity

15

Read papers, do a bit in garden if craving starts.
Take my turn at walking the dog for a change.
Already breathing better & Jill says I smell a lot
better too! So far so good. Now for next week...

'Cold turkey' is the simplest way to stop smoking but it is also the most difficult. You can make the break a little easier by preparing yourself for the big day, but don't use the preparation as an excuse to put off the big day altogether. It is sometimes easier to make the break when you are away from daily routine, for example, on holiday.

The relationship between no. of years as ex-smokers and death from lung cancer amongst males (*below*)

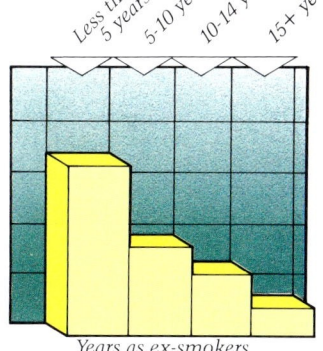

Less than 5 years *5-10 years* *10-14 years* *15+ years*

Years as ex-smokers

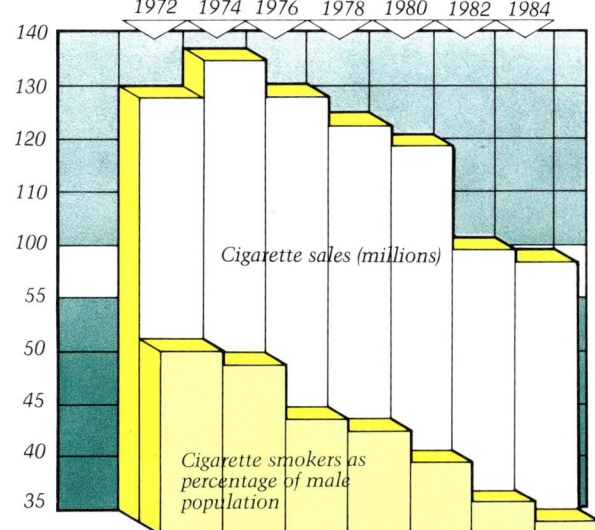

1972 1974 1976 1978 1980 1982 1984

Cigarette sales (millions)

Cigarette smokers as percentage of male population

The proportion of adult cigarette smokers has been falling since 1970 and in 1976 smokers became a minority. The sale of packeted cigarettes has shown a proportionally similar decline and has fallen nearly 25% since 1972. Sales of pipe tobacco have also fallen, and after a small rise between 1980 and 1982, handrolling tobacco sales are also on the decrease.

Continued from page 173

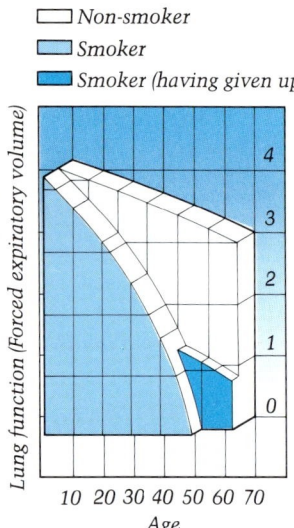

☐ *Non-smoker*
☐ *Smoker*
☐ *Smoker (having given up)*

Lung function (Forced expiratory volume)

4
3
2
1
0

10 20 30 40 50 60 70
Age

Lung function declines with age, but for the smoker the decline is rapid and severe. The moment the smoker gives up his curve mimics the normal decline, although obviously at the lower function level.

Chronic bronchitis, although not necessarily fatal, is probably the most serious effect of smoking. Together with the related disease, emphysema, it still kills some 20,000 people each year in England and Wales, and is so common that it is known elsewhere as the English Disease. Smokers are six times more likely to be killed by chronic bronchitis than non-smokers, and for those smoking 25 cigarettes a day or more, the risk is 25 times greater than for non-smokers. With chronic bronchitis and emphysema, which are described more fully in chapter 4, there is severe loss of function of the lungs. Those sufferers who are not killed face years of progressively crippling shortness of breath. Many require oxygen therapy just to help them get around the house.

As the diagram shows, stopping smoking is always beneficial. The deterioration in lung function will be arrested; the lungs cannot be restored to the condition of a non-smoker.

The other major group of diseases associated with smoking includes coronary heart disease and other disorders of the circulation. It is fair to say that smoking is only one of the risk factors in these diseases; the others include obesity, high blood pressure, diets rich in saturated fats and over-indulgence in alcohol. But it is true that smoking is probably the most important and also the most easily avoidable single risk factor.

Smoking is thought to be the main cause in about a third of the deaths from heart attacks and in about a fifth of the deaths from other cardiovascular diseases. The reasons for this are not entirely clear, but it is known that smoking increases the amount of fatty acids in the blood and increases the tendency of the blood to clot. The blood becomes more viscous, and there is an increased tendency for atheroma to form. The arteries gradually 'fur up' and blood flow is impeded. Moreover, if a clot forms, it can block a vital artery, such as the coronary artery, and cause a heart attack.

There is little doubt that smoking is the culprit for much of this type of disease. In most coronary care units, 70 per cent of patients under 65 years of age are smokers. And in one British study of people being considered for coronary by-pass operations to relieve angina (caused by furred-up coronary arteries), 91 per cent of the patients were smokers.

As well as the problems outlined above, cancers of the mouth, throat, pancreas and bladder are more frequent in smokers, as is peptic ulceration caused by swallowing the irritants contained in smoke and tar. Pipe and cigar smokers, who do not as a rule inhale, are not at such risk from lung cancer, but at a much higher risk from cancers of the lip, tongue and mouth, due to direct contact with irritant tar and smoke.

WHAT ABOUT THE NON-SMOKER?

For the non-smoker, tobacco smoke is an irritating nuisance. The smell is unpleasant and can irritate the nose and eyes. And in addition to the nuisance factor, smoking is also being criticized because of its possible threat to the health of non-smokers.

This potential threat is related to the phenomenon of side-stream smoke, which is the smoke produced by a cigarette or other tobacco while it is not actually being inhaled by the smoker. This smoke is different in composition from the inhaled/exhaled smoke, for it contains higher levels of carbon monoxide and several irritants.

The effects are not easy to prove, but some studies suggest that non-smoking members of the families of smokers are more prone to lung cancer and bronchitis than are other non-smokers. There is, however, no doubt that the children of parents who smoke have more respiratory infections than the children of non-smokers, especially in the first few years of life.

ALCOHOL – THE REALITY

Alcohol is another of the universally recognized and almost universally used 'social' drugs. It is also one at which, when used in moderation, little criticism has been levelled, except where its use is proscribed by religious or moral custom, as in orthodox Muslim communities and in some Christian groups.

Alcoholic drinks contain a variety of substances, but what we usually describe as alcohol is actually ethanol or ethyl alcohol. It is present at different levels in different types of drink.

- **Beer**
2.5-4% *(% by volume)*
- **Strong beer**
8%
- **Wines**
8-12%
- **Sherry/port**
20%
- **Spirits**
40%*

The alcohol content of spirits is declared in degrees of proof spirit on the label. This is a different scale of measurement.

One real difference between smoking and alcohol consumption is that while *any* degree of regular smoking is demonstrably harmful, used in moderation alcohol does not appear to have any permanent bad effects. The real question is, when does moderation become over-indulgence and lead to alcoholism?

More than 90 per cent of the adult population drinks to some extent. The average daily consumption for men is about 1½ pints of beer a day, or the equivalent in other forms of drink. But for young males, in their late teens and early 20s, average consumption may be 50 per cent higher. Surveys have shown that nearly half of all men will admit to having been drunk at some time during the previous three months. So this almost universal habit does have the potential for causing harm, and alcohol is obviously used to excess quite frequently.

Why do people drink alcohol? As with any drug, the primary motivation, at least at first, is to conform with a group. The social pressures to drink are strong, and many men would think it churlish to refuse a proffered drink. Moreover, unlike drugs such as nicotine, our first experiences with alcohol are usually pleasant, as alcoholic drinks have a pleasant taste.

Alcohol is absorbed very quickly, and has a measurable effect within five or ten minutes of being taken. Carbonated or fizzy drinks are absorbed more rapidly than 'flat' drinks. The effects vary with the amount drunk, and you should reckon that, in terms of their alcoholic content, a half-pint of beer or cider = one glass of wine = one measure of spirit.

Most people think of alcohol as a stimulant, which makes them more confident, talkative and vivacious. In fact, alcohol is a relaxant and a depressant, with a strong effect on the nervous system, removing the inhibitions. Thus the old saying that a drinker's true personality emerges when he is drunk does contain a germ of truth. However, as the amount taken increases, the effects of alcohol are also to impair judgement and physical co-ordination.

In general, after two pints of beer, or the equivalent, you will be feeling pleasantly relaxed. With a further two pints, the effects will be obvious to

A half-pint of beer contains the same amount of alcohol as a single whisky or a glass of wine and, poured in normal measure, can be thought of as one 'standard drink'. The table shows how many such standard drink units are found in different drinks. Measures poured at home tend to be more generous, and may well contain the equivalent of two or three standard drinks.

TABLE WINE		SPIRITS		LAGER & BEER	
Measure	**Standard Drink**	**Measure**	**Standard Drink**	**Measure**	**Standard Drink**
Standard glass	*1*	Small measure ($\frac{1}{6}$ gill)	*1*	Regular strength *1 can* *$\frac{1}{2}$pt* *1pt*	*$1\frac{1}{2}$* *1* *2*
Bottle	*7*	Large measure ($\frac{1}{4}$ gill) (standard in US)	*2*		
Bottle (litre)	*10*			Strong *1 can* *$\frac{1}{2}$pt* *1pt*	*3* *2* *4*
SHERRY, VERMOUTH, APERITIF		Bottle	*30*		
				Extra strong *1 can* *$\frac{1}{2}$pt* *1pt*	*4* *$2\frac{1}{2}$* *5*
Measure	**Standard Drink**				
Small measure	*1*			Export *1 can* *$\frac{1}{2}$pt* *1pt*	*2* *$1\frac{1}{4}$* *$2\frac{1}{2}$*
Bottle	*12*				

another person, as you begin to be uncoordinated and to slur your words. From then on, the effects of further alcohol depend very much on the individual as, like most drugs, tolerance develops after repeated use.

Alcohol is broken down in the liver, and its end products are carbon dioxide and water. The carbon dioxide is exhaled from the lungs, and the water passes out in the urine, which is one of the reasons why, after drinking, we always seem to urinate more than the volume of drink consumed. The other reason is that alcohol has a diuretic effect, causing the body to excrete extra water. Habitual drinkers break down alcohol more rapidly and efficiently than the occasional drinker.

The rate at which alcohol is broken down by the body is, even in habitual drinkers, a slow process. If a man drinks 10 pints of beer, he will have a dangerous blood alcohol level of 300mg when he leaves the pub, but by the next morning, his blood alcohol level will still be 150mg, and will continue to be over the legal limit for driving until the middle of the day.

Drinking several cups of black coffee or taking other 'magic' cures will not have the slightest effect on the rate at which alcohol disappears from the bloodstream. Drinking at this level causes serious long-term physical effects, apart from the risk of alcoholism, and the liver becomes damaged, reducing its capacity to break down alcohol. Thus the syndrome begins of the heavy drinker who gradually becomes less able to 'hold his drink'.

Alcohol, in whatever form of drink, contains empty calories. For example, there are 180 calories in each pint of beer or its equivalent (even more in sweetened drinks). But there is no nutritive value, which is one reason why those alcoholics who neglect to eat a sensible diet suffer from various forms of malnutrition, especially from serious vitamin deficiencies.

Another possible effect of the breakdown of alcohol in the liver is that the normal disposal of waste uric acid is interrupted. Uric acid accumulates in the blood and can precipitate an attack of gout, a disease traditionally associated with heavy drinkers.

THE IMMEDIATE EFFECTS
AND THE AFTERMATH

Alcohol absorption varies, depending on the type of drink consumed and the stomach contents. The presence of food in the stomach delays absorption, as does the traditional glass of milk before a drinking session.

Hangovers are partly caused by congeners — small amounts of tannins, esters and other related substances produced during fermentation. Darker coloured drinks contain the most congeners.

•**High hangover rating**
Stout
Bitter
Sherry
Port
Brandy
Dark rum
Red wine

•**Low hangover rate**
Gin
Vodka
White wine
White rum

However, they have no effect on the total amount of alcohol that will eventually be absorbed or on the end result, although the onset of drunkenness may be delayed when drinking is combined with a substantial meal. One interesting paradox is that strong drinks such as spirits are not absorbed quickly. They are retained in the stomach until diluted to a safer level by food or liquids, before they are discharged into the small intestine where the alcohol is absorbed. The dangerous effect of this is that the final brandy or aperitif taken before going home may have no obvious effects until it is suddenly diluted by a cup of coffee, which releases it to do its worst.

Delayed absorption or the slow breakdown of alcohol also causes serious hazards, and can cause the effects of the drug to be cumulative. A lunchtime drink followed by drinks after work can add to existing blood alcohol levels and push you over the limit for driving.

The after-effects of drinking are known to most of us: violent headaches and nausea. These have varying causes. Dehydration, which is mainly responsible for the dry mouth and headache, is due to the diuretic action of alcohol, and it can be eased by drinking about a pint of water or milk before you go to bed to sleep it off.

Much of the other components of the hangover are caused by congeners, which are small amounts of tannins, esters and other related substances produced during the fermentation process. They are present in the largest amounts in darker coloured drinks, and so may be avoided.

Unfortunately there is no such thing as a hangover cure. Aspirin tends to aggravate the nausea by irritating your stomach, which may already be inflamed. Paracetamol is preferable as an analgesic because it avoids this. And the 'hair of the dog', although it may make you feel better, simply makes you drunk again. As already mentioned, fluids will counteract the dehydration and the caffeine in tea or coffee will help to perk you up.

THE DRINKING PROBLEM

The occasional 'binge' seldom does any harm, provided that you don't drive or get involved in behaviour that could have legal or social repercussions. There is even some evidence to show that a small amount of alcohol each day may be beneficial to your health. But alcohol is a drug that should be taken in moderation, and its use should be watched carefully to make sure that dependence does not develop and that other alcohol-related problems do not follow.

Alcohol tolerance develops quite fast, so the single drink it took to produce a feeling of pleasant relaxation soon increases to two drinks, then three, and so on. There is a gradual slide from drinking for pleasure to eventual dependence. If you take more than the occasional drink, ask yourself these questions:

● Do you drink alone?
● Do you finish your drink before your friends have finished?
● Do you drink for the effect rather than because you like the taste?
● Do you drink after a stressful situation?
● Do you drink more than you used to?
● Do you feel uncomfortable without a drink?

If the answer to two or more of these questions is yes, you must be careful. You are in danger of becoming emotionally dependent on alcohol, and you may have to make a conscious effort to cut down before you become physically addicted.

The slide into alcoholism is gradual. There is no sudden threshold and no time limit; it could take six months or six years to become an alcoholic - the transition from heavy drinking to helpless alcoholism is imperceptible. The alcoholic never feels 'normal' unless there is alcohol in his bloodstream. He is affected both emotionally and physically. Alcoholics begin to suffer from memory lapses, depression and anxiety, which increase their tension and cause them to drink all the more. The effects on family life can be devastating. Although most alcoholics are adept at concealing their addiction, at least in its early stages, the end result is the severe disruption of family life. Child abuse and physical attacks within the family are frequently associated with alcoholism.

The greatest problem is for the drinker to admit that there *is* a problem. Once the need for help is admitted, there is a very good chance that a recovery can be made, although it is doubtful that any former alcoholic can be regarded as 'cured'. However, there is also a body of opinion that suggests that, rather than *never* taking another drink, previously physically dependent drinkers can learn to drink in a controlled way.

OVERCOMING ALCOHOLISM

Alcoholism is a medical condition, which needs professional medical help. An alcoholic may be acutely aware of his emotional dependence on drink, but the physical aspects of the dependence need careful monitoring. Some alcoholics only admit their condition once they have reached the dangerous phase when they experience hallucinations, nightmares and delirium tremens (the 'DTs'). By this stage the liver will be damaged, and there may even be some physical deterioration of the brain itself.

'Drying out' may take place at home, under medical supervision, or it may require treatment at a clinic. The withdrawal symptoms for alcohol are unpleasant and include muscle pain, nausea and sometimes further bouts of DTs. Tranquillizers are often given until the worst of the withdrawal passes. Subsequently, a drug may be given to cause violent vomiting if any alcohol is taken.

Alcoholics need constant support throughout the 'drying out' or detoxification period, and during the following months while their lifestyle is changed to accommodate alcohol-free life. Family and friends must be supportive, as must the doctor. Most alcoholics are helped greatly by patient groups such as Alcoholics Anonymous, which provide continuing support and can give encouragement when the will weakens. They can also help the ex-drinker explore the emotional problems that led to excessive drinking and show how other people succeeded in overcoming them.

TROUBLE WITH MEDICAL DRUGS

Although probably every drug that has been developed produces side effects in some people, very few are abused in the sense that people take them for pleasure, although it should be remembered that morphine, heroin and cocaine were once widely used medicinally.

At present the most widely abused drug is probably aspirin, which many people take to ward off headaches and musculoskeletal pains. Such people can become dependent on aspirin, taking many times the proper daily dose, and in so doing, they experience quite serious gastric bleeding. They may also suffer withdrawal symptoms when they stop. Oddly, however, there is strong medical evidence that taking a daily dose of aspirin can help protect against heart attacks or, at least, help protect those people who have already survived a first attack.

The medicinal drugs currently causing most concern because of their potential for abuse are tranquillizers belonging to a chemical group called benzodiazepines. Tranquillizers and some so-called 'sleeping tablets' are, in fact, identical. They contain the same drugs and have the same effects, but are used in different dosages and at different times of day. Tranquillizers are used for their calming effects, and in high doses they are very strongly sedative. Their properties are useful in the medical treatment of people suffering from chronic anxiety, which can be very disabling. They are also used to provide a temporary 'emotional crutch' to people suffering a life crisis such as bereavement or divorce.

These drugs are very effective; too effective, in fact. They are used, or misused, to calm the nerves before an occasion that is likely to be stressful, like an examination or interview, and when they are used in this way, emotional dependence can follow very quickly. Tranquillizers have to be prescribed by a doctor, but the problem usually starts after they have been prescribed, quite properly, for an emotional disorder. The fear that the initial anxiety will recur leads to their being taken whenever stress is anticipated. The use and abuse of tranquillizers can be correlated with people in high-stress occupations and with people who suffer the stress related to such problems as unemployment or family difficulties. They are still widely prescribed, although doctors are now less willing to do so, knowing their potential for causing emotional *and* physical dependence.

Physical dependence or addiction follows in the usual way. As tolerance increases, the user steps up the dosage, and, after long-term use, sudden cessation can cause typical withdrawal symptoms: dizziness, anxiety, insomnia, shaking and nausea. The withdrawal effects can mimic the original anxiety condition, tempting both doctor and patient to continue with the drug. Tranquillizers are sometimes taken purely for their pleasurable effects too, and they produce a mild intoxication, similar to alcohol, which lowers inhibition but also interferes with skills such as driving. However, as they are not supplied by the usually illegal sources in the 'drug culture', the user does not normally come into contact with the law, but obtains them quite legally on prescription.

Because tranquillizers are prescribed as a medicine and are legal if properly prescribed, the treatment of dependence is also a medical problem. It is usually overcome quite easily by a gradual reduction of the dosage, under medical supervision.

It is important for any user to consider his attitude to tranquillizers and to be aware of any undue dependence. Your doctor should be alerted and may need to discontinue or change the treatment. There is no need to fear the 'weaning process'. This can be done very effectively and with the minimum of discomfort - but only if your doctor is fully aware of any impending problems.

UPPERS AND DOWNERS

The abuse of amphetamines and barbiturates (commonly called 'uppers' and 'downers' respectively) is an unfortunate consequence of their original use. They have now been almost entirely superseded medicinally and are generally only used as drugs of abuse, manufactured and obtained illegally. As such, they introduce many more hazards than the original, legal forms of the drugs. Their popular names accurately describe their effects.

Amphetamines (also referred to as 'speed') are very powerful stimulants, which cause both mind and body to operate at fever pitch. The user feels full of energy, alert and creative, and he can stay awake for long periods without feeling tired. Unfortunately, this is a subjective view. To others, someone on an amphetamine high seems excited and confused, often talking or writing gibberish, as many students using the drugs as an aid to study or overcoming exam nerves have found to their cost.

Tolerance develops very quickly, and the dose is stepped up to the point where the user becomes irritable and restless, and may go for days without sleep. The end result is an 'amphetamine crash', with deep depression and blackouts. Amphetamines are physically mildly addictive, but produce a very powerful emotional dependence.

Barbiturates - or downers - are the exact opposite to amphetamines. They are very powerful sedatives, formerly used as sleeping tablets. In small doses they have similar effects to alcohol, causing relaxed, cheerful behaviour. But as the dose increases they soon cause lack of co-ordination, stupor and unconsciousness. They interact powerfully and very dangerously with alcohol, as each works in a similar way and this combination has led to many accidental deaths.

Barbiturates are among the most strongly addictive of all drugs, producing powerful physical as well as emotional dependence. Withdrawal from barbiturates is prolonged and highly unpleasant.

In the United Kingdom both types of drug are controlled under the Misuse of Drugs Act, and there are heavy penalties for their misuse. Almost all supplies offered are manufactured by illegal drug factories, and they are liable to be accidentally adulterated or deliberately 'cut' with supposedly harmless ingredients to make them go further. They are therefore highly likely to cause other medical problems. They are especially dangerous when injected, as is the practice of many hard-core drug users.

The worst aspect of uppers and downers is their concurrent use, often by apparently respectable people. Uppers are usually taken in the morning, to get the user through the day; downers are taken at night, to neutralize the effects of the morning dose. If taken with alcohol, they can be a lethal combination.

COCAINE - FASHION OR THREAT?

Cocaine, or 'coke', is enjoying a vogue in much of the world. Its use is illegal, and the possession of, and dealing in, cocaine carry heavy penalties. Despite this, cocaine does not yet appear to have the evil reputation of heroin and other illegal drugs, partly perhaps because it is used by different types of people from the traditional heroin-user.

Cocaine has acquired a glamorous image, and it has been widely used by people in the entertainment industry as well as others who do not (at first, at least) show the physical dependence and deterioration we have come to expect of the users of heroin. But now, with a world glut, the price of cocaine has tumbled, and the drug is cheaply available from all the usual sources of illegal drugs, and is no longer so expensive that it is reserved for the high-income users.

Cocaine is a stimulant drug belonging to the same group of local anaesthetic drugs as Procaine and Novocaine - widely used in dentistry. It produces a euphoric 'rush' when it is taken, usually by sniffing the powder. Mental stimulation follows, but the effects are short-lived, and the dose must be repeated quickly. However, since tolerance does not develop, the dosage is not stepped up.

With regular use, the euphoria is no longer experienced but is replaced by an excited and restless state, which may deteriorate into a condition of confused paranoia resembling schizophrenia. Regular cocaine 'snorting' - sniffing the white powder - may also cause physical damage to the membranes lining the nose.

Emotional dependence on the pleasurable effects of cocaine is strong, but until recently it had been thought that physical dependence does not occur. However, new evidence shows that there can be very strong physical dependence in some individual users, which may require treatment at a drug dependency clinic.

Despite its fashionable image, cocaine use undeniably risks mental and physical ill-health. It is not a harmless 'fun drug' and is to be avoided, especially in view of the legal implications of its possession or use.

THE USE OF CANNABIS

Cannabis, known in its various forms as hash, grass and pot, is found in the gum of the cannabis plant and is an illegal drug.

In Britain it is controlled by the Misuse of Drugs Act, but possession, although still a punishable offence, is regarded less seriously than that of 'hard' drugs. This 'soft' attitude reflects the medical views of the effects of cannabis, which probably does not produce physical dependence and only a mild emotional dependence.

Cannabis is usually smoked, mixed with tobacco in the form of reefers or 'joints', and is absorbed quickly in the lungs. Its effects depend on the expectations of the user and on the quantity and type of cannabis taken. Usually it induces cheerfulness and talkativeness at first, followed by a feeling of calm pleasure, with moments of reflection and introspection. Cannabis has demonstrably bad effects on concentration and manual skills. It also alters the perception of time and thus the perception of reality. Performing practical tasks like driving a car are therefore very dangerous, the more so if smoking cannabis is mixed with alcohol. In high doses it leads to stupor and even semi-coma, with an after-effect of depression.

Regular users taking high doses may get panic reactions, and some doctors think that heavy use can lead to mental illness. The physical effects are not generally serious. Smoking cannabis causes reddening of the eyes, and probably, in the long term, will carry the same risk of bronchitis and lung cancer as cigarettes. The drug has been criticized as leading inevitably to involvement with hard drugs, but this is a false assumption. There is no evidence that people experimenting with cannabis necessarily want to try other drugs, nor that they are particularly likely to be offered any.

Although cannabis remains illegal almost everywhere, it is by far the most widely used of the illegal drugs, and among some social groups, its use is regarded as casually as alcohol or cigarettes. In recent years, there has been a tendency for the authorities to turn a blind eye to the taking of cannabis, although not to dealing in the drug, or the growing or smuggling of the raw materials.

LSD — THE EFFECTS

Like cannabis, LSD is a drug for which it has not been possible to demonstrate any serious physical effects or physical dependence. Lysergic acid diethylamide, LSD, or acid, was a highly fashionable drug in the 1960s and 70s, but it is now not only less fashionable but much less freely available. It is an unusual drug, highly active in almost immeasurably small amounts and having dramatic effects on the brain. Its effects are primarily on the senses, and a user on a 'trip' sees and hears distorted and intensified versions of reality. In other words, it is a hallucinatory drug. For many, this makes use of the drug a spiritual experience.

Some users experience a 'bad trip', during which they get the 'horrors' and need immediate sedation. Despite earlier suspicions, there is no firm evidence that LSD causes brain damage or genetic damage, but it certainly can cause a transitory form of mental schizophrenia-like disturbance, which may be severe enough, or last long enough, to require hospitalization. It also causes 'flashbacks' in some users, when the LSD high may be repeated without warning months or even years after taking the drug.

The long-term use of LSD may cause some emotional dependence, but the primary reason for the drug being regarded as 'dangerous' is the fear that users may damage themselves or others while on a high. It is currently classified along with heroin and cocaine in the 'most dangerous' group.

GETTING HELP FOR DRUG PROBLEMS

For all the wide range of drugs discussed in this chapter, from coffee to LSD, medical treatment and counselling can be obtained.

Many agencies and organizations deal with drug addiction, and some helpful addresses are listed at the back of this book. But with all forms of addiction, a committed personal effort must be made to break the habit. The user must first recognize that he has a problem, then pluck up the courage to seek help. The earlier this decision is taken, the easier the process will be.

Support from family and friends is critically important, and if the dependency involves an illegal drug, it is essential to avoid the so-called 'friends' in the drug culture who can supply and encourage the habit. Of all forms of abuse of the body, drug abuse is the easiest to avoid. It takes a conscious effort to start the abuse, and in the early stages only a small effort is needed to control or avoid the habit. Dependency will develop only if the use is allowed to progress.

●For organizations offering specialist advice, see *Further Information*, page 200

The treatment of drug dependency, particularly for such dangerous drugs as heroin, is a highly specialized affair, outside the scope of this general book. Although the broad guidelines given here may help, they will never be a substitute for professional medical advice.

MATURE HEALTH

Old age is not a topic that young, vigorous men care to dwell upon. Like death and cancer, old age is an unmentionable subject. But if you follow the guidelines for a healthy lifestyle contained in this book, you will have every expectation of staying young for as long as possible. So how will you make it to a healthy old age?

Aging populations are not a result of a rise in life expectancy. Individuals do not live twenty years longer than they used to. The aging population is caused by more people living to their three score years and ten and the consequence is a higher proportion of elderly people in our societies.

There are already a very large number of elderly people in our communities, and as our average life span increases, the numbers will grow. By the year 2025, old people - that is, those over 65 years of age - will be a very large proportion of the whole population: 18.6 per cent in Britain and France, 20 per cent in West Germany and 15.8 per cent in the United States. This group will represent a substantial element of voters, who should cause conditions for the elderly to improve steadily, by ensuring adequate pensions and health and recreational facilities. In practical terms, therefore, the future is not to be feared. What is now necessary is to ensure that you continue to enjoy adequate health, and to use your retirement in a positive way.

Retirement is not a milestone marking the onset of old age; rather, it is the culmination of a hard-working and responsible life, for which you should have been preparing and looking forward for many years.

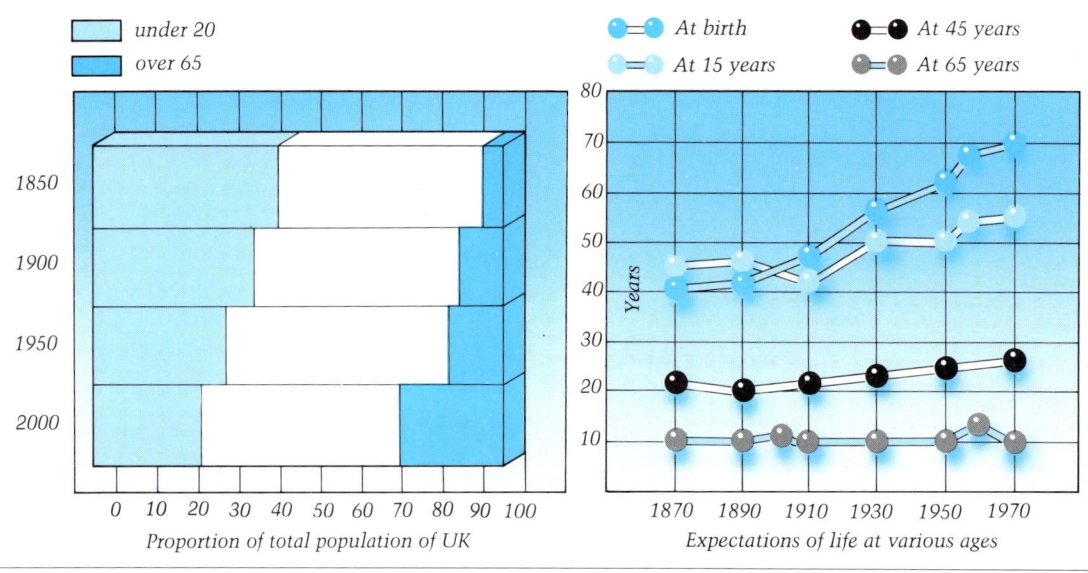

under 20 / over 65

At birth / At 45 years / At 15 years / At 65 years

Proportion of total population of UK

Expectations of life at various ages

The later middle years, when you are in your fifties, are a period when incomes usually peak and most men have reached the maximum level in their chosen career. Money worries have eased and responsibilities diminished as children marry and leave home to start their own lives. Most men enjoy the freedom of this period of their life, yet feel retirement creeping up on them. It is natural to resent the younger man who will take over your job eventually, especially if it is a job you feel you have built up and shaped into its present form. It is also natural to feel anger at the system or company that decrees that you will retire on an arbitrary date, whether or not you are tired of work or need the break.

Most men still feel mentally alert and believe that they have a great deal to give. They are quite correct. But what a man has to give now has to be shaped according to the different demands that will be made upon him. After a lifetime's work, you can expect to be set in a particular work pattern and conduct your life to a strict timetable of commuting, mealtimes and weekends. All this is going to have to change, and you have to accept this well before your retirement. But it does not all have to stop. What you must do is redirect your energies, both physical and emotional, to exploit your retirement to the full.

A PRODUCTIVE RETIREMENT

Surveys in many countries have shown that most retired people would like to continue to work, and many companies offer the option of part-time working as part of a pre-retirement wind-down. There are very good reasons for this, for there is no doubt that working in retirement can improve life expectancy and health, provided it is the right sort of work.

Getting a job is not easy. Most types of work are closed to the elderly, especially with the pressure from the unemployment among younger age groups. Finding work is best achieved by stepping outside the usual channels and job agencies. You may have to accept that you will be working for little money or perhaps even offering your services free of charge. But if you feel the need to work, that must be your main objective. You are not setting out to create a new career, with all the strains and tensions that would involve.

If you have an executive job, your choice of part-time retirement work may be relatively easy. Almost all charities need helpers, whether at a clerical level or as part-time accountants or book-keepers. You will have to sit down and prepare lists of possible contacts, then write and telephone them to offer your services. Don't be afraid to use friends and acquaintances to make contacts - this is no time to be proud. Let them all know that you are on the market and eager to use the skills you have acquired.

Of course, you don't need to have been an executive to make yourself useful in retirement. If you had a manual job, you will probably still be vigorous enough in retirement to carry on with the same sort of work. Once again, ask all your contacts and phone or write to anyone you think might need some part-time help.

Perhaps you can't think of anything special you would like to try. But you now have the opportunity to indulge yourself and try something different. You may be too late to train to be a pilot or doctor, but you certainly won't be too late to re-train for a different job or take up a new interest. Further education for the elderly is popular and with good reason. Some men take Open University courses after retirement; others train for leisure pursuits or hobbies. Whether your retirement interests are in academic or vocational courses, or in leisure pursuits, you will find a course to suit you. And these are usually free or available at only nominal costs.

THE RETIREMENT PLAN

Over the last ten years of your full-time working life, there are various ways in which you can help to ensure a secure retirement. You are not going to have a very large income on retirement, but your current earnings should be at their peak. Now is the time to think about increasing the payments on your mortgage, so it will be cleared up when you retire. Or you could organize an investment or private pension scheme if you have not done this already. Think about any major house repairs or building work that can be carried out now, while you can afford it.

A few years before you retire, think carefully about your home and the possibility of moving. This is probably the biggest decision you will ever make. Will you stay in a familiar community, with friends and relatives within easy reach, or will you retire to the dream home on the coast or in the country? Many thousands of old people live in unfamiliar towns, far from their families and friends, and are bitterly unhappy and lonely, particularly after the death of a marriage partner. But there are also thousands of very happy old people living in similar areas, who are enjoying a new lease of life, having adapted to the change and to the freedom from responsibilities.

Probably the main drawback to such a move is that it tends to mean living in a community of other older people in retirement, away from the stimulation of a community of mixed ages. And of course, if you do live in a 'retirement area', you are faced with the depressing prospect of the progressive loss of your new friends.

If you do decide to move, plan carefully. Visit the area you propose to move to and explore it thoroughly. Visit it in winter to see what is going on. Check the local library and community centre to discover what activities there are. Find out about public transport and medical care. And when you do find your dream home, think again. Could you still manage to look after it when you are older and possibly infirm? Planning and double-checking are essential.

PERSONAL RELATIONSHIPS

For most couples, the marriage partnership has meant a sharp division of responsibilities. For many years, you will have been going your separate ways in work and at home. Your time together at home has probably been limited to evenings and weekends, when there are chores like decorating or gardening to be undertaken. Now you are going to be thrown together for 24 hours each day.

Sadly, long marriages can founder at this point. Without the sense of direction that comes from the need to strive to further a career, some men find that their apparent marital contentment was merely a habit and that they cannot cope with the reappraisal of their married state. There is no need to concentrate on grown-up children any more, although some elderly people do this to the point of obsession. Now is the time to concentrate on yourself and your partner and enjoy family and friends without feeling responsible for them.

A man is particularly vulnerable in the early years of his retirement. It is common to feel un-needed. The house runs quite well without you, and you may feel in the way at first. Small wonder that many retired men suffer from depression and apathy. This is all the more reason for following your retirement plan. Few things cause mental and physical failure more rapidly than sitting dejectedly at home wondering how to pass the time, and the high mortality among the recently retired is notorious.

The problem can be greater for a man living alone. Often he must cope with learning to run a home as well as loneliness. Making friends and reinforcing existing friendships is absolutely essential, and, of course, it is never too late to make new partnerships. New friends are just as important for couples, providing new topics of common interest.

Sometimes it is more important to let go and forget about work or part-time jobs, than to try and preserve a former way of life. Instead, explore new friendships and leisure activities. Don't be afraid to push yourself too hard into a new leisure interest. After all, if you get tired, there's nothing to stop you lying in for a few hours in the morning or having an after-lunch nap.

• A satisfying sex life is not difficult to maintain, whatever age you are. See *Mature Health*, page 167

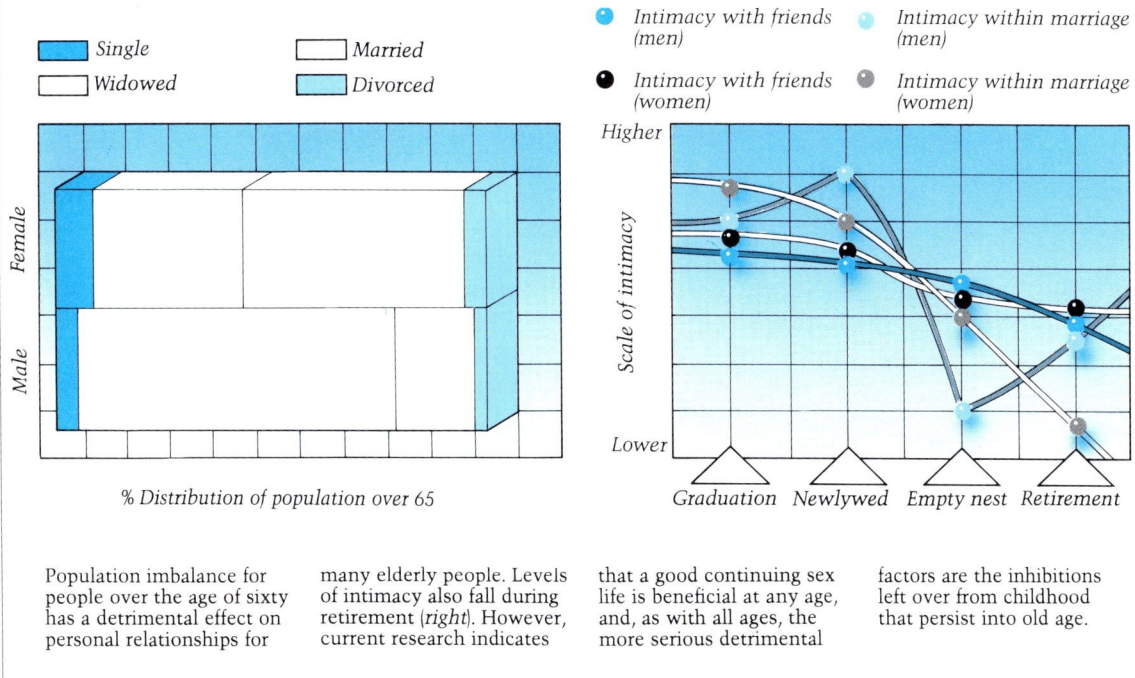

Single   Married
Widowed   Divorced

% Distribution of population over 65

Female / Male

Intimacy with friends (men)   Intimacy within marriage (men)
Intimacy with friends (women) Intimacy within marriage (women)

Higher / Scale of intimacy / Lower

Graduation   Newlywed   Empty nest   Retirement

Population imbalance for people over the age of sixty has a detrimental effect on personal relationships for many elderly people. Levels of intimacy also fall during retirement (*right*). However, current research indicates that a good continuing sex life is beneficial at any age, and, as with all ages, the more serious detrimental factors are the inhibitions left over from childhood that persist into old age.

BEREAVEMENT

The loss of one's wife, or anybody emotionally close, is a devastating blow. This is a problem which becomes commonplace when you are old.

Mourning is a natural process. If you allow it to happen as it comes and don't bottle up your feelings, then it is over eventually, even though it may take five to seven years. If you avoid it, then deep depression is the inevitable result.

There is an initial period of stunned shock when you usually feel nothing. This is because the feelings are so painful, that your mind cuts off from them - a very useful mechanism. It does not mean that you have no feelings, only that you can't face them at that time.

After two weeks or so these feelings start to come out. There are three main ones: guilt, anger, and a devastating sense of loss, finality, and loneliness. All these feelings are normal. You should not be afraid to talk about them, or show them when they occur. Eventually the pain will go. If after a year you are still wanting to hide away and avoid company, then you must make a huge effort to seek help from your doctor or from a counselling service.

PHYSICAL AGEING

The quality of your life in old age is going to be greatly improved if you remain physically healthy and have not abused your body over the preceding years by smoking, over-indulging in alcohol or eating the wrong foods. Time spent now in conditioning your body and keeping it healthy means that you will embark on your retirement with every right to expect many more years of healthy and productive life.

This doesn't mean that you will always be able to continue with your current level of physical activity or avoid the inevitable processes of ageing. But keeping your body at its peak *for your particular age* means that the ageing process can be delayed in certain respects. What you must accept is that your expectations of what you can achieve must be modified in the face of increasing age.

For example, arteries naturally become hardened in old age and they may gradually fur up as cholesterol is deposited on their walls. But we already know that a sensible low-fat diet can help to keep the arteries supple and reduce the rate at which atheromatous deposits form.

The heart pumps less efficiently in the elderly and, coupled with narrowing blood vessels, tends to cause the blood pressure to rise. Once again, a faulty diet is a factor, and the problem can be minimized. Obesity and cigarette smoking are directly linked to high blood pressure and thus to heart disease. Similarly, the risks of diseases such as bowel cancer, which become more common in the elderly, can be reduced by a low-fat, high fibre diet.

Some of the physical problems of old age are caused by the gradual running-down of the repair processes. This causes the muscles to become smaller, weaker and less efficient. In addition, some of the calcium in the

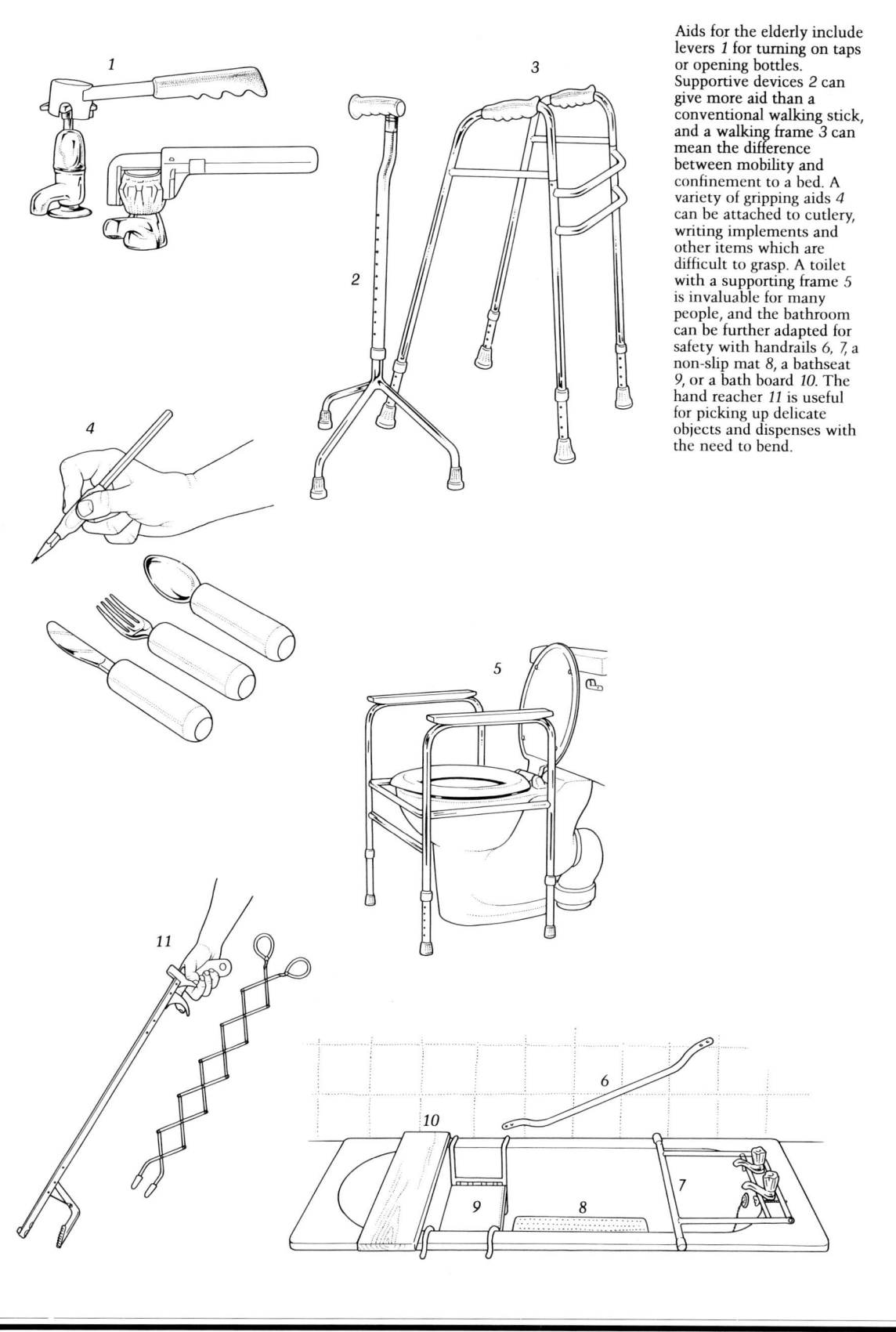

Aids for the elderly include levers *1* for turning on taps or opening bottles. Supportive devices *2* can give more aid than a conventional walking stick, and a walking frame *3* can mean the difference between mobility and confinement to a bed. A variety of gripping aids *4* can be attached to cutlery, writing implements and other items which are difficult to grasp. A toilet with a supporting frame *5* is invaluable for many people, and the bathroom can be further adapted for safety with handrails *6, 7*, a non-slip mat *8*, a bathseat *9*, or a bath board *10*. The hand reacher *11* is useful for picking up delicate objects and dispenses with the need to bend.

Most elderly people do not need a medical check-up before starting regular exercise, but see your doctor if:

• you've ever had high blood pressure or heart disease
• you have chest trouble, e.g. asthma or bronchitis
• you're troubled with joint pains, severe back pain or arthritis
• you're getting over an illness or operation or
• you're worried that exercise may affect another aspect of your health.

bones is lost, making them more brittle. But these processes can be delayed and even reversed by taking regular exercise to strengthen muscles, joints and bones. While it is true that physical exercise cannot be carried out at the level achieved in earlier years, it does not mean that physical exercise is not advisable or possible. Quite the opposite; exercise is extremely important and highly beneficial but you must learn to recognize your new limits.

The British Sports Council stated that:

"It has been shown many times that the capacity of elderly people for physical exercise can be improved with training just as with young people. Muscle power, tendon strength and the economy of the cardiovascular system can be restored and maintained with exercise. These beneficial effects have been demonstrated for both the aged in the community and geriatric patients in hospital."

Elderly people may lack strength and suppleness, but this should not inhibit exercise; indeed, it is a very good reason for taking exercise. However, the expectations and personal targets set need to be modified in the older men. The exercises described in chapter 1 are all relevant, but because the amount of effort needs to modified to take account of a reduced capacity in older men for vigorous exercise it is especially important to work only within the limits of comfort. Start gently and build up gradually.

It is not essential to check with your doctor before you start on a course of improved fitness - whatever your age. In certain cases, however, it may be sensible to do so, and these conditions are listed here.

Even for disabled people, there is nearly always some suitable form of exercise. Your doctor may be able to give some specific advice on this. Swimming is probably the best all-round activity for older people, as it involves most of the joints and muscles, and can be as vigorous as you care to make it. Because the water supports your weight, it is easy to exercise sufficiently to improve suppleness, without the tug of gravity which could strain a painful back or joints. It is also especially good for those suffering from arthritis, as is cycling, where it is important to strengthen the muscles around unstable arthritic joints. Walking is also an excellent exercise, and where possible it is sensible to walk rather than drive or use public transport. After all, now you've retired, what's the hurry?

Gardening is a form of exercise that can range from gentle pruning to hard digging, so you should find a comfortable level and avoid over-doing things by lifting too heavy objects or over-exerting yourself. Ideally, exercise should be steady and regular; the occasional heavy exertion may not be good for you.

During any form of outdoor exercise, and in your home in winter, be careful to wrap up in warm clothes. The blood supply to the skin is less efficient in the elderly than in young people, and some of the insulating fat beneath the skin is lost. Hypothermia, or a drop in body temperature, is a constant peril in cold weather, and it is particularly dangerous because it comes on imperceptibly, causing drowsiness and eventually, unconsciousness. If you recognize the symptoms, you can quickly warm up by using plenty of blankets and sitting by the fire; do not take brandy, however. It is better to avoid the problem by dressing warmly at all times and making sure that your home is adequately heated. Body heat is more efficiently preserved by proper clothing than by a fire or central heating. A string vest traps pockets of warm air next to the skin and insulated, thermal underwear is very efficient. Keep the extremities warm with proper snow boots and gloves; a woolly hat will prevent heat loss from the scalp. After this, hot drinks will have twice the effect.

FOOD AND THE ELDERLY

A proper diet can do a lot to preserve your health in old age. It is all too easy to lose interest in food when you are old, and to pick at a diet that eventually leads to mineral and vitamin deficiency. This is partly because the senses of taste and smell become less efficient, so food seems less appetizing. You can always use more seasoning to compensate - but watch the salt!

If you are on your own, it is a temptation to live on some convenience foods, which are quick to prepare and can be obtained in single portions. But you must be careful, if you are to have a healthy, balanced diet. You must still eat plenty of fresh fruit and vegetables, even if they are difficult to chew. You need the fibre, the vitamins and the minerals they contain. Fibre is particularly important in helping to avoid constipation, a common problem in elderly people who frequently have diets very low in roughage. The general dietary rules outlined in chapter 3 are even more appropriate for the elderly, whose bodies are less able to cope with an unbalanced diet, than for younger and more vigorous men.

You must be careful too that your weight does not creep up. Inactivity and a poor diet quickly cause obesity. This is made worse by the fact that the metabolic rate falls in the elderly and less food is needed to supply daily energy needs. The excess is converted to fat, which places extra strain on the heart and circulatory system and adds to the weight on the joints. Obesity further reduces mobility, setting up a vicious circle of inactivity and overweight, and inactivity.

You will need to drink more fluids than in your younger days, to keep your kidneys working well. Some elderly men suffer from incontinence and cut down on their fluid intake in an attempt to reduce this. This can be dangerous, and you should refer the problem to your doctor. There are several common causes; perhaps the best known is prostate gland enlargement which is cured by surgery.

GENERAL WELL-BEING

Often your doctor will be able to identify a developing problem before you are aware of it, and take corrective measures. Depression, for example, is particularly common among old people, but it is usually the physical effects accompanying depression that cause a man to visit his doctor. If the underlying depression is cleared up, aches and pains and insomnia often go at the same time.

RESTING TIME

The amount of sleep you require gradually diminishes throughout life, and there is a tendency to have several short naps throughout the day. The body demands sleep when it needs it, so this tendency should not be restricted.

Many elderly men become upset because they find they cannot get a 'full' night's sleep, but the fact is that they don't need it. Worrying about insomnia won't improve your mental and physical well-being. If you find yourself waking very early, try going to bed later and cutting out the day-time naps. You may find that coffee or tea keeps you awake at night, as the ageing body is less able to cope with the stimulant effect of the caffeine in these drinks, so they should be avoided at bed-time if you cannot get off to sleep. A malted drink or perhaps a glass of sherry, whisky or brandy can help you get a good night's sleep, and if you still have problems, try reading for a while to tire yourself out. Don't take any form of sleeping tablets unless they have been prescribed by the doctor; even then, double-check to make sure you really need them. The elderly should treat all drugs with great caution, as they are less able to deal with their side effects than younger, healthier men. Sleeping tablets are especially dangerous because they may cause confusion and even excitement, so avoid them.

Sleep patterns can be altered by many external factors. Modifying these may solve sleep problems without the necessity of drug therapy.

- **Tea, coffee, drinking chocolate**
Influence: more restless sleep caused by caffeine
- **Malted milk or light snack**
Influence: sounder sleep
- **Heavy meal**
Influence: more restless sleep caused by full stomach
- **Smoking**
Influence: more restless sleep caused by nicotine
- **Stress**
Influence: periods of wakefulness
- **Daytime naps**
Influence: periods of wakefulness
- **Exercise**
Influence: sounder sleep

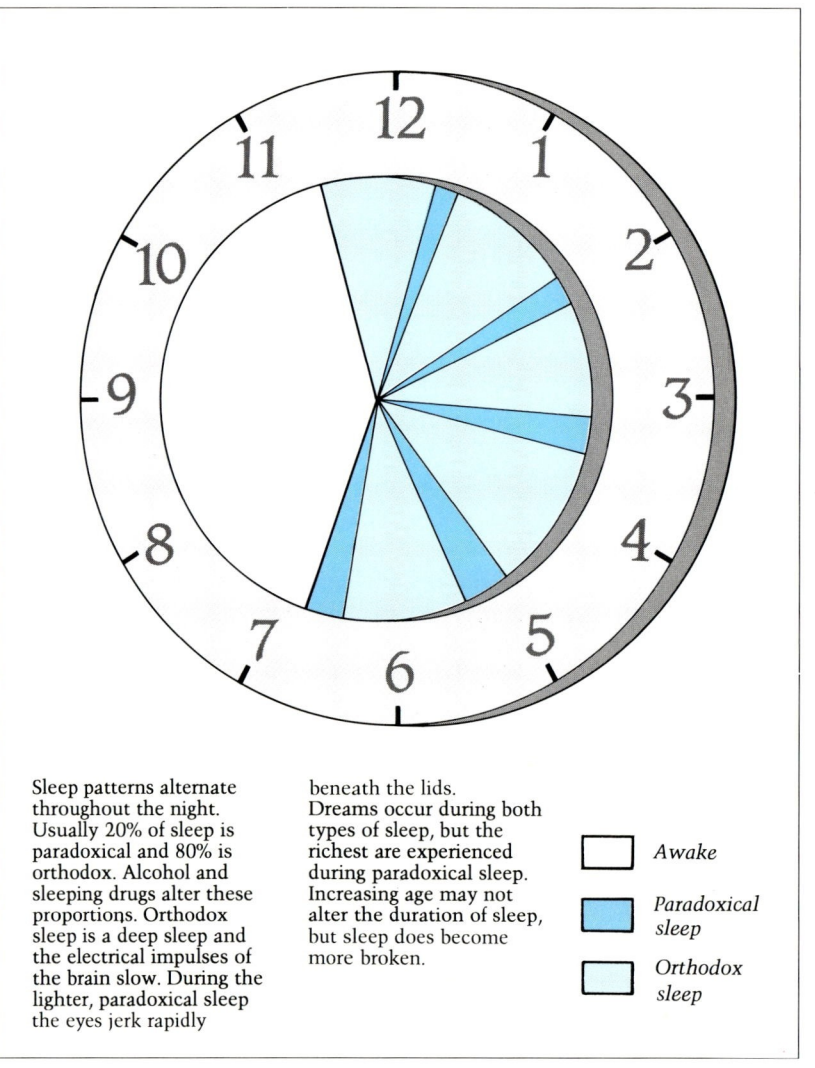

Sleep patterns alternate throughout the night. Usually 20% of sleep is paradoxical and 80% is orthodox. Alcohol and sleeping drugs alter these proportions. Orthodox sleep is a deep sleep and the electrical impulses of the brain slow. During the lighter, paradoxical sleep the eyes jerk rapidly beneath the lids. Dreams occur during both types of sleep, but the richest are experienced during paradoxical sleep. Increasing age may not alter the duration of sleep, but sleep does become more broken.

☐ Awake

☐ Paradoxical sleep

☐ Orthodox sleep

Doctors are consulted by older men about chest pain or respiratory problems, but even quite distressing chronic conditions affecting the urinary tract or a man's ability to get around easily are often suffered in silence.

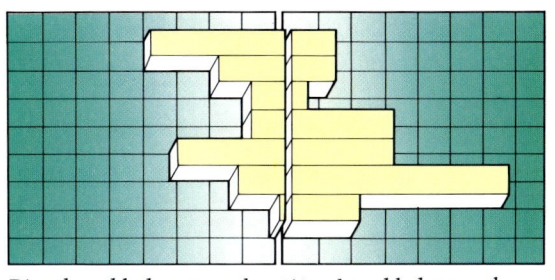

Respiratory
Cardiac
Nervous
Urinary
Locomotor
Feet
Depression

Disorders elderly men seek medical advice for   *Disorders elderly men do not seek advice for*

Taking care of your teeth is very important. Well-fitted dentures contribute a lot to happiness and well-being in the elderly, but now that most people retain their teeth into old age, it is still important to have regular dental check-ups and treatment. Similarly, your eyes must be looked after. Sight deteriorates as the lens in the eye hardens and loses its ability to focus properly, so most older people need glasses, at least for reading. These may need changing periodically, as your vision continues to alter. Get regular check-ups at your optician.

Equally important is being aware of possible failing hearing. Like the other senses, the sense of hearing usually deteriorates with age, and this may make it very difficult to understand speech. The unfortunate results are that many older people are treated in a patronizing way by well-meaning people who behave as if they were dealing with the senile. In reality, they are perfectly alert, merely unaware that they are being addressed. Proper medical care and possibly a hearing aid can often improve the situation. If deafness becomes severe, then lip-reading skills can be learnt. Courses are run by the Royal National Institute for the Deaf.

Many of the measures discussed above are ways in which you can conserve your health into old age. But there are some occasions when medical help is important. Don't be afraid or too proud to go to the doctor if you have a medical problem, or if you just want a check up to reassure yourself that you are remaining healthy, with every right to expect many more years of happy and productive life.

●For this and other useful addresses, see *Further Information*, page 200

CONCLUSION

Enjoying a happy, healthy, and stimulating old age is not just a matter of adding years to one's life. It's getting the best out of those years, including the best of health. And that has really been the message running throughout this whole book — how to maximize your potential for health and life. How to make the most of the good health you are given as a young man. How to invest in it wisely, and not fritter it away.

In this modern high-tech world of bodyscanners and bypass operations, of ECGs, laser scalpels and fibrescopes, of pacemakers and pills for every ill, you could be forgiven for thinking that looking after yourself is no longer very important. After all, if you have that coronary or develop that tumour, surely the doctors will bail you out and patch you up. Surely, you'll be as good as new, won't you?

Well, unfortunately there's no guarantee of that. Indeed, although great advances have been made in the early diagnosis and treatment of such killer diseases as heart disease and cancer, we are still a long way short of being able to cure the underlying pathological processes that lead to these all-too-common causes of premature disease and death.

But whilst the cure of such conditions continues to elude us, we are learning a great deal about prevention. We are learning that much of today's ill-health is caused by the way we lead our lives — what we eat, whether or not we take exercise, smoke cigarettes, drink excessively, suffer from stress, and so on. We are learning that it is foolish to rely too much on medical check-ups and major surgery on the assumption that almost anything can be dealt with if the need arises. Instead we are learning that by paying attention to lifestyle — no smoking, sensible eating and drinking, regular exercise, coping with stress — we can do a great deal to prevent many diseases from developing in the first place.

The body is remarkably resilient. It can do much to defend itself against the onslaught of bacteria and viruses, recover from serious illness, heal severe injury, cope with extremes of climate, digest a wide variety of different foods, detoxify potential poisons like alcohol and nicotine, adapt to physical demands, and cope with stress. But there's a limit to how much adversity your body can handle without developing trouble. With all these threats to health, and many others, it's important to know your limits and stay within them. This way, much illness can be avoided.

But true good health is more than simply avoiding illness, disease, disability or death. It is something much more positive. It is a state of maximum potential for life and well-being, physical and mental. And it feels good.

Like all good things in life it requires some effort to achieve and maintain — but the potential benefits are well worth it.

The choice is yours. To take your health for granted and squander it away with an attitude of 'don't care' until it is too late. Or to make the effort to invest in it wisely, adding years to your life and life to your years with 'mancare'.

Dr Alan Maryon Davis

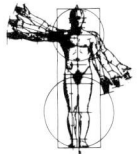

The following books, publications and organizations have been listed according to their relevance to a particular chapter in this book. Some of the associations provide general information, often in the form of helpful leaflets and booklets, while others offer more specific information within their particular area of concern.

CHAPTER ONE
MANPOWER

Ashton, D & Davies, B, *Why Exercise?* Blackwell, 1986
Bassey, EJ & Fentem, PH, *Exercise: The facts,* Oxford University Press, 1981
Diagram Group, *Man's Body: An Owner's Manual,* Paddington Press, 1976
Gillie, Oliver (ed.), *The Sunday Times New Book of Body Maintenance,* Mermaid Books, 1982
Mitchell, L, *Simple Relaxation,* John Murray, 1977
Open University, *The Good Health Guide,* Pan Books, 1982
Reilly, T (ed.), *Sports Fitness and Sports Injuries,* Faber & Faber, 1981
Wright, Beric, *The BUPA Manual of Fitness and Well-Being,* Macdonald, 1984

ADDRESSES

College of Health,
18 Victoria Park Square,
London E2 9PF
Health Education Council,
78 New Oxford Street,
London WC1A 1AH
'Look After Yourself'
Centre,
Christchurch College,
Canterbury CT1 1QU
Physical Education
Association,
162 King's Cross Road,
London WC1X 9DH
Sports Council,
16 Upper Woburn Place,
London WC1H 1AH

CHAPTER TWO
EATING FOR HEALTH

Burkitt, D, *Don't Forget Fibre in Your Diet* (4th ed.), M Dunitz, 1983
Cook, R & E, *Sugar Off, A Practical Guide to Sugar-free Living,* Pan Books, 1986
Coronary Prevention Group, *Healthier Eating,* CPG, 1985, *(Address below)*
Hanssen, M, *E for Additives: The complete 'E' number guide,* Thorsons, 1984
Health Education Council, *Guide to Healthy Eating,* HEC, 1986 *(Address below)*
Maryon Davis, A & Thomas, J, *Diet 2000,* **Pan Books, 1984**
Ministry of Agriculture, Fisheries and Food, *Manual of Nutrition* (9th ed.), HMSO, 1985 (from HMSO Bookshops)
Robbins, C, *Eating for Health,* Granada, 1985
Tudge, C, *The Food Connection,* BBC, 1985

ADDRESSES

British Nutrition
Foundation,
15 Belgrave Square,
London SW1X 8PS
Coronary Prevention Group,
60 Great Ormond Street,
London WC1N 3HR
Health Education Council,
78 New Oxford Street,
London WC1A 1AH
Vegetarian Society,
Parkdale,
Dunham Road,
Altrincham,
Cheshire WA14 40G

CHAPTER THREE
HEALTHY AND HAPPY

Coleman, Vernon, *Stress Control,* Pan Books, 1980
Cronin, D, *Anxiety, Depression and Phobias, and How to Cope with Them,* Granada, 1980
Livingston Booth, Audrey, *Stressmanship,* Severn House, 1985
Madders, Jane, *Stress and Relaxation,* M. Dunitz, 1980
Mitchell, L, *Simple Relaxation,* John Murray, 1977
Stanway, A, *Overcoming Depression,* Hamlyn, 1981
Pincus, L, *Death and the Family: The importance of mourning,* Faber, 1981

ADDRESSES

Cruse (for the Bereaved),
Cruse House,
126 Sheen Road,
Richmond,
Surrey TW9 1UR
The National Association for Mental Health (MIND),
22 Harley Street,
London W1N 2ED
Relaxation for Living,
29 Burwood Park Road,
Walton-on-Thames,
Surrey KT12 5LH

CHAPTER FOUR
BODY BASICS

Forrest, John, *The Good Teeth Guide,* Granada, 1985
Hart, Dr Frank Dudley, *Overcoming Arthritis,* M Dunitz, 1981
Stoddard, Dr Alan, *The Back: Relief from pain,* M Dunitz, 1980
Wilkinson, Marcia, *Migraine and Headaches,* M Dunitz, 1982

ADDRESSES

Action Against Allergy (AAA),
43 The Downs,
London SW20 8HG
Arthritis & Rheumatism Council,
41 Eagle Street,
London WC1R 4AR
Back Pain Association,
31-33 Park Road,
Teddington,
Middlesex, TW11 0AB
Health & Safety Executive,
St Hughes House,
Stanley Precinct,
Bootle,
Merseyside L20 3L2
Medical Advisory Services for Travellers Abroad (MASTA),
Bureau of Hygiene and Tropical Diseases,
Keppel Street,
London WC1E 7HT
Tenovus Cancer Information Centre,
11 Whitchurch Road,
Cardiff CF4 3JN

CHAPTER FIVE
SEXUAL REALITIES

Barlow, D, *Sexually Transmitted Diseases: The facts,* OUP, 1979
Butler, RN & Lewis, MI, *Sex After Sixty: A guide for men and women for their later years,* Harper & Row, 1976
Cauthery, P & Stanway, A & P, *The Complete Book of Love and Sex: Guide to understanding sexuality,* Century, 1984
Decker, A & Loebl, S, *We Want to Have a Baby: A sympathetic guide to the causes and cures of childlessness,* Penguin, 1980
Llewellyn-Jones, D, *Herpes, AIDS, and Other Sexually Transmitted Diseases,* Faber, 1985
Mayer, K & Pizer, H, *AIDS Fact Book,* Bantam Books, 1983
Shapiro, HI, *The Birth Control Book: A complete guide for men and women,* Penguin, 1980
Tatchell, P, *Surviving the AIDS crisis,* Gay Men's Press, 1986

ADDRESSES

Brook Advisory Centres,
Education & Publications Unit, 10 Albert Street,
Birmingham B4 7UD
Campaign for Homosexual Equality,
274 Upper Street,
London N1 2UA
Family Planning Information Service (FPIS),
27/35 Mortimer Street,
London W1N 7RJ
Terence Higgins Trust
(Information Service on AIDS),
BM/AIDS,
London WC1 3XX

CHAPTER SIX
STIMULANTS, RELAXANTS & YOU

SCODA (Standing Conference on Drugs and Alcohol), *Coping with Drugs, (from address below)*
Davies, I & Raistrick, D, *Dealing with Drink,* BBC Publications, 1981
Grant, M, *Same Again: A guide to safer drinking,* Penguin, 1984
Gregory, DN, *Become an Ex-smoker,* Worth Publications, 1982
ISDD (Institute for the Study of Drug Dependence), *Drug Abuse Briefing: A guide to the effects of drugs and to the social and legal facts about their non-medical use in Britain,* ISDD, 1984 *(from address below)*
Miller, WR & Murioz, RF, *How to Control Your Drinking,* Sheldon Press, 1983

ADDRESSES

Alcohol Concern,
305 Grays Inn Road,
London WC1X 8QF
Action on Smoking and Health (ASH),
5/11 Mortimer Street,
London W1N 7RH
Health Education Council,
78 New Oxford Street,
London WC1A 1AH
Institute for the Study of Drug Dependence (ISDD), & Standing Conference on Drugs and Alcohol (SCODA),
1-4 Hatton Place,
Hatton Garden,
London WC1X 8QF

CHAPTER SEVEN
MATURE HEALTH

British Dietetic Association & British Nutrition Foundation, *Healthy Eating for the Elderly,* British Dietetic Association
Gibbs, Russell, *Exercise for the Over-50s,* Jill Norman, 1981
Help the Aged in association with Health Education Council, *The Time of Your Life. A handbook for retirement,* Help the Aged, 1979
Kemp, F & Buttle, B, *Focus on Retirement,* Kogan Page, 1979
Mitchell, L, *Healthy Living Over 55: A getting on guide,* John Murray, 1984
Muir Gray, A, *Better Health in Retirement,* Age Concern, England, *(from address below)*

ADDRESSES

Age Concern England,
Bernard Sunley House,
60 Pitcairn Road,
Mitcham,
Surrey CR4 3LL
British Dietetic Association (BDA),103 Daimler House,
Paradise Street,
Birmingham B1 2BJ
Help the Aged,
PO Box 460,
St James' Walk,
London EC1R 0BE
Pre-Retirement Association,
19 Undine Road,
Tooting,
London SW17 8PP
Royal National Institute for the Deaf (RNID),
105 Gower Street,
London WC1

INDEX

Bold page numbers refer
to main entries. Page
numbers in *italic* refer
to captioned material.

ACKNOWLEDGEMENTS

The author and contributors would like to thank the following for their assistance in the preparation of this book:

ASH (Action on Smoking and Health); The Health Education Council; Homecraft of London and Nicholls and Clarke Ltd, suppliers of aids for the handicapped and the aged; MASTA (Medical Advisory Services for Travellers Abroad); The National Ankylosing Spondylitis Society, 6 Grosvenor Crescent, London SW1X 7ER; O'Reilly Marketing and Promotions, London; The Pleasure Drome, London for the use of the gymnasium and Welbeck Public Relations, London.

Photo credits:
Page 9, John Whatney Photo Library; 31, Colorsport; 33, All-Sport (UK) Ltd, and Colorsport (top); 32, White City Pool; 36, Bolton Stirland International Fitness Equipment; 91, Spectrum Colour Library; 107, 118, Science Photo Library Ltd; 122, Marshall Cavendish Picture Library.